Sixth Edition

Patient Practitioner Interaction

An Experiential Manual for Developing the Art of Health Care

Sixth Edition

Patient Practitioner Interaction

An Experiential Manual for Developing the Art of Health Care

Carol M. Davis, DPT, EdD, MS, FAPTA
Professor Emerita
Department of Physical Therapy
University of Miami Miller School of Medicine
Coral Gables, Florida

Gina Maria Musolino, PT, MSEd, EdD
Associate Professor and Director of Clinical Education, Leadership Team
University of South Florida Morsani College of Medicine
School of Physical Therapy & Rehabilitation Sciences
Tampa, Florida

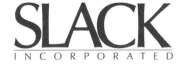

SLACK
INCORPORATED

www.Healio.com/books

ISBN: 978-1-63091-046-4

Instructors: *Patient Practitioner Interaction: An Experiential Manual for Developing the Art of Health Care, Sixth Edition* Instructor's Manual is also available from SLACK Incorporated. Don't miss this important companion to *Patient Practitioner Interaction: An Experiential Manual for Developing the Art of Health Care, Sixth Edition*. To obtain the Instructor's Manual, please visit http://www.efacultylounge.com.

Published by: SLACK Incorporated
                  6900 Grove Road
                  Thorofare, NJ 08086 USA
                  Telephone: 856-848-1000
                  Fax: 856-848-6091
                  www.Healio.com/books

Contact SLACK Incorporated for more information about other books in this field or about the availability of our books from distributors outside the United States.

Library of Congress Cataloging-in-Publication Data

Names: Davis, Carol M., author. | Musolino, Gina Maria, author.
Title: Patient practitioner interaction : an experiential manual for
  developing the art of health care / Carol M. Davis, Gina Maria Musolino.
Description: Sixth edition. | Thorofare, NJ : SLACK Incorporated, [2016] |
  Includes bibliographical references and index.
Identifiers: LCCN 2016006751 (print) | LCCN 2016007304 (ebook) | ISBN
  9781630910464 (hardback : alk. paper) | ISBN 9781630910471 (ebook) | ISBN
  9781630910488 (web-ready)
Subjects: | MESH: Physical Therapy Specialty | Professional-Patient Relations
  | Health Communication | Cultural Competency | Helping Behavior
Classification: LCC RM705 (print) | LCC RM705 (ebook) | NLM WB 460 | DDC
  610.69/6--dc23
LC record available at http://lccn.loc.gov/2016006751

Printed in the United States of America.

Last digit is print number: 10   9   8   7   6   5   4   3   2   1

DEDICATION

To Susan Emily Davis Doughty—friend to all, master women's health nurse practitioner, and my twin sister.

To Geneva R. Johnson, PhD, DPT (hon), FAPTA—beloved mentor and friend.

And again, to my friend Jamie, for the sixth time, with gratitude 6 times as great as with the first edition in 1989.

Carol M. Davis

To Carol M. Davis, DPT, EdD, MS, FAPTA for sharing her treasured gift with me—I am forever humbled.

To all colleagues in health care, near and far, who dedicate themselves to teaching both the intangible and tangible, in support of the patients and clients we serve in health care.

To my dear and daring clinical and academic educators in health care who never stop learning, never stop asking questions, never stop truly listening, and lead by example; for those who embrace an open mind and positive attitude, even when facing the impossible, and remember that the art of healing and the affective domain is as important as the science of practice.

For all in advocacy, may we never lose perspective and continue to tirelessly work to keep the care in health.

For my students and graduates, from whom I continue to learn—may you each continue to learn what matters most to your patients and clients, take the time to find out what the patient understands and what his or her goals are, and continue to do your best as partners in health care. May you have empathic ears in the face of discomfort and not be discouraged by the negativity. Health care is gratifying, and you have made the right choices. Learn from all your patients—keep asking *why?* And *why not?* Dare to dream of possibilities. Keep an attitude of gratitude in all you do.

For my patients—thank you for all you have taught me and changed in me for the better, and for entrusting me with your care. May your stories serve to help others seeking care.

And to my dear parents and beloved family members—you have made all the difference in my life, and I thank you immensely for my delightful formative years that allowed me to be self-aware and taught me faith, hope, and values in life, love, and profession. Thank you for the many blessings we have shared and wishing you all ten-fold in return.

Gina Maria Musolino

CONTENTS

Dedication . . . . *v*
Acknowledgments . . . . *ix*
About the Authors . . . . *xiii*
Contributing Authors . . . . *xv*
Preface . . . . *xvii*
Foreword to the Fifth Edition by Helen J. Hislop, PT, PhD, ScD, FAPTA . . . . *xix*
Foreword to the Sixth Edition by Shirley A. Sahrmann, PT, PhD, FAPTA . . . . *xxi*

Chapter 1   Basic Awareness of Self 1
Carol M. Davis, DPT, EdD, MS, FAPTA and Gina Maria Musolino, PT, MSEd, EdD

Chapter 2   Family History 13
Carol M. Davis, DPT, EdD, MS, FAPTA and Gina Maria Musolino, PT, MSEd, EdD

Chapter 3   Values as Determinants of Behavior 29
Carol M. Davis, DPT, EdD, MS, FAPTA and Gina Maria Musolino, PT, MSEd, EdD

Chapter 4   Identifying and Resolving Moral Dilemmas 49
Carol M. Davis, DPT, EdD, MS, FAPTA and Gina Maria Musolino, PT, MSEd, EdD

Chapter 5   Stress Management 73
Carol M. Davis, DPT, EdD, MS, FAPTA and Gina Maria Musolino, PT, MSEd, EdD

Chapter 6   The Nature of Effective Helping: Empathy and Sympathy Versus Pity .91
Carol M. Davis, DPT, EdD, MS, FAPTA and Gina Maria Musolino, PT, MSEd, EdD

Chapter 7   Effective Communication: Problem Identification and Helpful Responses 103
Carol M. Davis, DPT, EdD, MS, FAPTA and Gina Maria Musolino, PT, MSEd, EdD

Chapter 8   Assertiveness Skills and Conflict Resolution 117
Carol M. Davis, DPT, EdD, MS, FAPTA and Gina Maria Musolino, PT, MSEd, EdD

Chapter 9   Readiness for Reflective Practice: Peer and Self-Assessment 139
Gina Maria Musolino, PT, MSEd, EdD

Chapter 10   Leadership and Advocacy for Health Care 159
Gina Maria Musolino, PT, MSEd, EdD

Chapter 11   Communicating to Establish Rapport and Reduce Negativity 181
Helen L. Masin, PT, PhD

Chapter 12   Communicating With Cultural Sensitivity 199
Helen L. Masin, PT, PhD

Chapter 13   The Helping Interview 223
Carol M. Davis, DPT, EdD, MS, FAPTA and Gina Maria Musolino, PT, MSEd, EdD

Chapter 14   Spirituality in Patient Care 243
Darina Sargeant, PT, PhD

Chapter 15   Health Behavior and Effective Patient Education 263
              Kathleen A. Curtis, PT, PhD

Chapter 16   Communicating With Persons Who Have Disabilities. 285
              Kathleen A. Curtis, PT, PhD

Chapter 17   Sexuality and Disability: Effective Communication 301
              Sherrill H. Hayes, PT, PhD

Chapter 18   Communicating With People Who Are Dying and Their Families. 323
              Carol M. Davis, DPT, EdD, MS, FAPTA and Gina Maria Musolino, PT, MSEd, EdD

Afterword. 339
Financial Disclosures 341
Index. 343

Instructors: *Patient Practitioner Interaction: An Experiential Manual for Developing the Art of Health Care, Sixth Edition* Instructor's Manual is also available from SLACK Incorporated. Don't miss this important companion to *Patient Practitioner Interaction: An Experiential Manual for Developing the Art of Health Care, Sixth Edition.* To obtain the Instructor's Manual, please visit http://www.efacultylounge.com.

ACKNOWLEDGMENTS

My immeasurable gratitude goes to Dr. Gina Maria Musolino, who skillfully took the helm for this latest edition of *Patient Practitioner Interaction*, and to Tony Schiavo from SLACK Incorporated, editor of our dreams. The two of you together have produced a wonderful addition to this lineage, which began with the first edition in 1989. Thank you both for your outstanding work, and for the richness of our interactions and our friendship.

Carol M. Davis

The completion of *Patient Practitioner Interaction: An Experiential Manual for Developing the Art of Health Care, Sixth Edition* (PPI6) was far from an individual undertaking. There are many students, faculty, colleagues, family members, and friends with whom we share credit.

The SLACK Incorporated staff have done it once again and remain a dedicated and classy team. I am truly thankful for the opportunity to work so closely with Anthony (Tony) P. Schiavo Jr, Acquisitions Editor. Tony seamlessly took up the baton for PPI6 from the dedicated and charismatic Brien Cummings. I must admit I was a bit trepidatious due to the hand-off. Much to my delight, Tony was always responsive in his guidance and made the transition so seamless. Tony was patient with the process and kept me thinking one step ahead, although he was new to the project and I but a novice editor. Thank you, dear Tony, for always being willing to have deep discussions, giving truthful guidance, and always being willing to lend a listening ear. Thank you also for sharing your family with me; your 6 children and wife are truly blessed to have such a dedicated father and husband. Being one of 6 myself, your sharing your family with me took me back in time to the wonderful and carefree days of childhood. To dear John Bond, Senior Vice President: my only regret is not having known you sooner, as we wish you all the best continued success on your next journey consulting for publishers and associations. Twenty-eight years with SLACK Incorporated is an incredible contribution, and it shows in those you have mentored and influenced and in the success of SLACK. I will forever cherish the 1 year I spent with you, the very memorable Bond 45. You shall be dearly missed, my friend. I thank you for the joy you have shared; for your astute wisdom, sound counsel, and decision making advice; and for being forthright. I hope our paths shall intersect again. To April Billick, Managing Editor, who made contact early and followed us through to production in style. Thank you, April, for always assuring that we were visualizing things as they were and guiding us through the process. Your efforts in keeping aesthetics contemporary and complementary for the content did not go unnoticed. Thank you to Sarah Becker-Marrero, ELS, Project Editor, for your detailed work and caring as much for PPI6 as we do and for ensuring we did not miss an important component in the exciting production phase. Thank you also to Danielle Yentz, Marketing Coordinator, and Michelle Gatt, Vice President of Marketing, for your time, effort, and dedication to assure that PPI6 reaches all those in need throughout the nation and internationally. I hope to have the privilege to work on PPI7 and new projects with the outstanding and dedicated SLACK Incorporated team. Thank you for making my publication experience a pleasure!

I would like to specially acknowledge my coauthor, Carol M. Davis, DPT, EdD, MS, FAPTA, for sharing her treasured gift of PPI with me. Dr. Davis is a celebrated leader, remains a tireless advocate for the profession, and fearlessly addresses the affective domain of learning for developing health care professionals for the patients and clients we serve. Although Carol's text has been around since 1989, I did not discover PPI until later editions. I have used the PPI textbook since the mid-1990s with new and developing programs, where having no near peers makes the professional acculturation even more challenging. Early in my career as a faculty member, I never would have survived teaching the content without the book's guidance to facilitate the eye-opening exercises and often amazing teachable moments in the classroom and clinics and to prepare future health care providers to connect with themselves and their patients. I never dreamed I would have the honor to carry the torch, and I hope that I have done your work justice. Thank you for your trust in me and allowing me the freedom to expand the text beyond the formative years. PPI has made a difference in so many lives, and I trust my contributions shall carry on your celebrated work to continue to produce changes in professional behaviors and to develop sensitive, caring, and empathic health care professionals who serve as strong advocates for their patients and as dedicated leaders in health care teams. Thank you, Carol, for seeing in me what I did not even see in myself! Thank you for listening attentively, encouraging me without reservation, gently redirecting me when necessary, and being at-the-ready at key junctures. Thank you for using your energies to help me to soar to heights I had never dreamt of reaching. Thank you for entrusting this work to me to carry on your legacy. I hope I continue to make you proud.

To our contributing authors, Dr. Helen L. Masin, Dr. Darina Sargeant, Dr. Kathleen Curtis, and Dr. Sherrill H. Hayes—what a pleasure it has been to work with each of you. Your exceptional works have been revitalized, and you each remain deeply dedicated to PPI; for this we are all thankful. You are not only superb teachers and inspiring leaders and scholars, but you are all willing to consider new perspectives and help others to not only learn best practices but to enjoy them and have a thirst for more learning! Being able to teach by example, share your experiences through story, and facilitate through guided exercises is a true gift, and each of you has this gift and is able to stimulate others in the desire to learn and apply. We are deeply grateful for your lasting influence in challenging content areas, and that you have chosen to continue to answer the call for PPI6. Without your continued dedication to the work of PPI, it would not be possible, and your responsiveness along the way has made my work as coauthor a sheer delight! I commend each of you for your dedicated time, diligent efforts, and professionalism along the way, even when facing your own real-life challenges and transitions. Thank you for sharing your compassion and caring insights so graciously.

We cherish the Foreword previously provided by our dear departed Helen Hislop, PT, PhD, ScD, FAPTA. She now belongs to the ages and shall always be missed and remembered.

My sincere thanks to our esteemed colleague, Dr. Shirley Sahrmann, PT, PhD, FAPTA, for her contribution of the Foreword to PPI6. We all know Shirley is the one, and she has done it once again. We appreciate her taking time out from retirement and from her own high-impact, internationally renowned scholarly works to provide her insights for PPI6. One glorious fall semester, when I was but a neophyte student physical therapist, I had the incredible honor of spending Wednesday afternoons with Dr. Shirley with one of my peers at Washington University School of Medicine, Program in Physical Therapy (WUMS PT) in the then–Irene Walter Johnson Institute of Rehabilitation. Dr. Shirley was patient with us as novice learners (we were shaking in our lab tunics, yet wore the name badges that said we had the right to be there), at least as much as any seasoned professional ought to be with true rookies. Dr. Sahrmann provided needed encouragement and spirited critique and was certain to cajole when we thought we had it all figured out already. She enlightened us on her patients' movement imbalances and movement impairment syndromes and taught us to truly think on our feet. Thank you, Dr. Sahrmann, for sharing your discerning eye and words of wisdom on the important aspects of movement in every facet of health care and your personal patient-practitioner interaction insights! Your recognition of the significance of the role of the biopsychosocial influence for movement is genuinely appreciated. Your wisdom is highly valued, and we thank you for taking the time and effort to assure that we, as lifespan practitioners, keep the Human Movement System at the forefront for the benefit of our patients and clients.

Special thanks to the many dedicated educators in my life who provided important professional foundations, especially those at Washington University, School of Medicine, Program in Physical Therapy, St. Louis, Missouri; Nova Southeastern University, Abraham S. Fischler College of Education, Ft. Lauderdale, Florida; and Quincy High School, St. Peter School and Church of St. Peter, Quincy, Illinois.

Thank you to the countless dedicated colleagues who have given me the incredible opportunities to serve with the American Physical Therapy Association, Education Section, Florida Physical Therapy Association, APTA House of Delegates, California Physical Therapy Association, Florida Consortium of Clinical Education, Northwest Intermountain Consortium of Clinical Education, The University of Utah, and The University of South Florida, Morsani College of Medicine, School of Physical Therapy & Rehabilitation Sciences. Much gratitude as well to the many staff members with these fine organizations who do so much to support our endeavors. To my many dear colleagues in academics and in the trenches of clinical education—thank you for sharing your stories and allowing us to influence your works. I am indebted to the tremendous support and dedication of nationwide clinical instructors and clinical coordinators of clinical education who hold their protégés accountable for compassionate care and empathic patient-practitioner interactions—keep making a difference! You are the ones who continue to ensure that we translate PPI for patient care, advocacy, and leadership. Thank you!

We are in a blessed profession when we can call our colleagues our friends, and so it is in physical therapy. With enormous heartfelt gratitude to my cherished colleagues who continue to believe in me and connect with me at important touchpoints in my life and career: Dr. Alecia Thiele, PT, DPT, MSEd, ATC/L, ACCE; Dr. Catherine Page, PT, MPh, PhD; Dr. Dennis W. Fell, MD, PT; Dr. Michael Mueller, PT, PhD; Ronna Delitto, PT and Dr. Anthony Delitto, PT, PhD, FAPTA; Dr. Gail M. Jensen, PT, PhD, FAPTA; Dr. Elizabeth Mostrom, PT, PhD; Dr. Karen Hayes, PT, PhD, FAPTA; Dr. R. Scott Ward, PT, PhD, FAPTA; Dr. Charles Magistro, PT, FAPTA; Dr. Mary Rogers, PT, PhD, FAPTA, FASB; Dr. Kathleen Rockefeller, PT, ScD, MPH; Dr. Katherine J. Sullivan, PT, PhD, FAHA; Dr. Susan S. Deusinger, PT, PhD, FAPTA; and Dr. Shirley Sahrmann, PT, PhD, FAPTA. You have each encouraged me in abundant ways! Your professional influence and friendship are so appreciated.

Memorable thanks to those mentors gone too soon: the dearly departed Dr. Steven J. Rose, PT, PhD, FAPTA; Dr. Linda M. Howard, RN, PhD; and Beatrice F. Schulz, PT. Dr. Rose taught me the value of discerning the useful, useless, and harmful aspects of health care and research and taught me that putting our pencils down is not a bad thing! Linda shared her undying enthusiasm, effervescent inspiration, and dedication to students, along with change-hardy leadership. Bea taught me that it was always OK to have joy in your work and to keep smiling.

I remain especially grateful to my graduates, students, and patients, who have taught me more than I ever imagined possible! Thank you for your enthusiasm, support, and willingness to share your journeys with me and for the privilege to assist you in yours. Thank you for giving back and continuing your dedication to professionalism.

I especially thank my first teachers—my parents. My father, the late Dr. Joseph L. Musolino, DVM, had the true gift of being able to listen to his patients. Thank you, Dad, for allowing me to go on "country calls" with you, and being a true supporter of my every endeavor. For my wonderful M.O.M. (Mother of Many), who dedicates herself daily to the challenges of movement—you never cease to inspire and motivate. Thank you both for making sure I continue to reach my full potential. Thank you for your undying love, kindness, respect, tolerance, patience, playfulness, hope, faith, and understanding; you have never hesitated to share them all. I thank you both for your dedication to your children, whom you gave eagle's wings. Thank you to my family members and nieces and nephews who are always there, sparkling, constantly listening, supporting, sharing, and laughing, facing the unfortunate in life and love, doing the hard work of living and loss, and being passionate while dedicating yourselves to others, and pulling out all the stops in your learning and lifetime endeavors; you remain my deepest of inspirations. Stay courageous!

For each of you who cares to deeply dive in with PPI6: may your health care experiences bring you joy, and, when they are challenging, may you rely on PPI6 to guide and enrich you once again to cherish the human spirit and ensure care is in the forefront of your health care patient-practitioner interactions. We wish you courage and strength on your journey.

Gina Maria Musolino

ABOUT THE AUTHORS

Carol M. Davis, DPT, EdD, MS, FAPTA, is Professor Emerita of the Department of Physical Therapy in the Miller School of Medicine at the University of Miami and past Vice Chair for Curriculum. She retired from her academic responsibilities in 2015. Dr. Davis is an internationally known speaker and consultant in teaching and developing curriculum in professional behaviors, attitudes, and values and in complementary therapies in rehabilitation for physicians and all health professionals. In addition to being the author of *Patient Practitioner Interaction: An Experiential Manual for Developing the Art of Health Care, Sixth Edition,* she is the editor of *Complementary Therapies in Rehabilitation: Evidence for Efficacy in Therapy, Prevention, and Wellness, Fourth Edition,* also published by SLACK Incorporated, and co-editor of *Therapeutic Interaction in Nursing.*

Dr. Davis continues to teach doctor of physical therapy (DPT) students at the University of Miami Miller School of Medicine as volunteer faculty. She is an international invited lecturer on the structure and function of fascia. She has published several research articles in peer-reviewed journals and is the author of 18 book chapters. She served 6 years as a commissioner on the Commission on Accreditation for Physical Therapy Education and was a team leader and site visitor. She also served on the Ethics and Judicial Committee for the American Physical Therapy Association (APTA) and was Chair in 2004-2005. She was awarded the Outstanding Teacher award by the Section on Geriatrics of the APTA in 2003, was named the 2005 Linda Crane Lecturer by the Sections on Cardiovascular and Pulmonary and Education, and was awarded the Lucy Blair Service Award in 1991 and the Catherine Worthingham Fellow award in 2003 by the APTA.

In addition to teaching and consulting, Dr. Davis maintains an active clinical practice, primarily treating patients with pain using J. F. Barnes sustained myofascial release and exercise.

Gina Maria Musolino, PT, MSEd, EdD, is Associate Professor and the Director of Clinical Education, Leadership Team, University of South Florida (USF) Morsani College of Medicine, School of Physical Therapy & Rehabilitation Sciences (SPTRS), Tampa, Florida. She received her BS in Physical Therapy from Washington University School of Medicine, Program in Physical Therapy (WUMS PT; St. Louis, Missouri); her MSEd from Southwest Baptist University (Bolivar, Missouri); and her EdD with specialization in Curriculum Design, Development, and Evaluation from Nova Southeastern University (NSU), Fischler College of Education (Ft. Lauderdale, Florida). Dr. Musolino's published works and scholarship focus on service learning, cultural competence, health policy, and academic and clinical education. Dr. Musolino has been awarded grants and fellowships from numerous organizations in support of her research. She received the Beatrice F. Schulz Award for Outstanding Clinical Achievement, WUMS PT; the Southeast Division Center of the Month and Outstanding Customer Service Awards as a clinical administrator with Rehability Corporation (Florida); the Research Excellence Award from NSU, Fischler College of Education for her dissertation works; the Award of Merit in Technology Delivered Instruction from The Utah System of Higher Education, Utah Electronic College Consortium (Salt Lake City, Utah) for her instructional design and development of online education courses; the Feitelberg Journal Founder's Award, APTA Education Section, Journal of Physical Therapy Education, acknowledging excellence in publication by a first-time author for the research article "Enhancing Diversity Through Mentorship: The Nurturing Potential of Service Learning"; and the Alumni Award, WUMS PT. She was also corecipient of Outstanding Abstract with her colleagues by the APTA Annual Conference Program Committee for the abstract, "Physical Therapist Tests and Measures for a Patient with Parkinson's Disease for Consultation with Referring Neurosurgeon."

Dr. Musolino serves the APTA Education Section as President (was Vice President for 2 terms) and the Editorial Boards for *Journal of Physical Therapy Education* and *Journal of Allied Health.* Dr. Musolino is senior reviewer for APTA's journal *Physical Therapy.* She also served on APTA Appointed Work Groups: Honors and Awards, Education Awards Committee, Screening Proposals/Abstracts, and Annual Conference Program Committee. Dr. Musolino also serves as Chair, Research Committee, and Board of Directors member of the APTA Health Policy & Administration Section: The Catalyst. Dr. Musolino has served the Florida Physical Therapy Association (FPTA) as Assembly Representative for the West Central District of Florida, Delegate; APTA House of Delegates, member Florida Consortium of Clinical Education; on Task Forces for Temporary Licensure and Continuing Competence; and as former Vice Chair of the Southwest District of Florida. In 2012, Dr. Musolino was honored with the prestigious Lucy Blair Service Award from the APTA for exceptional service to the association. She is currently FPTA Chief Delegate, Florida, to the APTA House of Delegates and Board Member of the FPTA. Dr. Musolino also chairs the APTA Neurology Section, Advocacy & Consumer Affairs Committee; and serves as Federal Affairs Liaison. Dr. Musolino is a clinical mentor for the USF SPTRS student-run BRIDGE clinic for underserved/uninsured patients/clients. Dr. Musolino is an APTA Advanced & Basic Credentialed Clinical Trainer, educating clinical instructors throughout the nation and Florida for physical therapy and interprofessional health care instruction.

Contributing Authors

Kathleen A. Curtis, PT, PhD (Chapters 15 and 16) is currently Professor and Dean of the College of Health Sciences, Charles H. and Shirley T. Leavell Chair in Health Sciences at the University of Texas at El Paso. Dr. Curtis brings more than 30 years of leadership experience in clinical, education, research, and higher education administration roles in the health and rehabilitation sciences. Her background includes clinical appointments at Tufts–New England Medical Center, Santa Clara Valley Medical Center, and Cedars-Sinai Medical Center. She has held faculty appointments at Mount Saint Mary's College, the University of Southern California, the University of Miami School of Medicine, and California State University–Fresno, where she was honored with the university President's Award of Excellence.

She is the author of many research publications and 3 physical therapy textbooks. Her research in the area of prevention of secondary disability in persons with spinal cord injury has been internationally recognized.

Dr. Curtis recently received the Public Citizen of the Year award for her work in the El Paso community in support of the development of a master of social work program. Dr. Curtis received her BS in Physical Therapy from Northeastern University (Boston, Massachusetts); her MHS from San Jose State University; and her PhD in education from the University of California (Los Angeles, California).

Sherrill H. Hayes, PT, PhD (Chapter 17) is Professor and Chair Emeritus of the Department of Physical Therapy at the University of Miami Miller School of Medicine. She was Assistant Dean for Women's Health in the Miller School of Medicine and has had a long career of involvement in women's issues and physical therapy and obstetrics. She has a bachelor's degree in physical therapy, an advanced master's degree in allied health/neuroscience education from the University of Connecticut, and a PhD in higher education/administration from the University of Miami. She is a former president of the Education Section of the American Physical Therapy Association and an international consultant in physical therapy education. Her clinical specialties are in neuroanatomy and neuropathology, acute care practice, neurological dysfunction, and women's health. She has been teaching sexuality and rehabilitation for more than 30 years. She teaches in the entry-level doctorate (DPT) and PhD programs at the University of Miami.

Helen L. Masin, PT, PhD (Chapters 11 and 12) is an Associate Clinical Professor of Physical Therapy in the Department of Physical Therapy and the Department of Pediatrics at the University of Miami Miller School of Medicine. She currently teaches in the DPT and PhD programs. In her teaching role, she has taught Communications in Physical Therapy, Pediatric Physical Therapy, Professional Socialization and Leadership, and Self Defense for Women. In her research role, she has investigated cultural aspects of patient care and taught a wide variety of health professionals how to enhance their cross-cultural communication skills. In her service role, she has provided consultation to the Deaf and Hard of Hearing program at the Mailman Center for Child Development in the Department of Pediatrics at the University of Miami. She also serves as an Academic Coordinator of Clinical Education and supervises DPT students during their clinical internships. To assist her in her resolving challenges in the clinic, she became a certified practitioner in Neurolinguistic Psychology (NLP). Using her NLP background, she developed and published several articles on participant-centered problem solving (PCPS) as a method for resolving challenges in the clinic. In addition, she teaches PCPS to professionals interested in enhancing their problem-solving skills with patients, families, and colleagues.

Darina Sargeant, PT, PhD (Chapter 14) is Professor Emerita in the Department of Physical Therapy and Athletic Training in the Doisy College of Health Sciences at St. Louis University. Her areas of research include spirituality in physical therapy practice, interprofessional education, and clinical education. Dr. Sargeant has published articles and contributed to textbook chapters on spirituality in patient care and has published on interprofessional education and clinical education development in physical therapy and family practice medicine. Dr. Sargeant continues to teach spiritual care in physical therapy and professional development. Dr. Sargeant received her BS in Physical Therapy from St. Louis University in 1975 and has practiced in the acute inpatient, orthopedic outpatient, and home care settings. Dr. Sargeant earned her MEd in Curriculum in 1983 and her PhD in Educational Studies in 2003 with an emphasis on spirituality from St. Louis University.

PREFACE

"There is nothing to writing. All you do is sit down at a typewriter and bleed." –Ernest Hemingway

"Good writing is supposed to evoke sensation in the reader—not the fact that it is raining, but the feeling of being rained upon." –E. L. Doctorow

How does one improve on a bestseller? Since the First Edition of *Patient Practitioner Interaction: An Experiential Manual for Developing the Art of Health Care*, the text has remained a bestseller. With each new edition, the text has been improved with updates and progressions, and the Sixth Edition is no exception. All chapters are significantly updated with contemporary evidence, legislative updates, and additional chapter exercises for both basic and more progressive applications of the skills for patient-practitioner interaction (PPI). There are 2 new chapters, one devoted to peer and self-assessment and the other to leadership and advocacy for health care. A companion electronic format for exercises is included. While keeping with the low-tech need for developing PPI skills, multimedia, website resource links for applications to provide broader perspectives for a digital generation, are provided as key resources to enhance the content.

As in the last 5 editions, 3 chapters are devoted to students' self-awareness and understanding of their own history in developing their values and communication skills, along with exercises to analyze the effectiveness of those skills. The chapter on differentiating personal values and professional values remains and is updated with contemporary evidence and exercises. A new chapter exploring peer and self-assessment has been added to plant the seeds for developing reflective practice capabilities for the health care professional, for it is in education that the process of education is so closely tied to the process of healing. The word *education* derives from the Latin *educare*, meaning to mold, rear, or bring up; and/or *educere*, meaning to lead out, pull out, or lead forth. Genuine education for our students, patients, clients, families, and caregivers fosters self-awareness, self-knowledge, creativity, and self-trust, along with a realization of one's own abilities and identity. The barriers and challenges to peer and self-assessment are discussed, and current evidence and practical applications are incorporated to begin to develop the capabilities in thoughtful and meaningful ways. Learners are guided not only in habitual effectiveness, but in how to write goals for their own personal and professional development, to facilitate the development of mindfulness, which is important as a foundation for expertise and decision making.

The chapter on identifying and resolving ethical dilemmas with problem-solving processes is enhanced and includes conceptual frameworks and suggested new models to consider for more in-depth ethical applications. This chapter emphasizes the awareness that traditional biomedical (principled) ethical reasoning is not a sufficient process for those of us caring for patients day to day as we become embroiled in their histories and stories. Empathy, sympathy, and an ethic of care and discernment are described as virtue tools to assist in making sound ethical decisions within the framework of traditional ethical discourse that supports this process. Data are included elucidating the relationship of health care errors and everyday ethics in real-world health care examples. The chapter examining stress management has been expanded because the increasing demands of health care have led to the need to further examine cases of risk management, fraud, and abuse and ensure that developing health care providers are aware of the relationship of stress and integrity in practice.

We have built upon the most recent edition's updates and address the frustrations of the generations by continuing our conversation and discussion of the much-needed development of face-to-face skills while encountering 5 generations in the health care workplace. We more deeply examine each of the generations and share perspectives for healthier work environments with an effort toward mutual understanding.

The remaining chapters teach actual skill development in communicating with people who trust the professional to offer therapeutic presence as well as skills in clinical reasoning, diagnosis, prognosis, and treatment progressions. The ever-popular exercises in assertive communication and challenging scenarios remain, with clear frameworks to assist the novice's development. A new focus on modern-day bullying is added to confront and identify the targeted problem, with an exploration into how these behaviors undermine the culture of safety and meaningful progress in health care environments.

In addition, and by popular request, the chapter added for the Fifth Edition on communicating about spiritual needs is enhanced with a new exploration of the relationship with the Human Movement System. This is not a chapter on religion but a chapter focusing on helping health care professionals to better assess the needs of patients and families in dealing with hope, faith, and despair. New suggested frameworks are included as guides for the novice health care professional, as well as additional case examples incorporated throughout the text chapters.

The chapters on patient education and communicating with cultural sensitivity have been enhanced with updates on the application of the transtheoretical model of change and expanded patient/client education activities. The chapters further consider the appropriate use of interactive technology for patient/client education, along with tips and resources for health literacy considerations and fostering health promotion.

We have added a much-needed chapter on leadership and advocacy for health care, which asks developing professionals to understand the importance of incorporating leadership skills with patient health care, with links to the societal generations. Through guided reading and writing pre- and post-chapter exercises, learners are asked to proactively consider one's future as a leader while also appreciating the benefits of knowing when to lead and when to follow. Team work and advocacy are also highlighted, with key exercises to facilitate application for action.

Additional chapters explore mindful practice and well-being activities while examining the influence of neuro-linguistics, culture differences, cultural awareness, and special populations, contexts, and environments. New exercises exploring a patient's progression within the health care system are included, as well as an extensive list of media resources to supplement learning and reflection.

There is a changing face to health care. Increasing numbers of our students come from other cultures. Our patients and clients represent a variety of cultures and backgrounds. This text helps students to develop assertiveness skills for those who are shy or from another culture that may emphasize more passive ways of communicating. Instructors can use this text (and its accompanying Instructor's Manual) to teach skills such as how to communicate therapeutically with patients from a different culture, those who are depressed, those trying to cope with increasing disability, those who are facing death, those who have learned that they will not be able to be the same sexually as before injury, those with changed lives due to changed family dynamics from caretaker to caregiver or care receiver, those who are raging with anger and hostility, and those who are inappropriate sexually with the professional.

And, as always, exercises at the end of each chapter encourage an essential element in the inculcation of these fundamental skills—reflection and personalization of the material to one's own story. These exercises are also available online at www.healio.com/books/davisforms. Your password to the site is provided on the insert included inside the front cover.

Those who have used this text sometimes email, call, or send letters expressing gratitude for PPI. Some of the unique benefits and features of this text are that it helps to develop self-awareness and communication skills for those situations with patients and colleagues where the health care professional would say to him- or herself, "What in the world do I say now? They never taught me in school how to deal with THIS situation." PPI remains the answer to every curriculum's need to develop interpersonal professional behavior in its students, and we are grateful to say it has been so effective at this task that it has been a bestseller for nearly 3 decades.

This is material that is not easily or happily taught but is required by accreditation standards in all programs because effective professional health care requires these skills. An Instructor's Manual accompanies the text to teach faculty how to best use this text to facilitate learning the material in a student-friendly way. Hints are provided on how to facilitate group interaction, helping students grapple with the information personally and make the necessary changes in long-standing, practiced communication styles that will not serve them well with patients.

We all want to enjoy ourselves, and we should be able to as we learn and grow as professionals. One of the forces that interferes with that enjoyment is not knowing what to say in an uncomfortable or highly emotional situation with patients, colleagues, or students. Once you start practicing the self-awareness and skills that this text is designed to teach, life will be much more enjoyable. And that's as it should be, and is our wish for all who read it and put these words into practice.

FOREWORD TO THE FIFTH EDITION

It was an unexpected joy to read this book and write the requested foreword. Though I have always known that this subject was of importance to practitioners in the health professions, my major interest has been in the basic sciences. As Chairman of a physical therapy program since before this book came into being, I assigned the general subject as part of a broader course to members of the faculty more in tune with this broad topic. They were capable of teaching and inculcating the importance of values, attitudes, and so forth as elucidated so beautifully and completely by Dr. Davis in this book.

Now I have read the book in its entirety, and what a delightful experience it has been! The author and contributors have made the topic not just a walk through social and personal issues and professional and personal behaviors, they have encased it in a scientific format of mainstream humanity, within each individual, between a caregiver and a care receiver, between friends or adversaries. Even more notably, Dr. Davis has provided health professionals with a road map to personal growth and worth and a source of human behavior that will engender faith, trust, and open and honest interactions between patients and therapists—in short, a thesaurus and encyclopedia of the sacred trust that must exist for a successful humanitarian experience in the health care arena.

This book has made its content part of the mainstream of health care, not just an adjunct to the process of that care. Anyone who reads and studies this book and gives him- or herself to the exercises that open very personal doors to behavior recognition and possible modification will find great satisfaction and gratification in the broader framework for successful and rewarding practice.

For persons now beyond retirement age, many will recall the time of the 1950s and some into the 1960s when there was a movement called sensitivity training. This was developed and offered as an organized course, or experience, in which individuals would attend seminars in an environment devoid of intrusion or extracurricular activities. Attendees were put through an experience designed to increase their sensitivity to others and to their own behavior (psyche) by self-reflection and exercises where the group delved deeply into each person's most personal behaviors. My description is most inadequate, because I never participated.

What I do know is that many who attended these training group sessions returned from them as very different people. Some carried on as before and stated that they felt helped. More of the persons I knew returned very different: Unable to sustain their daily lives as before, some who had been leaders in their profession had difficulty making decisions that before had been a major asset of their lifestyle. Their interaction with long-time colleagues changed and their considerable leadership skills and interpersonal relations had become woeful. Thus, I became skeptical and derisive of such efforts and suspicious of any sort of tinkering with personal behavior.

Then along came a new generation, with new ideas, better education, better social skills that had validity, and programs based on evidence. This book is the apotheosis of a new science, call it behavioral or social. Dr. Davis's work represents the best of that science and its evidence in this book speaks for itself.

When we become health care professionals, we commit ourselves to a sacred trust to care for people who need our special skills. *Patient Practitioner Interaction: An Experiential Manual for Developing the Art of Health Care, Fifth Edition,* will add significant substance to that trust, for it is not just what we do but how we share ourselves with those for whom we care, their families, and their friends—and the role models we can become for colleagues and students.

This book should be a required text in every school of physical therapy and for every program that expects superior performance in patient care whatever the discipline. Congratulations, Dr. Davis.

Helen J. Hislop, PT, PhD, ScD, FAPTA (1929-2013)
Former Chair, Division of Biokinesiology and Physical Therapy
University of Southern California
Los Angeles, California

Dr. Hislop was a pioneering chair at USC and visionary for the profession. She spent 23 years at USC, and during her tenure she engineered the growth of the program's size and prestige. She developed the first PhD program in Physical Therapy and embraced evidence-based practice. She innovatively created clinical specialization within the Division curriculum and transformed physical therapy residencies while at USC. She successfully launched one of the first DPT programs, graduating the first class at USC in 1998 and retiring that same year. Dr. Hislop provided the often-cited 1975 Mary McMillan lecture, "The Not So Impossible Dream." You may learn more about Dr. Helen Hislop's life and work in her tribute video (http://pt.usc.edu/Helen_Hislop_Video/) and oral history (http://pt.usc.edu/About_The_Division/Division_History/).

FOREWORD TO THE SIXTH EDITION

I wish that my selection to write this Foreword were based on my expertise in the topic, but unfortunately that is not the case. If the invitation is because of my belief of the importance of the topic, then the choice is accurate. Fifty-seven years ago, during my physical therapy educational program, the type of information contained in this book was not even considered for the curriculum. A basic course in psychology was a prerequisite requirement, and that was the extent of anything close to social science being included in the curriculum. I truly believed, for all too long, that if I got the treatment right, that was the key issue to a successful outcome. Entering the profession during the last stages of practice involving polio patients and the early stages of patients with upper motor neuron lesions provided for a very different environment than is currently present. Patients were hospitalized or in rehabilitation centers for many months. I remember very well therapists becoming emotionally involved with their patients, particularly the young spinal cord–injured patients, and trying to be counselor, social worker, and best friend. When you were working with individuals for hours a day, at least 5 days a week, for anywhere from 6 to 10 months, maintaining the proper relationship was often difficult. Also, in those days, acceptance of individuals with physical disability was far from ideal, just as the physical barriers also made life outside the hospital or rehabilitation facility difficult. My world and that of most of fellow staff members was small, with limited exposure to different types of people.

Because treatment was in a big gym-type room, I learned how different ways of relating to patients made a difference in their participation by watching other therapists. Bit by bit, I realized that knowing the best treatment was certainly important, but of almost equal importance was establishing the necessary rapport with the patient. I had to learn by trial and error about myself and how I reacted to different patients. There were challenges, such as convincing the formerly highly independent farmer, now partially paralyzed, that I could safely help him transfer and walk. I had to learn how to be serious with the no-nonsense types and how to lighten the atmosphere for those who were devastated by their loss of body function and independence. After many years of patient care, which also involved personal maturity, I was able to pride myself on how well I could establish rapport with my patients so that they knew we were in this together and maximum effort would be expended to help them as much as possible.

Students and practitioners are so fortunate to have this book to provide the guidance and insights to help them gain, in a short period of time, what took me all too many years. In the intervening years, the world has gotten large for all of us. People of a variety of cultures are present not just in large cities, but also in small towns. Communication skills have been enhanced and compromised by the availability of the Internet and smart phones. I believe several factors are increasing the importance of this type of information. First, physical therapists are among the few health professionals who actually work with their patients. Clearly, patient participation in the treatment program is essential and, for the majority of patients, being guided and inspired by their therapist is key to adherence. As physicians continue to shorten their time with patients and care is spread among a variety of specialists, the therapist can become the constant and trusted professional for the patient. I believe that the change in reimbursement is going to lead to a larger number of patients who pay out of pocket, or more vested payments in other ways, who will be seeking even greater value from a practitioner that they can truly trust. We will need to be sure to understand patients' movement problems, and, therefore, to establish an appropriate, therapeutic relationship. In the future, we will not discharge patients, but will instead just end an episode of care. We are already working within this model in some settings for patients with neuromusculoskeletal, integumentary, endocrine, and cardiopulmonary movement disorders, affected by diseases for which we are still seeking cures in the 21st century. As the profession continues to develop the concept of the Human Movement System, the importance of precise movement in preventing musculoskeletal health syndromes, and the essential role of exercise for health, we will be lifespan practitioners.

The way you move affects every aspect of your life, and the way you decide how to interact with your patients and clients to facilitate their success for movement is key for actively engaging your patients and clients for their health. All of these aspects of practice require professionals who have learned the most about themselves and how best to relate to patients and clients. This is the book that can provide the knowledge and ability to be that professional. The included exercises are particularly valuable for learners. I cannot recommend this book and the information it contains more highly for the sake of professionals and the profession.

Shirley A. Sahrmann, PT, PhD, FAPTA
Professor Emerita Physical Therapy
Washington University School of Medicine
St. Louis, Missouri

1

BASIC AWARENESS OF SELF

Carol M. Davis, DPT, EdD, MS, FAPTA and
Gina Maria Musolino, PT, MSEd, EdD

"Nobody sees a flower, really—it's so small—we haven't time, and to see it takes time..." –Georgia O'Keefe

OBJECTIVES

- To introduce the concept of the self.
- To emphasize the importance of self-knowledge in relation to the quality of one's life and the choices one makes.
- To begin to understand potential barriers to self-awareness and helpful resources for self-awareness.
- To facilitate self-awareness through reading, completing exercises, and journaling about oneself.

WHAT IS THE SELF?

How well do you know yourself? Why would anyone ever ask that question? Some would say that the better you know yourself, the more aware you are of your thoughts and feelings, your strengths and weaknesses; the more you feel in control of your life, the less stressed and helpless you feel, and the less surprised you are by your responses to life. Thus, it might be said that the quality of one's life is, in part, measured by the amount of personal control one feels over day-to-day happenings and choices.

People who are forced to live in institutions and be cared for by others especially feel the negative effect of powerlessness in being forced to succumb to the rules of the larger order—the system. For example, few personal choices are preserved in nursing homes and hospitals. Today, more efforts are being made to incorporate a person's life story in their care, but this involves a paradigm shift for health care professionals (HCPs) who are less inclined, unfortunately, to take the time to get know their patient as a person first. This chapter asks you to get to know yourself better as a person first so that you may better care for yourself and your well-being and, therefore, be more available and present to care for others as a health care professional. You are becoming a professional, so it is important to know who you are and who you are becoming.

What is the self? How is the self different from the body? What are people asking when they ask, "Who am I, really?" and "Why am I here?" These are timeless questions that seem to become more the focus of concern during the second half of life than during the first. It has been said that, for many of us, the first half of life is the "doing" half and the second

Davis CM, Musolino GM. *Patient Practitioner Interaction: An Experiential Manual for Developing the Art of Health Care, Sixth Edition* (pp 1-12).
© 2016 SLACK Incorporated.

half is the "being" half. When we are busy achieving and working for security and happiness, questions such as "Who am I?" seem distracting. Once we grow beyond our mid-30s, these questions take on greater importance as we reflect on the meaning of life as we begin to recognize and realize our own mortalities.

Young children are unable to be truly self-aware. But, you may remember that delicious moment when you first discovered, all by yourself, that you were uniquely different from anyone else in the whole world. You were probably 6 or 7. Richard Zaner, in his text *The Context of Self*,[1] described a colleague's recounting of this moment:

> *As far as I can tell, I must have been younger than 8 years old when I began having what I now call I-am-me experiences. On such occasions I would tell myself insistently, "This is me, me ..." The inner pronouncing of these words and especially the repetition of the personal pronoun were accompanied with the feeling of a cave-in, a dropping down from a surface level of self-awareness to a more and more personal me-myself. Along with it went a feeling of being sucked down as by a whirlpool into a bottomless depth. As I repeated the pronoun "me" I felt as if one mask after another fell off, until the actor behind these masks was stripped to his naked core.*

To be able to reflect upon the full nature of one's self, however, seems to require the cognitive skills and experiences of a person with a mature nervous system. To become aware of oneself, one must go outside of one's self and ponder the self and, for example, analyze one's motives for behavior. This only becomes possible, according to Piaget,[2] at the stage of formal operations.

THE DESIRE FOR SELF-AWARENESS

The wish to become self-aware often has to do with the search for meaning in life and the desire to experience a choice in the process of whom one is becoming. In other words, the question "Who am I?" is necessary before one can truly be who one chooses to be. Parents tell children how to act most often with good intention. Most children are socialized into becoming what their parents or guardians believe are good human beings who will live happy and productive lives. The influence of the family on one's self-esteem and self-concept is a very important topic that will be covered in more depth in Chapter 2.

The goal of education for health care professionals is to assist students in becoming a certain way: **professional**. What does it mean to be professional? Much has been written elsewhere about that question. Suffice it to say that any description of a professional would contain the integration of a body of knowledge and skills and the proficient and effective delivery of the same. In the profession of health care, proficient and effective delivery requires a therapeutic use of one's self while interacting with clients. Superior skill in the technology of the profession *must* be balanced with the *art* of relating to those who request our services in such a way that healing is facilitated, rather than interfered with, in the provision of care.

If health care consisted of working on bodies alone, perhaps a consideration of the self would not be necessary. But the fact remains that health care involves people and interacting with people in such a way that what is not right is correctly analyzed and appropriately influenced so that it is changed to approximate more closely what is right. This analysis and influence takes place between human beings who have not just brought their bodies to us but have also brought their feelings, fears, hopes, frustrations, and pain. Illness is meaningful only as it is lived, moment to moment. When we care professionally, we care for people living with their illnesses, not for broken bodies. Let us take a closer look at the nature of the self: what it is; what it is not; how it grows and is influenced; and how it performs as we mature into healthy, more self-actualized human beings.

THE SELF

Human beings are tremendously complex organisms, capable of portraying various identities or roles, depending on what the situation calls for. Much study has been devoted to the manner in which we can divide ourselves into various parts or take on different roles and remain essentially the same person, or whole. Transactional analysis literature teaches about the "parent, adult, and child" in each of us.[3] We each portray various roles throughout the day, such as employee, boss, sister, brother, and friend. Carl Jung, in his attempt to explore the nature of the unconscious, described archetypal elements present in all personalities. Among them were the persona, the shadow, and the self. Freud is famous for his explications of the ego, the id, and the superego. All of these now-common terms were created to help explain the complex behavior of human beings.

The psychology literature informs us about the nature of the self and its role in human growth (Figure 1-1). The nature of self figure represents the various layers of a person or the various aspects of a personality. The outermost layer is best described as the *persona*, or the public face, each of us puts on in the world to appear in control, intelligent, witty, sensitive, and lovable. We act in the ways that we believe are going to bring us love and recognition. But, deep inside, we know that

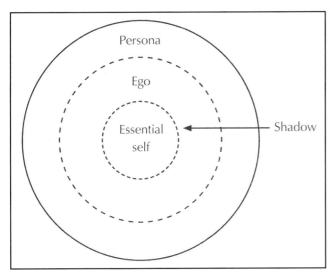

Figure 1-1. The nature of self.

the persona is really a mask. Underneath that mask is another aspect of ourselves that is filled with doubts and insecurities. Almost all of us are dissatisfied with living our lives totally from behind the mask. Each of us desires to drop our false fronts and to become who we truly are, to express ourselves more honestly, to be more truly ourselves, and to be loved for who we truly are inside.

The second layer is composed of the *ego*, or the center of the conscious mind as described by Freud, and the *shadow*, the unconscious, natural side of our personalities. The ego is the part of us that gets the job of living done. It is the force that gets us through school and makes choices for us that are designed, as best we know, to bring us happiness. It problem solves for us and helps us have the courage to act and the patience to wait. But the ego is made up of all kinds of misinformation about ourselves and about the world. Egos tend to be very protective; they tend to move us toward safety, toward the status quo. The ego believes in its own omnipotence. But it has to sustain that belief by using a lot of energy and by ignoring many messages that would refute that omnipotence. The feeling of a god-like ego is an illusion. In fact, the ego is filled with erroneous ideas and fears about the world and about ourselves. Our egos tell us we are very intelligent one minute and totally naïve and stupid the next. First they tell us the world is a wonderful, loving place, and then that it is a dangerous place.

Each of us tends to listen to the still, small voice of the ego when we have to make important choices, but we become very confused about what is important and true. This is because we tend to allow the voice of the ego to reflect what we have heard from important people in our lives about ourselves. If we heard, "You are so stupid, you'll never amount to anything" when we were young, we believed that for a time until we had the power to prove that it was not true. As we achieved success, we told our egos, "See, I really am bright. I can succeed!" But instead of dropping the old data and incorporating the new, the ego holds onto the whole package and spits both messages at us at times when we feel most unable to modify that quiet voice.

Eckhart Tolle,[4] in his well-regarded book, *A New Earth: Awakening to Your Life's Purpose*, tells us that we need others to give us a sense of ourselves. How we are seen by others evolves into how we come to see ourselves:

> *If you live in a culture that to a large extent equates self-worth with how much and what you have, if you cannot look through that collective delusion, you will be condemned to chasing after things for the rest of your life in the vain hope of finding your worth and completing of your sense of self there. … The ego isn't wrong, it's just unconscious.*

The *shadow* is Carl Jung's term for another aspect of the unconscious part of this second layer. It is our inferior side, the part of us that wants to do all the things our ego tells us we cannot do. When we say things like, "I wasn't myself" or "I don't know what came over me," we are acknowledging the presence of our unconscious shadow that tricks us into behaving in ways we say we abhor. Underneath these outer 2 layers, at the center of the person, lies the rest of us, the "more" that the outer 2 layers cannot fully incorporate: the *self*. The self is the essence of the person and incorporates conscious and unconscious elements of the person into itself. I have my persona, I have my ego, I have my personality, I have my body, I have my possessions in life…I am my self. The self is the irreducible energy of my uniqueness. It is the thing that makes me absolutely unique in the whole world despite the fact that, for example, I have an identical twin sister and probably thousands of people share my name. It is that marvelous essence of me that I approach as the masks are, one by one, stripped away in the search for what is undividable, what is at my core. It is the unfolding answer to the eternal question, "Who am I, really?"

The self is that energy that can linger for days before the moment of the "crossing over" into death of the physical body. Those who care for the terminally ill have often experienced the phenomenon that, for a time before the body stops functioning totally, it is more accurate to say that all that remains in the bed is a shell that looks like the person's body. The essence of the person seems to come and go, little by little, spending more time gone than present.

The self has to do with the energy inside each human that reincarnationists say is a piece of the deity that is never created or destroyed.[5] It is my "higher self." Christians would call it the "Christ self" within each of us, and Buddhists would call it the "Buddha self." It exists for all time; it always has and always will, and the task of human beings on Earth is to house this energy as we grow and change, lifetime after lifetime, with the end goal of becoming more like God, like truth.

Jung said this about the nature of the self[6]:

> *The self...can include both the conscious and the unconscious. It appears to act as something like a magnet to the disparate elements of the personality and the processes of the unconscious, and is the centre of this totality as the ego is the centre of consciousness, for it is the function which unites all the opposing elements in man and woman, consciousness and unconsciousness, good and bad, male and female, etc, and in so doing transmutes them. To reach it necessitates acceptance of what is inferior in one's nature, as well as what is irrational and chaotic. This state cannot be reached by a mature person without considerable struggle; it implies suffering, for the Western mind, unlike the Eastern, does not easily tolerate paradoxes. [The self] consists...in the awareness on the one hand of our unique natures, and on the other of our intimate relationship with all life, not only human, but animal and plant, and even that of inorganic matter and the cosmos itself. It brings a feeling of "oneness," and/or reconciliation with life, which now can be accepted as it is, not as it should be.*

Thus, the self, once uncovered, seems to hold the real truth about us as human beings. It is our connection with the Truth, and it is out of this center of our existence that we come to feel at one with our fellow human beings. It is the self that is able to cross over in empathy and experience and feel what a moment in life must be like for another person. It is the self that we return to as we quiet our working minds in meditation. It is the self that allays our fears, that gives us true courage rather than braggadocio or false bravado; it is the self that feels the essential goodness of our humanness, in the face of our incompleteness; it is the self that grows in wisdom and becomes more as we mature, approaching the all-knowing goodness of Truth; it is the self that enables us to laugh at our egos and forgive the well-meaning unkindness visited upon us by parents and relatives as they tried desperately to get us to "act right" as children and thereby systematically helped to destroy our inborn connectedness with our true selves.

SELF-AWARENESS

Rogers[7] has said, "It appears that the goal the individual most wishes to achieve, the end which he knowingly and unknowingly pursues, is to become himself." How do we become ourselves? How do we discover our true natures? How do we access the self? How do we get close to it, get right up next to it? It begins when we recognize the burning desire to be known for who we are, not for who we believe others want us to be. It begins when we are willing to shed the roles we have assumed to win attention and affection and acceptance and instead commit to being truthful and honest. Often the first steps we take in this direction come with our challenges to our parents and the "rules of the house."

Self-awareness requires reflection to ascertain who we truly are. The ego will work overtime to tell you about yourself, but it takes time and effort of a different sort to reflect deeper to the messages of the true self.

Often, we need help in this process of becoming more self-aware because our perceptions are unavoidably colored by the messages we heard when we were very young. To sift through unchallenged truths that were reinforced for years (eg, all women are emotional, all men are insensitive) requires, for example, the perspectives of literature, art, and music and the professional preparation of counselors and psychologists to help us examine our habitual assumptions. The goal of growth of this sort is to expand the narrow, parochial views we held as children and become more aware of a wider world view that incorporates diversity and trades black-and-white, dualistic thinking for the wonderful colors of ambiguity, free from the need to be right and from the fear of being wrong. It is, in a sense, the search for truth that we are after as we mature in our world views. We want to enfold all possibilities, rather than leave out information that might be critical for comprehending the complexities of ourselves, our lives, and the world we live in. In the search for the self, the goal becomes to give up beliefs that entrap us in negativity, doubt, and self-centered behavior and replace them with beliefs that enlarge our consciousness and help us feel compassion for our oneness with all of life and sincere interest in the needs of those we serve.

EXAMPLE OF LACK OF SELF-AWARENESS

When we find ourselves distracted from the moment, or if we have never participated in self-awareness activities, patients can suffer from our insensitivity. Let us consider an example:

A recently graduated physical therapist was having a particularly difficult day and was not taking regular check on his emotions. He went into his patient's room and found the patient engrossed in a conversation with his nurse. The patient was trying to understand the various medications he was taking and their possible side effects. He was anxious and could not seem to understand what the nurse was repeating over and over to him. As the physical therapist waited for this discussion to be completed, he became increasingly impatient, recognizing that he was becoming more behind in his patient treatments for the day. He interrupted the conversation rudely and stated, "Look, I've been waiting patiently here for 5 minutes. I am on a tight schedule, and I have to see this patient next. Please wrap this chat up and let me get to work, will you?"

Had he stopped for a second and taken a deep breath, he might have realized, first of all, that he was annoyed and, second, that this was an important conversation and he had several choices available to solve his problem. Because he lacked self-awareness and tact, he saw the problem not as his, but as the nurse's.

This lack of self-awareness brought a negative energy into the entire situation, and this could have been completely avoided had the physical therapist, once he recognized his emotion of annoyance and impatience, reviewed his options and invited the nurse and patient to help him decide when would be a good time to return. This was obviously an important conversation between the patient and nurse that needed to continue, and the needs of the patient are more important than the therapist's schedule. Very often, the major goal of young people, as they become socialized into acting professionally, is to recognize that patient care is about patients, not about "me." Patients and their needs come first, and this may be a new perspective for young health care professionals to accept. It is all part of growth and development into maturation in becoming a health care professional.

SEARCH FOR THE SELF

This text is designed to help you examine your values, beliefs, and communication patterns in an effort to assist you in the search for your self and to broaden your world view. It is from the self that we give health care of the highest quality. It is the self that has the capacity to see clearly and to display compassion in the face of threat or fatigue, which crosses over into empathy. It is the self that sets appropriate boundaries and refuses to attempt to have personal needs met by patients. It is the self that has unlimited patience and great understanding. It is the self that comprehends the need to be ethical and act with integrity. It is the self that has the desire and the capability to feel unconditional positive regard and oneness with all living beings, which cancels out judgment and prejudice.

However, it is the frightened ego that pities and pretends that it is displaying compassion; it is the frightened ego that becomes impatient and defends itself rather than offering a healing response to the angry patient; it is the ego that needs to be puffed up and made to feel important at the expense of others' feelings. It is the frightened ego that *requires* our patients to do as we say, to get better, and to thank us for helping them.

All of us want essentially the same thing: to be respected and to be treated with unconditional positive regard. But all of us want that positive acceptance of our whole being, not just of our persona (ie, our ego). We want others to love and accept us as we are wholly, in all of our incompleteness. The more the ego tries to defend itself, the more difficult it is to catch a glimpse of ourselves and our essential natures. If you have been told that you tend to respond defensively to people, you developed this coping skill out of necessity. However, it is not very useful in patient care. This will be a good opportunity for you to examine the messages you are receiving that make you feel as if you must defend yourself. Defensiveness always obliterates the truth. It is noisy and useless and has no sense of humor at all. It is the mark of a person responding to life from an insecure ego, not the sign of a whole and integrated self who might respond to criticism with, for example, "I didn't know I was coming across that way. I'll take a closer look at my behavior now."

As health care professionals gain expertise, they find that it becomes important to regularly take stock of one's feelings during the day. The emotions are key to what we experience, and sometimes we find ourselves disassociating from people in response to feeling overwhelmed with work or feeling insecure or angry with the system. Regularly experiencing our feelings as they arise during our day becomes an important component of practitioner well-being and keeps us connected with ourselves and able to focus on our patients and the task at hand. One must not lose track of normal emotional responses because this is what makes us sensitive and caring providers. Yet, as health care professionals, we must learn to cope and manage appropriately by taking the time to recognize and respond to our own feelings, too. Sometimes we must take a personal time-out to make sure that this happens in a healthy manner. Again, caring for others means first caring for your self.

Patients appreciate demonstrations of personal caring and responding with emotion to their stories and situations of the day. The expert clinician knows how to do this and set appropriate boundaries at the same time, which allows for therapeutic presence without burdening the patient with our feelings. The more connected we are with our own selves, the more connected we become with our patients and colleagues and the higher the quality of our caring and efforts.[8]

Signs of Growth in Self-Awareness

As people struggle to become more themselves, usually out of the painful realization that the masks they have been using are no longer bringing them happiness and love, they change in noticeable ways. As described by Rogers,[7] they seem to do the following:

- Drop the defensive mask with which they have faced life and begin to discover and to experience the stranger who lives behind these masks—the hidden part of self.
- Emerge with a tendency to be more open to all elements of experience, growing to trust in one's organism as an instrument of sensitive living.
- Accept the responsibility of being a unique person.
- Develop the sense of living in life as a participant in a fluid, ongoing process, continually discovering new aspects of one's self in the flow of experience.

When we live daily with an awareness of our true selves, negative feelings are confronted, and the beliefs behind them are analyzed and replaced with beliefs that are more positive and cosmic. Thus, we take responsibility for creating our own reality, moment to moment. No longer do we allow ourselves to get away with such beliefs as, "You make me so angry." We acknowledge that we make ourselves angry in response to someone because of a belief we have about that person or that behavior, and then we search for a larger, more hopeful and understanding belief that will replace feelings of negativity.

Tolle[4] reminds us that "[t]he primary cause of unhappiness is never the situation but your thoughts about the situation. … See the link between your thinking and your emotions. Rather than being your thoughts and emotions, be the awareness behind them."

Be aware in today's society that the use of technologies may prohibit us from fully realizing who we are or can be as a person. Do not allow technology to keep you from knowing your self. Do not "fall prey to the illusion of companionship through the gathering of thousands of Twitter followers and Facebook friends, and confusing tweets and wall posts with authentic communication."[9] As Turkle[9] described, this "relentless connection with technology leads to a new solitude." Technology may serve to connect persons who might not otherwise connect, but it is not a replacement for knowing your true self. We may be more connected but more disconnected. Take time to get to know your self and others in more connected ways. You will find greater happiness in life making true connections and using technology to enhance your relationships and expand your circle, but do not use it as a substitute for first-hand communication, whenever more appropriate. Do not allow technology to be another mask. As future health care professionals, we must make every effort to be as connected as possible in the 2-, 3-, and 4-dimensional world in which we live today.

As developing professionals, selecting the most appropriate means of communication to ascertain the most meaningful ways to communicate is key. Do not allow objects to replace who we are as a person; experience your humanness.[10] Be fully present with those you are with and engage in meaningful and deep conversations so as not to be depleted by the hype. Superficial communication shall leave you wanting. You will be more self-aware by not succumbing to a pure persona of social media, but by being yourself. Above all, as you develop as a health care professional and engage in the often hectic environments of health care delivery, take time in your life to do nothing, disconnect from technology, contemplate your navel, take a moment, take a minute, and pause for the cause of just being and for self-awareness. In this "stopping, we discover the vast spaciousness of life, of love, of connection."[11]

Conclusion

Following most chapters in the text, including this one, you shall find additional helpful resources and references to further explore the topical content for each chapter. As a developing professional, you will want to revisit the textbook chapters and additional resources as you progress in your development. It will be especially relevant for you to follow up and revisit the workbook learning in more depth as you begin and continue your patient-practitioner interactions (PPIs). Seeking out and exploring these resources, now or in the future, shall continue to catalyze your personal professional development and reinforce your continued self-awareness and learning. As a health care professional, it is important to maintain your sense of self and to stay centered so you are able to help others reach their full potentials. Even your posture, the way you carry yourself, and being able to truly pay attention to your own movement, emotions, and sensations is key to your own self-awareness.[12,13] Again, in this technologically driven society, people are losing touch with their bodies and may be compromising their own health status and self-awareness; as a health care professional, it is even more important for you to realize this in yourself, your patients, and your clients. Continuing to examine your own mind-body-spirit connections work and how we use technology to enhance or detract from the human interface is something we need to be aware of and tuned into for our preferred PPI. Our journey together is just beginning; in Chapter 5, we will look to explore stress management; in Chapter 8, we shall discover mechanisms to resolve conflict in PPI; and in Chapter 14, we shall specifically delve into aspects of spirituality in health care and the impact on PPI.

The goal of this entire text is to assist you in learning more about yourself so that the way in which you relate to patients and clients who come to you for help might be sensitive, compassionate, and free from prejudice and negativity. Central to this goal is the assumption that our true or essential selves reflect the essential goodness in all of us and can be covered up by the persona, the many masks we wear, and the ego that sees the world through lenses that were originally set when we were very young and helpless. The behaviors that facilitate healing, as we apply our technology, are those behaviors and underlying beliefs that bring about wholeness and oneness. Behaviors that interfere with healing result in fragmentation, discord, and negativity. I believe that it is possible to grow such that the nature of our essential selves is accessible to us and that, out of a connectedness with our essential selves, we are empowered to provide health care of the highest order. In that connectedness with our essential selves, we have the power to realize the fears and shortcomings of our egos, the falseness, and manipulation of our personas. Out of that connectedness with our essential selves, we can be the persons we were created to be—capable of *unconditional positive regard* for all humans[7] and especially those we serve as our patients and clients. This is the greatest calling of health care professionals. It is a tremendously challenging task to grow to this goal, but the rewards are indescribable. Be open to the possibilities on your journey to becoming a health care professional.

REFERENCES

1. Zaner RM. *The Context of Self.* Athens, OH: Ohio University Press; 1981.
2. Piaget J. *The Construction of Reality in the Child.* New York, NY: Basic Books; 1954.
3. Berne E. *Transactional Analysis in Psychotherapy.* New York, NY: Grove Press; 1961.
4. Tolle E. *A New Earth: Awakening to Your Life's Purpose.* New York, NY: Plume Books; 2008.
5. Challoner HK. *The Wheel of Rebirth.* Wheaton, IL: The Theosophical Publishing House; 1969.
6. Fordham F. *An Introduction to Jung's Psychology.* Baltimore, MD: Penguin Books; 1953.
7. Rogers CR. *On Becoming a Person.* Boston, MA: Houghton Mifflin; 1961.
8. Gordon GH. Giving bad news. In: Feldman MD, Christensen JF, eds. *Behavioral Medicine in Primary Care: A Practical Guide.* 2nd ed. New York, NY: McGraw Hill Medical; 2003:17-22.
9. Turkle S. *Alone Together: Why We Expect More From Technology and Less From Each Other.* New York, NY: Basic Books; 2012.
10. Boyer J. *This "Me" of Mine: Self, Time & Context in the Digital Age.* Bloomington, IN: Xlibris Corporation; 2013.
11. Kundtz D. *Quiet Mind: One-Minute Retreats From a Busy World.* York Beach, ME: Red Wheel/Weiser; 2002.
12. Rosen M. Rosen *Method Bodywork: Accessing the Unconscious Through Touch.* Berkeley, CA: North Atlantic Books; 2003.
13. Fogel A. *Body Sense: The Science and Practice of Embodied Self-Awareness (Norton Series on Interpersonal Neurobiology).* New York, NY: WW Norton & Company; 2009.

SUGGESTED READINGS

Fogel A. Body sense: restorative embodied self-awareness as a pathway to well-being. *Psychology Today.* https://www.psychologytoday.com/blog/body-sense.

Frankl VE. *Man's Search for Ultimate Meaning.* New York, NY: Basic Books; 2000.

Heatherton TF, Baumeister RF. Binge eating as an escape from self awareness. *Psychol Bull.* 1991;110(1):86-108.

Malik K. Collaboration between self and Self. *Bridges: International Society for the Study of Subtle Energy and Energy Medicine.* 2002;13.

Masterson JF. *The Search for the Real Self: Unmasking the Personality Disorders of Our Age.* New York, NY: The Free Press; 1988.

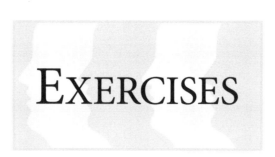

EXERCISES

REFLECTIVE RUMINATIONS: JOURNAL ACTIVITY

At the conclusion of the chapter exercises, begin a journal about yourself during this time. Journal entries are most useful in learning about yourself if they relate what you learned from the experience. Most of us confuse the concept of a journal with a diary. A diary is designed to record significant events in one's life. A journal is a letter to yourself that is designed to stimulate reflection about an experience, rather than just record the experience.

One way to keep from simply recording the event is to begin each entry with the following phrases:

- What I felt during the exercise.
- What I learned about myself.
- So what? Significance or meanings of my learning.

Your journal should be kept in a book with a cover and pages that do not easily become dislodged, or you may wish to keep an electronic journal. Ideally, entries are to be written following each chapter. Many find it useful to journal as a way of privately discussing the chapter and its personal significance as well. Your journal is what you make it. Most university students are unaccustomed to this sort of activity and some abhor writing. Make a commitment to this activity; it is the beginning of becoming a reflective health care professional, which we will discuss more in Chapter 9. Use the Feeling Wheel (Figure 1-2). Remember, this journal is by you for your personal use. Set aside the time on your calendar, and, once

Figure 1-2. The Feeling Wheel. (Reprinted with permission from Willcox G. The Feeling Wheel: a tool for expanding awareness of emotions and increasing spontaneity and intimacy. *Transactional Analysis Journal.* 1982;12[4]:274-276.)

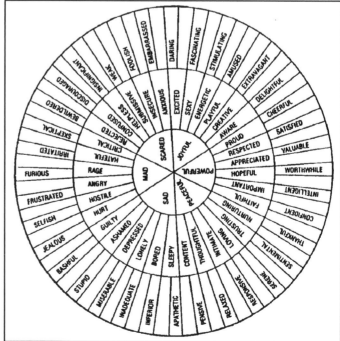

you get into it, the journal will become rewarding. Your course instructor may wish to see your entries now and again to be sure that you are keeping up. In that case, confidentiality may become more limited. You will not be graded on your journal. Because it is a collection of your feelings and reflections, a grade would be wholly inappropriate. However, the value of the activity is such that your instructor may collect it to check your discipline with the activity and may comment on how well you reflected on the experience rather than simply describing what happened.

EXERCISE 1: WHAT'S SO ABOUT ME?

On a separate sheet of paper that you can keep confidential, answer each of the following as honestly as you can for this moment. Allow at least half a sheet of paper for each question. Each question requires reflection, but jot down the first thing that comes to mind and then take time with each question to clearly communicate your awareness (or lack of it!). You may wish to complete the entire set over a period of a week or so, taking 1 or 2 questions at a time. Ask yourself as you reflect over your responses, "Is that my ego talking? Is this truly what I believe about myself, or is this what I have heard others tell me about me?"

1. I would describe myself as…
2. Others would describe me as…
3. People are essentially (good, bad, neutral)…
4. I am proudest of…
5. I was most embarrassed when I…
6. I am most annoyed about myself when I…
7. I get angriest when…
8. Under severe stress, I usually…
9. What I want others to understand about me is that…
10. I'm most anxious that…
11. Characteristics of other people that impress me most include…
12. I protect myself when…
13. I would be willing to die in 6 months if…
14. I don't know how to say…
15. Aspects of my communication that I want to keep and refine are…
16. Aspects of my communication that I want to change include…
17. Goals I want to achieve…
    a. With this course…
    b. In my lifetime…

Discussion

Once you have answered these questions, write a description about yourself from what you have discovered. Are you totally happy with yourself at this point? What would you change? What did you learn about yourself that will assist you in being a health care professional? What may detract from your effectiveness? How aware are you of the messages from your ego, of your shadow? How aware are you of your self? Identify responses that have a negative aspect to them. What is the belief that you hold that makes that answer true for you? What is an alternative belief that you also hold that would replace the negative one so that your response might be more positive and hopeful?

Example: I protect myself when I am criticized for being too unscientific, naïve, or idealistic. Negative belief: I lack the intellect to scientifically prove what I believe is true and important. Replacement belief: The scientific method holds one way of verifying what is true. The balance of logic and facts with intuitive knowing together frames a larger truth. I have proven skills as a scientist, and I have faith in my intuition. Both serve me well in my work.

EXERCISE 2: CLINIC WAITING ROOM EXERCISE

This exercise is designed to help you recognize nonverbal indicators of emotion and, thus, keys to inner values that are often subtle and overlooked but, when recognized, can be of valuable importance in communication. It also reinforces what Tolle[4] said about recognizing that we are more than our emotions, and our emotions reflect our thoughts, which often are not accurate or appropriate to a situation but are false beliefs, things that we tell ourselves over time that we never question but should, because the source of much unhappiness is often erroneous beliefs and emotions that simply feel bad and are not even true.

The instructor writes one word describing an emotion on a 3 × 5 file card—words such as impatient, lonely, sad, eager, peaceful, relaxed, satisfied (see the Feeling Wheel [see Figure 1-2] for suggestions). There is one card for each member of the class, and it is kept secret, known only to the holder of the card. Three chairs are placed side by side in the front of the classroom to represent the waiting room in a clinic. The exercise starts by having one person come forward spontaneously, and his or her task is to act out the word on his or her card. Then another person comes forward and joins the first person, acting out his or her word. You can use verbal expression but you cannot use the word on your card. The goal of the rest of the class is to guess what emotion or behavior each person is representing. A third person then comes forward spontaneously, and the first person gets up and leaves, so there are always 2 people interacting in the "clinic."

Once everyone has had a chance to act out their word, the entire class forms a circle for discussion and guesses each person's word. Discussion should be focused on the nuances that each person used to convey an exact meaning (eg, depressed in contrast to sad). Finally, discussion should center on how this would be helpful to students in interaction with their patients and, even more importantly perhaps, for self-awareness. How does each student convey feelings of joy? Anger? Impatience? Fear? What about being a health care professional is joyful, frustrating, and fearful, and how would that look in your behavior? How will you know this?

EXERCISE 3: COLLAGE

With the use of any material, construct a collage that represents you as you know yourself at this moment. Your collage may comprise pictures and colors as in a traditional collage, or you may wish to use other materials such as digital images or 3-D objects to construct a less traditional montage. Do not choose representations of your persona only. Search your heart for symbols of your true self, the part of you that you hold dear but that you do not readily reveal. Also, choose representatives of your ego and your shadow as well. You may want to use video or digital pictures to represent yourself. If you do decide to do that, be comprehensive. For example, the exercise would not be complete if you simply brought in one song on an iPod and played it and declared, "This is who I am," without going into more detail.

Bring your creation to class wrapped so that others cannot identify it. Gather in small groups. Place one creation in the center of the group and observe it carefully without speaking for 2 or 3 minutes. Gather a private impression of what the creator was trying to convey. Then, in turn, offer observations that you perceive about the person for 5 minutes or so. After this anonymous discussion, identify the creator. He or she then will respond to what was observed by classmates, what was on target, and where classmates missed the mark. Finally, group members should share what each learned about this classmate before bringing forth the next collage. Sample collages follow for your reference in Figures 1-3 and 1-4. Please feel free to use your own creative style and ideas. The University of South Florida, School of Physical Therapy & Rehabilitation Sciences current and former students provided permission to proudly share. Enjoy!

Figure 1-3. Collage by Dr. Christopher Kroger, PT, DPT, class of 2015.

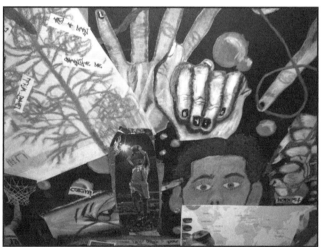

Figure 1-4. Class of 2016-2017 student physical therapists: Monica Seal, Katelin Foley, Elizabeth Tillman, Katie Sullivan, Nima Sobhani, and Kendra Smothers.

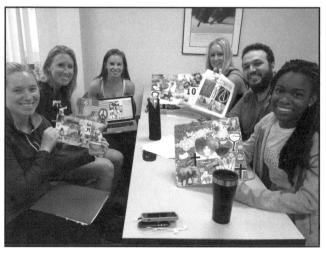

> **The exercises at the end of this chapter are also available online.**
> **Please refer to the sticker in the front of the book and enter the access code provided.**

2

FAMILY HISTORY

Carol M. Davis, DPT, EdD, MS, FAPTA and
Gina Maria Musolino, PT, MSEd, EdD

"Life is difficult. This is a great truth, one of the greatest truths. It is a great truth because once we truly see this truth, we transcend it. Once we truly know that life is difficult—once we truly understand and accept it—then life is no longer difficult. Because once it is accepted, the fact that life is difficult no longer matters." –M. Scott Peck

OBJECTIVES

- To describe, in general, the role families play in the formation of identity and self-esteem.
- To examine the development of a mature personality as described by Erikson.
- To introduce the concept of the false self in relation to the true self as it develops in dysfunctional families.
- To recognize the dangers inherent in being raised by overly attentive parents and those who, because of addictions to drugs, alcohol, or work, cannot truly parent.
- To introduce the concept of the generations in relation to families and the work system.
- To stress the importance of self-awareness to authenticity or the awareness of the true self as opposed to the false self.
- To stress the importance of authenticity to effective, mature helping.

It has been said that a clinician's most important tool is the effective use of self. Our personalities and our styles of relating have everything to do with how effective we are in facilitating the healing process. No one wants to be treated unkindly, least of all when we are not feeling well. Yet, unkindness abounds in health care settings. If we would ask health care professionals (HCPs) to assess their abilities to relate effectively with people, few would admit to the inability to establish good rapport and eye contact with patients, lapses in temper, prejudicial behavior, irritability, or cutting sarcasm. Yet, these and other negative behaviors occur with great frequency. More difficult to observe are such negative behaviors as lack of honesty, breaking confidences, lack of fidelity to one's colleagues, and causing a patient to become overly dependent on oneself.

You might ask, "Why be a health care professional if you cannot act in ways that are positive and assist healing?" Often, clinicians are unaware of their behaviors or their effect on others. Patients challenge our sensitivity and maturity in unique ways. Patients react out of the stress of their illness or pain, but practitioners also must work under stress and the stresses unique to health care. It requires great maturity and patience to respond in healing ways in less-than-ideal situations.

Davis CM, Musolino GM. *Patient Practitioner Interaction: An Experiential Manual for Developing the Art of Health Care, Sixth Edition* (pp 13-28).
© 2016 SLACK Incorporated.

In fact, Dutch researchers[1] have found that worse outcomes in physical therapy were linked to therapists' higher neuroticism scores on the Big Five Index (BFI) score.[2] A lower neuroticism score (emotional stability, impulse control, and the tendency to express unpleasant emotions) indicates being more "calm, relaxed, secure, and hardy." The study supports that concept that a therapist's not feeling mentally stable may have consequences for his or her attitude when interacting with the patient. Researchers support self-awareness and reflection training during the early stages of study.[1]

INFLUENCE OF THE FAMILY ON SELF-ESTEEM

Before reading any further, turn to Table 2-1 and skim through each column. Which column best describes your perception of the family dynamics you grew up with? Place a pencil check beside the phrase in column 1, 2, or 3 that best describes your family for each item listed.

Each of us views the world from a unique perspective. I like to use the analogy of a pair of lenses to illustrate one's world view. You and I can be looking at the exact same thing, but what I see, hear, feel, and experience will be different from what you experience because my lenses are set differently from yours. We receive our lenses as small children. One's world view evolves out of what one hears and experiences as a child growing up in a unique family unit. We develop in the ways that our parents would have us develop because we are, to them, an image on their lenses. Even twins, growing up under the same circumstances, will develop differences in their lenses based on what each chooses to attend to, ponder, and emphasize.

Children are not little adults, as Piaget first clearly described.[3] Children have underdeveloped nervous systems and lack the capacity to move, think, and act in the ways that adults can. Children live in a land of make-believe, enjoy fantasy, and are egocentric. They are unable to handle abstract logic and are present oriented and concrete. If you ask a child which of 2 parallel, identical pencils is longer, he or she will say, correctly, that both are the same length. But then, if you slide one pencil so that it is ahead of the other, although still parallel, and then ask, "Which pencil is longer?" he or she will say the pencil that is ahead of the other is longer. In other words, children cannot conserve information. Likewise, children are unable to come outside of themselves and view themselves, as we discussed in Chapter 1. Ask a child who has a brother if he has a brother, and he will say, "Yes." If you ask him if his brother has a brother, he will say, "No."[4] Finally, children idolize their parents. Feelings of helplessness and dependence are coped with by believing that Mommy and Daddy are perfect and no harm can come to me as long as they are with me in life.

Erikson[3] developed a useful description of the development of personality (Table 2-2) that centers on the successful resolution of tension, in a series of dialectical steps, encountered by the growing person from birth onward. A certain degree of accomplishment is required with each stage as it is encountered, or the child will have to master the goal later. This is similar to the child who skips crawling, wherein critical movements necessary for accomplished gait remain absent. There is a certain level of suffering or pathology that results even if one seems to function adequately. Table 2-2 summarizes Erikson's theory of development. We will return to this theory when we discuss the development of effective helping behaviors.

Human beings are among the few living creatures born without the capacity to crawl, wiggle, or walk to a source of food. It might be said that for 9 months in the womb and 9 (or more) months out, we are totally helpless to move about to a source of food or nourishment. We lie there like blobs and must wail and cajole to get the attention of the big people around us to get our basic survival needs met. The fact that we are born totally dependent on others for our survival is a critical aspect of the development of our world view because who we are and how the world is for us depends totally on how we are responded to, in our profound neediness, and on what we hear others say to us and about us. As a child, I have no identity save what others say about me. It is obvious that the maturity of the parent and the extent to which the child is wanted and anticipated have a great deal to do with how the parent responds to the child and thus fosters or inhibits the development of a sense of self-identity and self-esteem.

Few of us grew up in ideal homes. Perhaps you think you are the exception. The fact is that we experience denial, and many of us have difficulty remembering the negative things about our childhoods. Remember that little children all think that their parents are perfect. Adolescents give up those notions but replace them with strongly held mores to honor parents and respect them. If parents were emotionally or physically abusive to a child, the child will automatically believe that it was his or her fault because he or she must have been bad. Part of maturation is to give up our idealized views of our parents. No parents are perfect. Ironically, however, the more abandoned the child was, the more he or she clings to the fantasy of how perfect his or her parents were. To idealize your parents is to idealize the way they raised you.[2] It is important to look back at what was happening in your family when you were growing up as one mechanism to increase your awareness of your self and your world view. What do you remember about the circumstances of your birth? Were you a wanted child? How did you birth order influence things?

Each child is born into a unique and complex family situation and encounters various challenges, as described by Erikson,[3] as he or she develops day by day. If I, as a newborn, experience feelings of physical comfort, emotional calm,

TABLE 2-1

CHARACTERISTICS OF FAMILIES

OPEN/HEALTHY	TROUBLED	CLOSED/UNHEALTHY
○ Open to change ○ Flexible responses to each situation	○ Nothing can be done ○ What's the use?	○ Rigid, fixed, harsh rules ○ Right vs wrong, no exceptions
○ High self-worth ○ People are valued as individuals	○ Shaky self-worth ○ Covers feelings of low self-control	○ Evasive responses ○ Low self-worth, lots of shaming behavior ○ Low ownership—blaming
○ Functional defenses ○ Uses defenses as coping skill with insight	○ Uses defenses to hide pain ○ Defenses more often deny real feelings ○ Choice is lost ○ Always smile or cry or complain	○ No choice—reacts compulsively and rigidly out of fear ○ Short fuse ○ Lots of avoidance or rage
○ Clear rules discussed ○ Hours, respect for property, telephone use, chores, etc, regularly negotiated	○ Unclear—rules inconsistent ○ Depends on who is asked, what day, which child, etc	○ Edicts or no rules at all ○ Chaos—rules cannot be followed
○ People take risks to express feelings, ideas, beliefs	○ Not safe to express feelings or give opinions—"Don't rock the boat" ○ Can't disagree	○ Denial of problems ○ Ignores bizarre behaviors ○ No-talk rule, even about serious problems, especially drinking, drugs
○ Can deal with stress, pick up on other's pain ○ Nurturing and caring for each other ○ Seek out those in pain to support, encourage	○ Avoid pain ○ Do not see it in others ○ Sweep problems under the rug ○ Pretend all is okay	○ Denial of stress ○ Can't cope with any more—glazed eyes don't see pain ○ Ignore basic need to be seen, acknowledged ○ Children become early helpers
○ Accepts life stages, welcomes them ○ Celebrate growth—sexuality, new friends, accomplishments	○ Parents may compete with kids ○ Growth is accepted painfully—don't talk about sex, try to keep children dependent	○ Adults treated as children ○ Children may try to act like adults ○ Children ridiculed, teased but try to become helpful
○ Either clear hierarchy or egalitarian ○ Strong parental coalition ○ Less need to control ○ Can negotiate	○ Hidden coalitions across generations ○ Parental coalition weak ○ Rigid or shifting pattern of domination	○ Either upside-down family—children may run it, or chaotic, no giving out of rules—or one parent in charge of all and can't cope
○ Affect is open ○ Direct expression of feelings ○ All feelings are okay ○ Anger is in context of awareness of other person ○ Considerate of others	○ Negativism, low feeling, bickering, argumentative controlled mood, some feelings okay, some not, inconsistent acceptance of feelings	○ Cynicism, open hostility, violence, sadism—actually try to manipulate and hurt each other ○ Only happiness is allowed

---

TABLE 2-2

PSYCHOSOCIAL THEORY OF DEVELOPMENT:
A SUMMARY OF ERIKSON'S EPIGENETIC STAGES OF DEVELOPMENT

TRUST VERSUS MISTRUST (0 TO 12 MONTHS)

From birth to approximately 1 year, this stage is the basis for all future development of personality. A feeling of physical comfort accompanied by minimal fear and uncertainty results in a sense of trust for the infant. The quality of the relationship with mother or maternal figure is more important than quantity of food or love demonstrations. Experiences with one's body are the first and primary means of social interactions for the baby; thus, they provide the foundations for psychological trust. The issues involved in trust and mistrust are not settled for all time during this phase of life; they may arise again and again during development and later life. Later confrontation with trust may shake one's basic trust or provide another opportunity for further development if these needs were not met adequately the first time.

AUTONOMY VERSUS SHAME AND DOUBT (2 TO 4 YEARS)

As the child of 2 to 4 experiences the world around him, he begins to discover that his behavior can bring about certain results. Out of these encounters with reality grows a sense of autonomy. At the same time, the child has some conflicts about asserting or remaining dependent and in which situations. Exploring is a primary goal of this growing and increasingly coordinated physical being. It becomes increasingly difficult to remain in a confined place. The child is occupied with activities involving retaining and releasing—manipulating objects, expressing himself, making new friends and letting them go, and bodily functions. The degree to which the child will allow others to regulate his behavior is regularly tested, leading to a greater sense of self-understanding and responsibility or, in the case of being overly controlled, leading to shame and doubt.

INITIATIVE VERSUS GUILT (4 TO 5 YEARS)

During the fourth and fifth years, language development and locomotion have reached a sufficiently high level to permit expansion of imagination. Play activities are more interesting and companionship with peers is sought. There is curiosity and comparison with others around size and skill issues; who is the better tree climber, who is biggest or best at—almost anything. The child in this stage is into everything and seeks attention verbally and physically. Sexual curiosity and genital stimulation are apparent. Adult treatment of the curiosity will reinforce the initiative or result in shame and guilt. Because of a very active imagination, the child may feel guilty for the mere thoughts and for activities that no one has observed. The evolving conscience is becoming established and will ultimately control initiative. If the child's activities are perceived as a nuisance, whether motor or verbal, he may develop feelings of guilt over self-initiated activities that may last a lifetime. Healthy identification with parents, teachers, and peers help resolve some of the guilt problems.

INDUSTRY VERSUS INFERIORITY (6 TO 11 YEARS)

Between the ages of 6 and 11, the child moves seriously into the world of competition and the separation of work and play. Individuals who impact on the developing sense of self now include many other adults and a wider sphere of peers. As the lessons of work are learned, the child often needs to slip into the familial play world to bolster what may feel like flagging initiative. The developing industry evolves from efforts and achievement rewarded by significant others and leads to a sense of social worth. When the child learns that social worth is linked to background of parents, color of skin, or the label on his clothes, identity with those conditions rather than self may result. These first 4 stages form the base upon which the adolescent builds a sense of identity.

(continued)

---

and joy at my presence and if my needs are attended to with love and compassion, I will develop a sense of trust and the view that the world is essentially a warm and loving place. If, for example, something happens to my mother and I become a burden to others left to care for me, and people are mourning the loss of my mother and harbor resentment toward me for causing her loss, I will experience a different set of feelings and may believe that the world is uncertain and chaotic in nature. If I am born to a 15-year-old girl who still needs love and attention from her parents and who has little love to give and should be giving it to herself, the situation becomes cruelly different. Very likely, she cannot stand to hear me cry and may physically harm me when I do. If that is the case, I will experience the world as a hostile place, and I will mistrust

TABLE 2-2 (CONTINUED)

PSYCHOSOCIAL THEORY OF DEVELOPMENT: A SUMMARY OF ERIKSON'S 3 EPIGENETIC STAGES OF DEVELOPMENT

IDENTITY VERSUS IDENTITY DIFFUSION (12 TO 18 YEARS)

During this stage of changes, the consistent task is striving to be oneself and to share oneself with something else. The beginning of separation from parents finally becomes a serious agenda. The adolescent experiences the need to be master of his own affairs and to be free of dependency. The emerging young adult is eager to know his abilities and to have the adult world recognize them as well. The adolescent also fears that the demands of adulthood will exceed the capacities to meet them. Time perspective versus time diffusion becomes the dilemma. When the adult world offers the adolescent responsibilities and privileges at an appropriate pace, commensurate with capacity and desires, there is resolution of some of the issues with a sense of time perspective, as opposed to urgency and hopelessness. The derivatives of the second stage of "autonomy versus shame and doubt" are reworked in the adolescent in the form of establishing a sense of self-certainty. When adult(s) can offer reinforcement appropriately to build the adolescent's self-esteem, feelings of inferiority diminish. The remains of "initiative versus guilt" reappear with the need to discover individualized and unique talents and interests. There seems to be a need to experiment with different roles and express initiative in different ways. If stymied in this dimension, it may seem easier to resolve the conflict by seeking behavior or roles in conflict with parents or the community, thus achieving a negative identity, which is preferable to an "identity diffusion," which is experienced as being nobody at all. Most authorities agree that the period of adolescence brings with it an increase in psychic energy. The young person who uses these energies effectively can experiment in many ways and have experiences of achievement. If much of the energy is used to resolve feelings resulting from earlier unresolved crises, which often reappear at this time, the rather fragile sense of self may be seriously threatened, with introspection interfering with concentration. The successful resolution of adolescent tasks and the development of a strong sense of identity may require many years beyond age 18. During this time the young adult experiments with new behavior and may ignore some societal mores in the process. It is important for this process to work itself through, especially with talented and creative persons. Negative labeling may reinforce a temporary identity, which, given time, will work itself into something else.

INTIMACY VERSUS ISOLATION

The first phase of adulthood comes into being after the adolescent has worked out a sense of identity. Dealing with sexual and psychological intimacies between 2 people while retaining one's own identity is the primary task of this stage. This goal is sought through forms of friendship, leadership, and athletics— even combat. Unwillingness or inability to achieve intimacy will result in distancing oneself from others who pose a threat to identity. Achievement is characterized by the ability and willingness to share with another in mutual trust, to regulate cycles of work, and to participate in society in self-satisfying ways. This stage continues through early middle age.

GENERATIVITY VERSUS STAGNATION

The basic agenda of the middle years is aimed at guiding the next generation, whether in parenting or through employment and enjoyment situations. The critical question of this time occurs when the individual looks back to examine what has happened up to that time in life and whether it was good. If the individual turns inward and becomes self-absorbed, stagnation results.

INTEGRITY VERSUS DESPAIR

The primary task of the later years is the acceptance of one's self and one's life. When the individual has experienced the feelings that accompany a share of the good things of life without being overwhelmed by its tragedies, disappointments, and frustrations, ego integrity is the result. There is acceptance of one's existence with full responsibility and commitment to a certain way of life and its values. Having experienced what is felt to be a full life, the individual can accept giving it up with "integrity." If, on the other hand, the person feels that there has been little good from life and there are few prospects of any coming, there is a sense of despair often accompanied by fear of death.

Reprinted with permission from Ramsden E. Affective dimensions in patient case. In: Payton O, ed. *Psychosocial Aspects of Clinical Practice*. New York, NY: Churchill Livingstone; 1986.

from the very first days of my life. This scenario is the genesis of violent adolescents who are out of control, which is so prevalent in our contemporary society.

And so we develop inwardly; we set our emotional lenses in response to the way our maturing nervous systems take in the information around us. At about age 2, we are confronted with the need to be toilet trained. This is reflected in Erikson's[5] second stage, Autonomy Versus Shame and Doubt (see Table 2-2). Some children are placed on the potty at 6 months, before total head control occurs, let alone complete myelination of the nerves. As the description in Table 2-2 suggests, critical learning at this stage is the child's appropriate and balanced willingness to allow others to regulate and control his or her behavior. Autonomy results in the feeling of success, free from shame and guilt. Shame and guilt result when the child is unable to succeed and consequently allows the adult to be overly controlling of his or her behavior. Only shame, or the feeling that "I am bad," can result when a child is placed on a potty and told to urinate when she does not even know what that means or how it feels to control that function because she cannot yet feel sensation in those nerves. However, when the child is fully ready for this learning, a marvelous feeling of success and pride results with being able to "make bubbles" in the water on command.

It is unrealistic to believe that each stage of development might be totally successfully conquered. Children will have successful resolution at times and will suffer unsuccessful resolution at times. The point to stress here is that the balance toward more successful resolution, rather than unsuccessful resolution, has a great deal to do with parents and other adults who do not set children up to fail. Parents who do not parent well were, themselves, not parented well. Dysfunctional parents learned to be dysfunctional from the families in which they were raised.

Current self-awareness is assisted by an attempt to remember (and to ask the help of others who watched one grow through) critical stages in development over the years. How we respond to the world today is greatly influenced by our sense of ourselves and the adequacy of our self-esteem. The development of a healthy self-esteem requires more successful than unsuccessful resolution of the tensions described by Erikson,[5] either as we mature or later. As adults, we can examine our growing up experiences, gain insight into our dysfunctional views, and consciously change our distorted world views or correct our lenses to give us a more true and accurate focus of the world and of ourselves. However, we usually enter into this examination only because we are experiencing emotional pain or are bored with our lives.

HEALTHY OR OPEN FAMILIES

Healthy families interact in ways that have been described as open in contrast to the rigid or closed functioning of troubled or dysfunctional families (see Table 2-1). A family functions to provide a safe and supportive environment for all of its members, to help them learn basic values, grow, and become more fully human. In healthy families, members feel empowered to adapt to change and feel supported in coping with the stresses of the world outside the home and within. The stress inside the home is usually perceived to be less than the stress faced outside in the world, except in transient phases of family crisis. Individuals are recognized as being unique and having worth. There is value to the family unit, and there is open communication in which members feel free to speak their opinions but do so with concern and caring for others. In sum, family members feel safe, supported, encouraged, and appreciated. Roles and responsibilities of members are flexible but clear. People function well day-to-day and in crisis. Finally, quality time is shared by parents and children and is enjoyed.[6]

DYSFUNCTIONAL OR CLOSED FAMILIES

Whitfield[7] believed that many people grow up in families that stifle the development of the true self and, instead, cultivate in the child a false or codependent self. Children need to feel as if they are safe and protected at all times. They need to feel free to ask questions, to run and play, and to know that the boundaries that parents set for them are fair and consistent. Children need to feel as if they can be children, learning and growing without fear of being ridiculed or punished cruelly for making mistakes. Children need to be invited to feel their feelings and put words on them so they can learn gently how not to be impulsive and controlled by their feelings.

However, dysfunctional families in the last half of the 20th century responded to the neediness and dependence of children in ways that interfered with the development of authenticity. In the dysfunctional family of the 20th century, and perhaps even now, children were to be seen and not heard. They did not feel free to make mistakes but felt that if they were not right, they would be called stupid. "Children are virtuous when they are meek, agreeable, considerate, and unselfish."[7] Adults assumed the role of authoritarian masters intent on breaking the child's will at any cost, or they tended to be absent totally from parenting, escaping in alcohol, work, mental illness, or travel. Children, who want to think of their parents as perfect, soon began realizing that they were not free to act naturally or to be children and so adopted another way of being, usually that of comforting and nurturing the parent. The child thus became a parent to the parent. As a result, a false self emerged in the child. According to psychologist Alice Miller,[8] the persistent denial of the true self and true feelings takes its toll in the development of the coping mechanisms of depression or feelings of grandeur, neither of which is facilitative to a realistic view of the world or to healing. Such was the more common parenting pattern for current, mid-career, and later career professionals' parents and grandparents: the Traditionalists (born 1925 to 1945), the Baby Boomers (born 1946 to 1964), and the Generation Xers (born 1965 to 1981).[9] Many early career professionals (Millennials) have grown up with what is referred to as helicopter parenting.

PARENTING OF THE MILLENNIAL GENERATION

With the advent of the technology age and the ubiquitous presence of cell phones and instant communication, even at a distance, children born between 1982 and 2000, referred to as Millennials, were parented in ways that are 180 degrees opposite from the authoritarian ways of previous generations. Their parents are often referred to as *helicopter parents*, due to their hovering. Millennial children are encouraged to be unique and are often rewarded and celebrated for any and all accomplishments, no matter the level of achievement. As often happens, parents are loathe to inflict what they perceived as poor parenting on their children and, as often happens, difficulties in establishing healthy parent-child relationships continue to occur but with a different twist.

According to Mueller[10]:

> *The renewed enthusiasm and concern for the welfare of the nation's children that began in the late 1980s was a dramatic contrast to the prevalent "antichild" attitudes of the previous 2 decades. Millennial children were treated as precious commodities, protected at every turn. Beginning with their births, ubiquitous "Baby on Board" stickers adorned their parents' cars, loudly and proudly exhorting other drivers to be mindful of the priceless human cargo within. … the millennials' parents became known as the "helicopters," hovering, continually at the ready to answer every question at the speed dial ring of a cell phone.*

As a result, instant access to parental advice and guidance helps to enable children's dependency and unwillingness to stand on their own under difficult circumstances, which can, in turn, delay a young person's readiness to assume responsibility as an adult health care professional responsible for the well-being of patients entrusted to their care.[11] I have presented the extremes of older and newer patterns of parenting, but both can be envisioned to present difficulty in assisting with the maturation of children and adolescents to the point where they feel confident and self-reliant when it comes to assuming responsibility for those trusting in them for their care.

HEALTH CARE PROFESSIONALS' SELF-ESTEEM

It has been said that many people enter the health professions for a variety of poor, although unconscious, reasons. At the surface, most applicants to health care professions admit that they have a great desire to help people. Among more subconscious or unconscious reasons might be a need to be depended upon, a need to control people, and a need to get one's natural attention and affection needs met. Some may be looking for emotional healing themselves by way of making life easier for others. Few people are conscious of these motives, however. Nonetheless, they act in ways that are responsive to their unconscious needs and do things that are harmful in the long run to patients and are contrary to the healing process, as is characteristic of early helpers. In addition, young Millennial adults admit to a dearth of practice in establishing one-on-one communications with strangers, let alone family members, and feel somewhat inept at personal interactions.

The bottom line is this: dysfunctional families breed early helpers and dysfunctional interactions. One example of a dysfunctional family is a family in which one or both parents are addicted to alcohol. It is estimated that "76 million Americans, about 43% of the US population, have been exposed to alcoholism in the family. Almost 1 in 5 adult Americans (18%) lived with an alcoholic while growing up."[12] The literature that has developed from the Adult Children of Alcoholics movement in the United States has shed needed light on the distorted world view of the adult who grew up in a home where one or both of the parents were not able or willing to parent. This circumstance encourages the development of the false self, stifles the successful resolution of the tensions described by Erikson,[5] and contributes to chronic low self-esteem and feelings of being, if not very bad, then never good enough. All children experience shame, but children in dysfunctional families take on shame as part of their identity. Children in dysfunctional families are never free to be children; they have to be grown up and helpful. It seems as if, because this is a difficult task indeed, they are always doing something wrong. Shame is different from guilt. Whitfield[7] described shame as "the uncomfortable or painful feeling that we experience when we realize that part of us is defective, bad, incomplete, rotten, phony, inadequate, or a failure." Thus, guilt says, "I made a mistake" and shame says, "I am a mistake."

Self-esteem can be viewed as the extent to which we are able and willing to own our essential goodness (our true self) in the face of our own incompleteness or lack of perfection. More than simply self-acceptance, self-esteem includes pride in the promise of ongoing growth and change with maturity and the hope of a richer and more peaceful and congruent life as a result of honest, day-to-day struggle. Children reared in dysfunctional families feel the shame of never being quite good enough rather than confidence and pride in doing the best they can. Because they were ridiculed and punished just for being, they grow up repressing hurtful feelings, thus believing that they had a marvelous family life as a child. But underneath the repressed feelings lie severe self-esteem problems that must be admitted and talked about for one to identify the lenses. Feelings of shame must be identified, confronted, and replaced with a more humane, realistic acceptance of one's own imperfections and essential goodness.

Parental dysfunction may or may not be due to alcohol or drug dependence. The critical factor seems to be how well the parent was genuinely present for the growing child in such a way as to encourage the natural curiosity of the child and the natural desire to learn and grow and explore the world; how well the parent nurtured and protected the child; and how safe and free from potential harm the child felt.[7] When the parent absents him- or herself from those responsibilities, for whatever reason (drug dependence, workaholism, depression or mental illness, absence of a good model for parenting, too much concern with activities outside the home), the child starts parenting the parent, and an early helper emerges. A common description given by children from dysfunctional families is that they feel that they were a burden and that they were being bad when they simply showed natural curiosity or asked questions. In fact, it was their very existence that seemed to bring unending pain and suffering to their family.

Children are not meant to be parents. When they take on this role, they take on a false self, and authentic feelings of curiosity, fear, and need become repressed, covered by feigned feelings of bravery and affection in an attempt to please the needy parent. Common characteristics that materialize from the distorted world view and false view of the self that then emerge include the following[13]:

- Fear of losing control
- Fear of feelings that seem overwhelming
- Fear of conflict
- Fear of abandonment
- Fear of becoming alcohol or drug dependent
- Fear of becoming dependent on another person for survival
- Overdeveloped sense of responsibility
- Feelings of guilt and grief
- Inability to relax and have fun spontaneously
- Harsh self-criticism
- A tendency to lie, even when it's not necessary
- A tendency to let one's mind wander, lose track of a conversation, and figuratively leave the room
- Denial and/or the tendency to create reality the way you want it to be, rather than the way it is
- Difficulties with intimacy and getting close to people
- Feelings of vulnerability, of being a victim in a harsh world
- Compulsive behavior, tendency to become addicted to things that alter mood
- Comfort with taking charge in a crisis; panic if you cannot do something in a crisis
- Confusion between love and pity
- Black-and-white perspective (all good or all bad)
- Internalizing (taking responsibility for others' problems)
- Tendency to react rather than act
- Experiencing stress-related illnesses
- Overachievement

Despite this, "we have a marvelous ability to survive and cope."[13] Children from dysfunctional families are the heroes in health care, the ones who, at great personal sacrifice, go above and beyond the call to fix things for everyone else and are praised and admired for it. They thrive on rescuing others and on creating order out of chaos. And, very often, these are the people whom others admonish to lighten up because they take every aspect of their lives seriously.

As Miller pointed out, having a world view that necessitates the coping behaviors (noted previously)—the behaviors of a false self, not the true self—inevitably leads to depression and often to the desired comfort of addiction as well.[8] Addictive behavior is repeated, and habitual behavior that is designed to bring comfort and take attention away from experiencing what appears to be the negative, intense feelings of the true self attempt to break through in a given situation. For all the comfort that the addiction brings, the dependence it brings on chemicals (often depressants), on experienced highs, or on a kind of numbness simply reinforces a denial and continues to reinforce the false self, making the authentic or true self even more difficult to locate. Whenever the true self is blocked, our life energy, authenticity, and capacity to truly respond to the question "Who am I?" are blocked. We cannot grow and become who we were created to be. We are stuck like a mouse on an exercise wheel.

CODEPENDENCE AND THE GENERATIONS

For many young people, addictive impulses are focused not only on drugs and alcohol but on another person and/or virtual connections, a potential source of affection to help ease the pain of never feeling as if one received enough authentic recognition, affection, and unconditional love as a child. Discomfort emerges when one nervously admits that he or she cannot live without the other person because the dependency has become so great. Millennials often admit, with mixed feelings, that their parents are their best friends and they do not want to have to live without them. Because the true self of the person has been underdeveloped or lost long ago, it is a false self that has "fallen in love" and proceeds to do its best to please the other, indeed to live for the other, much as it did for the parents. This phenomenon of living for (being addicted to) the happiness and well-being of another person is termed *codependence*. In fact, codependency is experienced with more than just a person. It has been described as "an exaggerated dependent pattern of learned behaviors, beliefs, and feelings that make life painful. It is a dependence on people and things outside the self, along with neglect of the self to the point of having little self-identity."[7] The person demonstrating codependent behavior looks outside him- or herself to discover what he or she wants, needs, and believes in for identity, security, power, and belonging. He or she looks **outside** him- or herself to feel whole and get what is missing inside. The codependent person often says yes when he or she means no.

Greeting cards do us a great disservice when they express this pathological view with sentimentality, such as, "Even before I knew what my needs were, you were there to help me. You alone taught me the meaning of true love." These are leftover fragments, memories of immature needs from our totally dependent infant. Adults must mature and take responsibility for knowing what their needs are and setting an appropriate course to get them met beyond destructive dependence on others. The goal of maturation is to develop autonomy, self-control, self-reliance, and interdependence on others.[14] For life to be lived in an authentic way, one's identity, power, self-worth, and individuality must be experienced as coming from **within**.

Just as families are dysfunctional, the influence of the generations has an impact on the workplace and families. Today's contemporary workplace also asks us to be able to function as mature individuals with 4 different generations of influence. Lancaster and Stillman,[15] in their text, *When Generations Collide*, describe the fact that in today's workforce systems, we have 4 and sometimes 5 separate generations working side by side. Sociologically, the generational demographics have been trended and categorized by timelines, and some slight variations[9,15-18] exist in the timelines depending on whose classifications you are viewing, nationally and internationally.

A taxonomy of the generations[17] has been published (Figure 2-1) with slightly different year spans from the categories introduced earlier in the chapter, based upon contemporary trending and historical data. The generations are defined as the following: the Traditionalists or Builders (born 1925 to 1945), the Baby Boomers (born 1946 to 1964), Generation X or Xers (born 1965 to 1979), Generation Y or the Millennials (born 1980 to 1994), and the rising Generation Z (born 1995 to 2010).[17] The generation on the horizon is often referred to prospectively as Gen-D (for *digital*) and describes those growing up in the digital era. From a sociological perspective, the vast differences between iconic technologies alone are reason to recognize the need to bridge the divide, ranging from the Traditionalists using rotary telephones and radio to Boomers using television and audio cassettes and to the Millennials and Gen-D with Snapchat, FaceTime, Twitter, and iPads. Traditionalists have a hard time imagining why Millennials would want to communicate on a digital data center platform server, whereas Millennials can hardly imagine what a rotary telephone is or what to do when presented with one. Millennials may contact their best friend's parents via text in order to make a decision, whereas the Traditionalists would "stand on their own two feet" to make a decision.

	Builders 1925-1945 Aged 70s - 80s	Baby Boomers 1946-1964 Aged 50s - 60s	Generation X 1965-1979 Aged 30s - 40s	Generation Y 1980-1994 Aged 20s - early 30s	Generation Z 1995-2010 Aged kids - teens
Aust PM's	Robert Menzies John Curtin	Gough Whitlam Malcolm Fraser	Bob Hawke Paul Keating	John Howard Kevin Rudd	Julia Gillard
US President	Truman / Eisenhower	JFK / Nixon	Reagan / GH Bush	Clinton / GW Bush	Barack Obama
Iconic Technology	Radio (wireless) Motor Vehicle Aircraft	TV (56) Audio Cassette (62) Transistor radio (55)	VCR (76) Walkman (79) IBM PC (81)	Internet, Email, SMS DVD (95) Playstation, XBox, iPod	MacBook, iPad Google, Facebook, Twitter Wii, PS3, Android
Music	Jazz Swing Glen Miller Frank Sinatra	Elvis Beatles Rolling Stones Johnny O'Keefe	INXS Nirvana Madonna Midnight Oil	Eminem Britney Spears Puff Daddy Jennifer Lopez	Kanye West Rhianna Justin Bieber Taylor Swift
TV & Movies	Gone With the Wind Clark Gable Advent of TV	Easy Rider The Graduate Colour TV	ET Hey Hey It's Saturday MTV	Titanic Reality TV Pay TV	Avatar 3D Movies Smart TV
Popular Culture	Flair Jeans Roller Skates Mickey Mouse (28)	Roller Blades Mini Skirts Barbie®/Frisbees (59)	Body Piercing Hyper Colour Torn Jeans	Baseball Caps Men's Cosmetics Havaianas	Skinny Jeans V-necks RipSticks
Social Markers/ Landmark Events	Great Depression (30s) Communism World War II (39-45) Darwin Bombing (42) Charles Kingsford Smith	Decimal Currency (66) Neil Armstrong (69) Vietnam War (65-73) Cyclone Tracy (74) National Anthem (74)	Challenger Explodes (86) Haley's Comet (86) Stock Market Crash (87) Berlin Wall (89) Newcastle Earthquake (89)	Thredbo Disaster (97) Columbine Shooting (99) New Millenium September 11 (01) Bali Bombing (02)	Iraq / Afghanistan war Asian Tsunami (04) GFC (08) WikiLeaks Arab Spring (11)
Influencers	Authority Officials	Evidential Experts	Pragmatic Practitioners	Experiential Peers	User-generated Forums
Training Focus	Traditional On-the-job Top-down	Technical Data Evidence	Practical Case studies Applications	Emotional Stories Participative	Multi-modal eLearning Interactive
Learning Format	Formal Instructive	Relaxed Structured	Spontaneous Interactive	Multi-sensory Visual	Student-centric Kinesthetic
Learning Environment	Military style Didactic & disciplined	Classroom style Quiet atmosphere	Round-table style Relaxed ambience	Cafe-Style Music & Multi-modal	Lounge room style Multi-stimulus
Sales & Marketing	Print & radio Persuasive	Mass / Traditional media Above-the-line	Direct / Targeted media Below-the-line	Viral / Electronic Media Through Friends	Interactive campaigns Positive brand association
Purchase Influences	Brand emergence Telling	Brand-loyal Authorities	Brand switches Experts	No Brand Loyalty Friends	Brand evangelism Trends
Financial Values	Long-term saving Cash No credit	Long-term needs Cash Credit	Medium-term Goals Credit savvy Life-stage debt	Short-term wants Credit dependent Life-style debt	Impulse purchases E-Stores Life-long debt
Ideal Leaders	Authoritarian Commanders	Commanding Thinkers	Co-ordinating Doers	Empowering Collaborators	Inspiring Co-creators

Figure 2-1. Generations defined. (Reprinted with permission from McCrindle Research. © 2012 McCrindle Research.)

Social markers and landmark events vary greatly and traverse the generations. Learning and on-the-job formats for the generations range from the traditional top-down focus, with formal classroom-based instructions, to contemporary lounge room, café-style learning and work environments, mixed in with gaming, with a multimodal media and e-learning emphasis. Historical timeline events for the generations range from the Great Depression of the 1930s to World War II, the Vietnam War of the mid-1960s to early 1970s, the September 11 attacks in 2001, school shootings, and Operation Desert Storm and Shield and the Gulf Wars (Iraq and Afghanistan Wars). Suffice it to say that the need to bridge these generational divides in the workplace system[18] is similar to perspectives and variations within families. From traditional nuclear families to blended families, generational differences are evident in many aspects of life and personal and lifestyle characteristics: core values, reward systems, and expectations; family; education and media; methods of communication; and how we handle financial matters. Generational differences also take their toll on workplace systems and continue to be a great source of financial and management strain. Understanding the generational perspectives will help us become better health care professionals and improved team players in health care work environments, through more effective interactions with all generations. Our patients, too, shall be representative of all generations.

We will talk more about the generations in relation to leadership and health care teams in Chapter 10 and in terms of communication in Chapter 11. However, knowing your **self first** remains key to being able to relate more effectively with others, no matter the generation; this must come from **within**.

THE NEED TO KNOW OURSELVES

The mature health care professional must know him- or herself well, as emphasized in Chapter 1. He or she must be aware of behaviors that result in harmful dependence on patients, in having personal needs for intimacy met, or in behaviors that fail to facilitate therapeutic presence and listening due to undeveloped rapport-building skills that have taken a backseat to the impersonal nature of technology. When one spends a great amount of time communicating with the thumbs (ie, texting or emailing), face-to-face, deep listening skills are not learned and practiced. Multitasking is not an effective method to facilitate communication with your patients. The end goal of all healing is the restoration of independent function for the highest and deepest quality of life possible for the patient. Patients who never feel adequately listened to and patients who depend on us, rather than on themselves, for this independence struggle to make it on their own. We foster this destructive dependence when we ourselves depend on our patients to meet our needs for attention, affection, and/or power and authority. We do them a huge disservice when we fail to **establish good rapport** and **truly listen** to their unique stories.

Self-awareness helps us to identify whether our lenses need resetting, cleaning, or replacing. It is difficult to help others effectively if we need help ourselves. Help is available through the insights gained in this course; through feedback from your classmates and faculty; in the excellent literature now available for those who grew up in dysfunctional families; and through counseling and participation in stress and support groups and 12-step groups that meet throughout the United States, such as Al-Anon, Overeaters Anonymous, Narcotics Anonymous, Alcoholics Anonymous, and Adult Children of Alcoholics; or through other support measures. The goal of seeking help is always to become acquainted with the true self that was repressed many years ago. In this process, one gains insight into the distortion of one's lenses and then, often for the first time as an adult, clearly discerns that there are choices in behavior and that many of the choices one has habitually made in the past have contributed to a chronic feeling of chaos and victimization. Another goal would be to identify negative shame-based beliefs and replace them with more accepting, cosmic beliefs as described in Chapter 1.

The specific support groups listed previously were formed by people who realized that compulsive behavior and addictions serve to blunt one's awareness of the true self. In order to rid oneself of addictions, support is necessary. These groups are devoted to helping people heal from their addictive behavior and live authentic and genuine lives in the search for the true self, lost long ago in an effort to cope with the unfair stress of childhood. It takes courage to seek support, yet the return on that investment leads to self-awareness and finding the true self.

SELF-AWARENESS THROUGH ACTION

The exercises for this chapter are designed to help you review your family history, your growth and development, the messages you received, and the values you adopted from growing up in your particular setting and circumstances. Try to withhold judgment on what you remember and experience. Remember, feelings **are**—they exist. Feelings are neither bad nor good, appropriate nor inappropriate; they just are. However, what we do with our feelings and how we respond to them is open to our evaluation and choice. Being aware of our feelings is the first step. No family is perfect, and parents often parent the way they were parented. Use these exercises to gain insight into your experience and to set goals for your personal growth that will help you become a mature health care professional.

CONCLUSION

The next chapter discusses values in more depth. We develop our values initially by learning what to value from significant people in our lives, but a value cannot be said to be our own until we accept it for ourselves and act on it. In your journal, reflect on your values that you caught from significant people in your life. How many of them can you say you have truly reflected upon or tested and have adopted as your own? Do you hold any values that would be perceived as negative? By whom? How does that make you feel?

REFERENCES

1. Buining EM, Kooijman MK, Swinkels IC, Pisters MF, Veenhof C. Exploring physiotherapists' personality traits that may influence treatment outcome in patients with chronic diseases: a cohort study. *BMC Health Serv Res.* 2015;15:558.
2. John OP, Srivastava S. The Big Five trait taxonomy: history, measurement, and theoretical perspectives. In: Pervin LA, John OP, eds. *Handbook of Personality: Theory and Research.* New York, NY: Guilford; 1999:102-138.
3. Piaget J. *The Construction of Reality in the Child.* New York, NY: Basic Books; 1954.
4. Bradshaw J. *Bradshaw On: The Family: A New Way of Creating Solid Self-Esteem.* Deerfield Beach, FL: Health Communications; 1996
5. Erikson EH. *Identity, Youth and Crisis.* New York, NY: WW Norton; 1968.
6. Krysan M, Moore KA, Zill N. *Identifying Successful Families: An Overview of Constructs and Selected Resources.* Washington, DC: Department of Health and Human Services; 1990.
7. Whitfield CL. *Healing the Child Within: Recovery Classic Series.* Baltimore, MD: The Resource Group; 1986.
8. Miller A. *The Drama of the Gifted Child: The Search for the True Self.* 3rd ed. New York, NY: Basic Books; 1997.
9. Raines C. Managing millennials. In: Raines C, ed. *Connecting Generations: The Sourcebook for a New Workplace.* Menlo Park, CA: Crisp Publications; 2003:171-185.
10. Mueller K. *Communication From the Inside Out: Strategies for the Engaged Professional.* Philadelphia, PA: FA Davis; 2010.
11. Tyler K. The tethered generation. www.gendiff.com/docs/TheTetheredGeneration.pdf. Accessed May 13, 2015.
12. National Association for Children of Alcoholics. www.nacoa.org. Accessed May 13, 2015.
13. Malone M. Dependent on disorder. *MS Mag.* 1987;15:50.
14. Greenberg LS, Johnson SM. *Emotionally Focused Therapy for Couples.* New York, NY: Guilford Publications; 2010.
15. Lancaster LC, Stillman D. *When Generations Collide: Who They Are, Why They Clash, How to Solve the Generational Puzzle at Work.* New York, NY: Harper Collins; 2003.
16. Lancaster LC, Stillman D. *The M-Factor: How the Millennial Generation Is Rocking the Workplace.* New York, NY: Harper Collins; 2003.
17. McCrindle Research. Generations defined. http://mccrindle.com.au/resources/Generations-Defined-Sociologically.pdf. Accessed May 19, 2015.
18. Zemke R, Raines C, Filipczak B. *Generations at Work: Managing the Clash of Boomers, Gen Xers, and Gen Yers in the Workplace.* 2nd ed. New York, NY: AMACOM; 2013.

SUGGESTED READINGS

Kaslow FW. *Handbook of Relational Diagnosis and Dysfunctional Family Patterns.* Hoboken, NJ: John Wiley & Sons; 1996.
Kushner HS. *When Bad Things Happen to Good People.* New York, NY: Anchor Books, 1978.
Peck MS. *The Road Less Traveled: A New Psychology of Love, Traditional Values and Spiritual Growth.* New York, NY: Simon & Schuster, 1978.

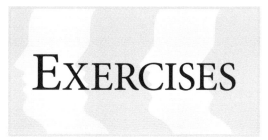

Exercises

EXERCISE 1: MAGIC CARPET RIDE

This exercise is best carried out with the instructor reading the instructions to a group. It is intended to help participants remember what it was like as they were growing up in their families. The magic carpet is a symbol for a ride back into time and memory. Thus, this is a type of guided imagery exercise followed by personal reflection on the content that concludes with a group discussion where participants are able to share with one another, at their own level of comfort, what insights they gained.

Instructor

"So, sit back in your chairs, feet flat on the floor, and breathe deeply 3 times, each time feeling more and more relaxed. Concentrate on your breathing, have your mind go blank as you focus on the air going in through your nostrils and back out through your mouth. With each breath you feel more and more relaxed." (Pause.)

"I want you to go back in time when you were a little child in elementary school." (Pause.)

"You are inside your house with your family all gathered together; your parents are there, or those who reared you, and any brothers and sisters are also there." (Pause.)

"People are having a conversation." (Pause.)

"What are they talking about?" (Pause.)

"Now, ask them to stop talking for a second because you want to ask each of them an important question. Starting with the adults, ask each one, in turn, to tell you something about you. You're so—what? Listen carefully to the descriptions each gives you and pay attention to the feelings each person seems to display as each answers your questions." (Pause for 2 or 3 minutes.)

"As you get ready to leave the group, say goodbye to each person and come gently forward in time to the present, opening your eyes slowly as you return." (Pause.)

"Before talking, write down the names of each person with whom you spoke, then jot down what each told you about yourself, the feeling or attitude conveyed in that message, and how that made you feel." (Pause for 2 or 3 minutes.)

"Now, choose one person with whom to share your experience. Remember, your fantasy was a very private adventure. Some of what you remembered you may decide to keep private. You choose, carefully, the extent to which you want to reveal things about yourself and your family." (Pause 5 minutes for discussion in groups of 2 or 3.)

"Now, return to your written comments. Search each message for the values that underlie each. For example, if you heard from your mother, "You're so messy! I wish you'd clean up your room," you might discern that she values neatness or obedience to her values. "You're so helpful" naturally leads one to the value of helping or perhaps altruism, unless said with sarcasm. Then search for the message behind the message. Perhaps what was meant was, "I wish you'd stop interfering in my life by always trying to do things for me.""

Large-Group Discussion

1. List and discuss various messages and feelings. How many heard essentially negative messages about themselves? How many essentially positive? How many half and half?

2. How many people live up to the description heard from one or both parents? Negative or positive? Give examples.

3. List and discuss values inferred from messages.

Conclusion

Record what you learned and felt about the exercise in your journal. Explore the impact that the messages you heard have on your current self-esteem. How do you feel about yourself today in general? How does that relate to the messages heard? Was this exercise a positive or a negative one for you? What made it so?

EXERCISE 2: FAMILY GENOGRAM

1. Draw your genogram for at least 3 generations (Figure 2-2). Label anything that seems important to you. See if you can locate pictures of family members to go with the circles and squares on your page.

2. Try to identify any addictions, family tension, conflicts, or incidents of children parenting their parents. What patterns emerge? What do you now know about yourself that you failed to see before? What stories are important enough to be handed down? Who/what is the family proud of? What secrets does the family hide from others?

3. Discuss your genogram with 2 other people in your class that you choose. Each of you should take 5 minutes to describe the people represented and 25 minutes to discuss the family dynamics as you understand them.

4. Perhaps questions came up for you about various family members' lives and habits. Write to relatives asking them to fill in the missing pieces to help you better understand your heritage.

5. Remember, with this exercise in particular, the importance of confidentiality. Nothing revealed should ever leave the classroom. Be worthy of the trust placed in you as others take the risk of discussing private and sensitive material with you.

6. Journal about your feelings and your awareness from this exercise. Can you identify behaviors that you've developed from your family that may interfere with mature healing? Comment on any, and problem solve ways in which you might be able to work through those behaviors.

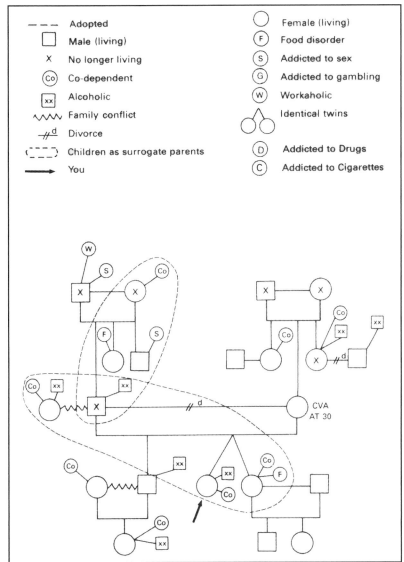

– – –	Adopted
☐	Male (living)
X	No longer living
(Co)	Co-dependent
(xx)	Alcoholic
∿∿∿	Family conflict
–//d	Divorce
(⎯⎯)	Children as surrogate parents
→	You
○	Female (living)
(F)	Food disorder
(S)	Addicted to sex
(G)	Addicted to gambling
(W)	Workaholic
○△○	Identical twins
(D)	Addicted to Drugs
(C)	Addicted to Cigarettes

Figure 2-2. A family genogram is a map of a family for several generations. It is a very useful picture that reveals multigenerational patterns.

EXERCISE 3: VALUE BOXES

1. Figure 2-3 is a diagram of 8 boxes surrounding a circle that represents you. Each box represents a significant person in your life. Envision a person who corresponds to the descriptor at the top of each box and place that person's initials in the upper right corner. If there is no one who meets that description right now in your life, cross out the descriptor and simply put another important person's initials there. One person should not appear in 2 boxes.

2. Now list 4 or 5 things you perceive each person would want you to value. What do they count on you for? What demands do they place on you? What do they want you to do, think, and be? What do they want you to value?

3. Now, look for similarities from various people. Are there values that are repeated often? List them in the lower right of the diagram as recurring values.

4. Underline each value that you want for yourself and place those values in the center circle.

5. Now, list the conflict areas to the lower left of the diagram. What do others want for you that you do not desire? What values seem most important to you?

Figure 2-3. Value boxes.

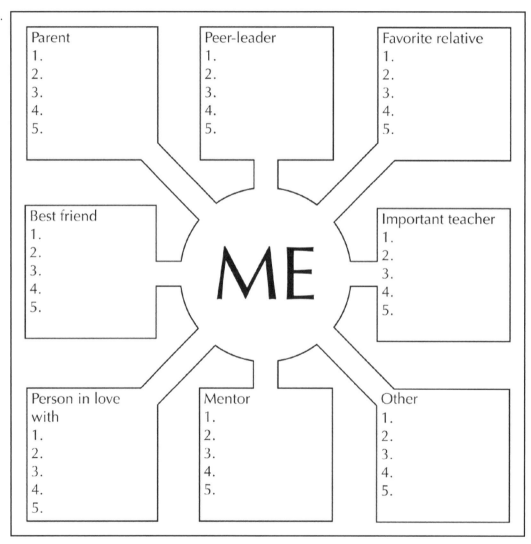

The exercises at the end of this chapter are also available online.
Please refer to the sticker in the front of the book and enter the access code provided.

VALUES AS DETERMINANTS OF BEHAVIOR

Carol M. Davis, DPT, EdD, MS, FAPTA and Gina Maria Musolino, PT, MSEd, EdD

"It's not hard to make decisions once you know what your values are." –Roy E. Disney

OBJECTIVES

- To define and examine personal and professional values.
- To explore the role of personal and professional values in determining one's behavior.
- To emphasize the importance of critical thinking and self-reflection to the formation of one's values.
- To examine the values that underlie behaviors that interfere with healing and those that enhance healing.
- To distinguish between being morally aware and morally conscious.
- To distinguish between nonmoral and moral values.
- To describe evidence that supports the importance of values for health care professionals (HCPs).

The process of professional socialization is a process of growth, of becoming a professional person. Ideally, that growth is holistic and permeates ourselves at deep levels. We realize that we have grown and that we have learned when we can observe changes in our thoughts and in our behaviors. Most obviously, we know more as we become a professional. We incorporate an entire new body of knowledge and skill and use much of it daily in our professional care. But we also develop different attitudes and values as we grow professionally. In other words, professional growth involves changes in our knowledge, skills, attitudes, thoughts, values, and beliefs. You may not realize it, but you are becoming someone different as a result of your professional development as a health care professional. You should be changed through the process, and you are encouraged to consider who you are becoming in your professional development.

We will get to the definition of what a value is in a moment, but first, here are some general observations. All people, after a certain age, can be said to have values. Some of those values we examined in Chapter 2. Consequently, you are now more aware of some of the values you learned and adopted or introjected from your family. It is appropriate for family members to help us grow as children by teaching us what to believe and value when we are too young to choose critically for ourselves. Babies are not born with values needed to live peacefully in the community. We appreciate this when we eat at a restaurant with a 4-year-old child who has not yet been socialized adequately and runs around the room playfully throwing food at people.

Davis CM, Musolino GM. *Patient Practitioner Interaction: An Experiential Manual for Developing the Art of Health Care, Sixth Edition* (pp 29-47).
© 2016 SLACK Incorporated.

Sometimes we introject the values of our parents so completely that we do not even know what we value or why. The story is told of a young couple starting life together cooking a special dinner for guests. As one partner prepared the roast, he cut the 2 ends of the ham off before putting it in the oven. His wife chided him for wasting so much meat, and he defended himself by saying that his mother taught him always to cut the ends off. "Why?" she asked. He responded that he did not know, but he thought it was important and probably had something to do with the proper cooking and circulation of juices.

The next time they visited his parents' home, the new wife asked her husband's mother about cutting the ends off the ham. "Oh, yes," she replied, "My mother always taught me to do that. It's critical to the cooking of the meat." Still not satisfied, the grandmother was called on the phone. "Grandma, tell our new daughter-in-law why it is so important to cut the ends of the meat off the ham before cooking it!" Grandma replied, "Oh, that old trick. It's just a habit I got into. When I first married, we did not have a big enough pot to fit the meat in, so I just trimmed the ends. After a while, it just became a habit, I guess."

And so it is with some of the values we catch from our parents, without thinking about them. Cutting off the ends of ham is not a good example of value-based behavior, but the analogy is important. A clear definition of value-based behavior follows.

Rogers and Stevens[1] indicated that immature people, in an attempt to gain or hold love, approval, and esteem, place the locus of evaluation of values on others. They learn to have a basic distrust for direct experiencing as a valid guide to appropriate behavior. They learn from others what values are important and adopt them as their own, although they may be widely discrepant from personal experience. Because these introjected values are not based on genuinely experienced personal feelings, they tend to be fixed and rigid, rather than fluid and changing.

Culturally accepted values change over time as society changes. The dawning of the age of information technology has brought with it a whole new set of values and a vocabulary to match. Rogers and Stevens[1] disclosed a list of what they termed the commonly adopted or *introjected* values and their associated beliefs found often in the subjects from the United States they studied in the 1950s and 1960s. Consider how times have changed over the years:

- Sexual desires are mostly bad. Source: Parents, teachers, the church.

- Disobedience is bad. To obey is good; to obey without question is better. Source: Parents, teachers, the church, the military.

- Making money is the highest good. Source: Too numerous to mention.

- Aimless, exploratory reading for fun is undesirable and lazy. Source: Teachers, the educational system.

- Abstract art is good. Source: "The sophisticated people."

- To love your neighbor is the highest good. Source: Parents, the church.

- Cooperation and teamwork are preferable to acting alone. Source: Companions.

- Cheating is clever and desirable. Source: The peer group.

- Coca-Cola, chewing gum, electric refrigerators, and automobiles are utterly desirable. Source: Advertisements (still reinforced by people in many parts of the world).

This list reveals that commonly held values reflect the cultural mores of the time a half-century ago. Now in the 21st century, it is much more difficult to find broadly held cultural values than it was 65 years ago when the United States was emerging from the great Depression and World War II. Individualism has become even more valued, sometimes to the detriment of the society as a whole. Next generations are more group focused, likely as a result. What values can you identify that are broadly held in this era? Surely the commonly held sanctions against killing and abuse hold true. The entrepreneurial spirit and creativity are robustly honored. Unfortunately, the value of making a lot of money as an end, no matter what means are used (as long as you do not get caught breaking the law), seems to prevail. However, the massive housing and financial crisis of 2009, the environmental disaster of the BP oil spill in the Gulf of Mexico of 2010, and the tragedies of September 11 and subsequent increasing global terrorism have caught the attention of our entire world and have demanded that we as citizens reevaluate prevailing value-based beliefs and behaviors that endanger the whole of society in ways not even imagined by most people 40 years ago.

"Having a lot" in these times is mistaken for self-worth and intrinsic value. The health care system saw a decline from a service profession to a business as an economic-driven health care system took shape in the mid-1990s. Universal access to health care in the United States has now become law, but not all agree on the values that were codified in the health care reform law that passed in Congress and continues to be discussed and debated with efforts to repeal or implement it differently at state and national levels. Perhaps we are getting ahead of ourselves. Let us take a closer look at what constitutes values.

DEFINING VALUES

What is a value? Values have been defined in many ways, but, in general, the term value refers to an operational belief that one accepts as one's own and that determines behavior. Morrill[2] was far more specific, however, and defined values as follows:

- Standards and patterns of choice that guide persons and groups toward satisfaction, fulfillment, and meaning

- Constructs that orient choice and shape action

- Concepts that call forth thought and conduct that have worth, that lead (under the right conditions) to the fulfillment of human potential or to the discovery of a variety of types and levels of meaning

- Concepts that are not themselves beliefs or judgments but come to expression in and through thought

- Concepts that are not themselves feelings or emotions but inevitably involve desires and fears and that cannot be defined as deeds but are always mediated through specific acts.

Thus, values orient our choices and inspire our actions. Because this is a text devoted to developing appropriate professional ways of being, it becomes critical to examine and clarify the values you now hold in relation to the values that form ethical and sensitive professional caregiving.

VALUES VERSUS NEEDS

Values can be distinguished from needs, which also influence our behavior. If you are thirsty, without thinking much about it, you get something to drink. Needs push us into behaving in certain predictable ways. A theory of human behavior based upon a hierarchy of needs has been outlined in detail by the psychologist Maslow.[3] However, for behavior to be value based, I must reflect upon the choices I have and act according to my reflection. Thus, need behavior is more automatic and driven, whereas value-based behavior takes place upon reflection.[4] Implied in this distinction is the idea that value-based behavior is more mature and less impulsive, especially when compared with behaviors that are based on the more basic or lower-level needs. People with chronic conditions that impact their endurance and ability to walk may want to get a drink when they are thirsty and value the need for hydration. However, they may be considering instead how much effort it will take them to get the water and how it will make them later need to urinate and, therefore, need to walk again, which is a challenge. Their values are affected and now changed dramatically by the influences of their chronic condition and may require assistance to meet their daily needs and reinforce their true values.

The example from earlier—cutting off the ends of the ham—does not represent value-based or reflective behavior but an introjected behavior based on the tendency to distrust one's own experience as a guide. Perhaps the value underlying this behavior was to follow the example of elders despite logic. Indeed, 2 generations of the family distrusted their own experience! It may be motivated out of respect or tradition, but the *why* was not really known or questioned. And so it goes in our families.

MORAL VERSUS NONMORAL VALUES

The professional socialization process requires the clarification and prioritization of currently held values and the adoption of new values that are consistent with the values of the profession. Deciding how to prepare ham or what clothes to wear to a party is a decision-making process of a different sort than deciding whether a patient is a good candidate to receive an above-knee prosthesis. The differences are important. The first category is an example of personal choice or preference; the second is a professional decision. Personal and professional choices can be based on reflection of values, but professional choices are not the same as value preferences. The first is a choice that bears little consequence for the chooser if the less-than-best decision is made. However, the decision about the prosthesis has profound consequence for another person if the less-than-best decision is made.[5]

Values that lead to personal preference are termed *nonmoral values*, whereas values that have to do with the way we relate to and interact with fellow human beings are termed *moral values*.[6] Moral values, such as compassion, trust, justice, honesty, love, confidentiality, and faithfulness to one's professional colleagues, form the heart of a profession's value structure. Moral values take on more importance than value preferences and must be regarded with greater seriousness because the needs of human beings are more important than what food, music, and hairstyle we prefer.

PROFESSIONAL VALUES

Professionalism is grounded in core values. In days past, professions assumed that new members would automatically pick up professional values and behaviors, but this is no longer the case.[7] The American Physical Therapy Association (APTA) has identified 7 core values that they feel compose professional behavior: accountability, altruism, compassion/caring, excellence, integrity, professional duty, and social responsibility.[8] The core values are accompanied by behavioral indicators that describe what one would see if the physical therapist was demonstrating the core values in his or her daily practice. Even a cursory look at these values reveals that they might be universally held values rather than unique to physical therapy alone. The APTA's core values are as follows[8]:

1. Accountability: Active acceptance of the responsibility for the diverse roles, obligations, and actions of the physical therapist, including self-regulation and other behaviors that positively influence patient/client outcomes, the profession, and the health needs of society.

2. Altruism: The primary regard for or devotions to the interest of patients/clients, thus assuming the fiduciary responsibility of placing the needs of the patient/client ahead of the physical therapist's self-interest.

3. Compassion/Caring: Compassion is the desire to identify with or sense something of another's experience, a precursor for caring. Caring is the concern, empathy, and consideration for the needs and values of others.

4. Excellence: Practice that consistently uses current knowledge and theory while understanding personal limits, integrates judgment and the patient/client perspective, embraces advancement, challenges mediocrity, and works toward development of new knowledge.

5. Integrity: The possession of and steadfast adherence to high moral principles or professional standards.

6. Professional Duty: The commitment to meeting one's obligations to provide effective physical therapy services to individual patients/clients, to serve the profession, and to positively influence the health of society.

7. Social Responsibility: The promotion of a mutual trust between the profession and the larger public that necessitates responding to societal needs for health and wellness.

As you review these 7 core values, do you believe that you have the ability to exhibit these as a developing professional? Can you imagine the challenges if you are not able to acculturate to these values that the profession has accepted? Developing health care professionals are often challenged by the values because they mismatch their personal beliefs and values for their generation. You can see how a clash of values might transpire, especially if you were not aware (see Figure 2-1) in comparison with the expected core values for the profession of physical therapy. Now that you are more aware of the values of the profession, where do you see that you might have areas that you may need to evolve or are the values congruent with your personal values and beliefs?

Peterson and Seligman[9] published a list of 6 overarching virtues that many people the world over aspire to achieve. These virtues and their accompanying character strengths can be viewed as values that would strengthen clinical therapeutic presence[9]:

1. Wisdom and Knowledge: Creativity, curiosity, love of learning, perspective

2. Courage: Authenticity, bravery, persistence, zest

3. Humanity: Kindness, love, social intelligence

4. Justice: Fairness, leadership, teamwork

5. Temperance: Forgiveness, modesty, prudence, self-regulation

6. Transcendence: Appreciation of beauty, gratitude, hope, humor, religiousness

VALUES CONFLICTS

There are times when the behavior of health care professionals comes into direct conflict with patients' behaviors. The moral or interpersonal values that the profession espouses, for example, in its code of ethics or its core values statements, and the behavior observed in many hospitals and patient/client care settings, often seem far removed from each other. Often, the behavior exhibited in conflict situations is not value based or based on reflection at all, but is highly impulsive and defensive.

Values conflicts are always rich in their lessons for learning, although many of us shy away from them because we are afraid of doing the wrong thing. In tense times, most of us want someone to tell us what to do. Debriefing when conflicts occur is also another rich learning opportunity for our own professional development and reflection.

A moral dilemma exists when we do not know what choice to make from 2 or more conflicting choices; thus, we have difficulty choosing which value should have priority. Chapter 4 focuses on the examination of ethical dilemmas and their resolution, but a brief example here will illustrate this point. Respect for life is the central value for advocates of a woman's right to choose abortion, as well as for those opposed to abortion. The difference in opinion and belief of these 2 groups is not the value of life, but the importance of the mother's life over the fetus's life. The antiabortionists claim the primacy of the fetus's life above all considerations, whereas the reproductive freedom advocates claim the primacy of the mother's choice for the quality of her life and resist outside interference with her right to choose.[5] Likewise, those who favor capital punishment value the lives of those who might become victimized over the life of the person convicted of murder.

The set of moral norms adopted by a professional group to direct value-laden choices in a way consistent with professional responsibility is termed a *code of ethics*. One might follow the code without internalizing it or introjecting it, just as one did in younger years with parents' values. For a code of ethics to function as a set of professional moral values, one must reflect on it and decide that it forms a values complex around which one is willing to organize professional choices. Thus, as stated previously, reflection is necessary to the internalization of values to make them truly one's own, whether personal or professional. Those who make the smoothest transitions into professional practice are likely to be those whose personal values and priorities greatly overlap with the values inherent in their chosen professional practice. Given that one's basic human survival needs are met, the more one reflects on one's choices and on which choices result in a good and meaningful life, the more one is apt to experience consistent reward from choices made.[6]

VALUES DETRACTING FROM THERAPEUTIC PRESENCE

Often, patients and clients end up needing the help of rehabilitation professionals because of impulsive, poor choices reflecting an immature and inconsistent set of values that have been introjected but not clarified or claimed as one's own. An example might be a young man who comes to physical therapy needing relief from low back pain incurred from lifting a heavy railroad tie while showing off in front of some young women and men he decided he needed to impress. Many patient and client problems in movement and function are not the result of fate but the result of a lifetime of choices that reveal little attention or value to behaviors that preserve physical and emotional health. Thus, it sometimes becomes difficult to avoid becoming judgmental, and, as professionals, we sometimes feel resistance to treating people who have not practiced wellness behaviors and have become, for example, obese or are chronic smokers.[5]

Professional ethics demand that, when a feeling of criticism and negative judgment of a patient occurs, we must be aware of it and consciously work to not let it interfere with our commitment to compassionate quality care. Common behaviors that reveal difficulty in this task include the following[5]:

- Acting cool or aloof, obviously paying more attention to other patients. **Underlying value:** Prejudice or indifference
- Overly criticizing the patient so that he or she feels as if nothing is right. **Underlying value:** Prejudice, perfectionism, rigidity
- Treating the patient as an object rather than a person with feelings of pain, worry, and insecurity. **Underlying value:** Depersonalization
- Treating the patient as if he or she were a child, incapable of understanding or making wise choices. **Underlying value:** Patronizing, adopting an air of condescension
- Being unable or unwilling to help the patient in treatment; leaving the patient alone most of the time. **Underlying value:** Indifference or prejudice
- Making fun of the patient in his or her presence and/or behind his or her back. **Underlying value:** Depersonalization
- Telling others things the patient shared in confidence. **Underlying value:** Breaking confidentiality
- Refusing to let the patient work on his or her own, constantly supervising and instructing. **Underlying value:** Fostering dependence, having own need to be needed met by patients.
- Guessing what is best to do, refusing to find correct and best treatment alternatives, and acting on habit. **Underlying value:** Refusing to recognize and act based on one's own limits of knowledge.
- Always fitting the patient in as if everything else is more important. **Underlying value:** Selfish interest over needs of patients
- Refusing to listen to a patient's story of pain and difficulties dealing with pain and dysfunction. **Underlying value:** Importance of defending oneself against personal feelings of fear and insecurity around pain and possible addiction.

Most of us would read this list of behaviors and say to ourselves, "I'd never act like that!" But as much as we would never want to act in ways that interfere with healing, when we are unclear of our values—or, more important, when we are not in touch with our feelings and when we don't know ourselves—we often end up doing and saying things, especially under stress, that we regret later. These regretful behaviors stem, in part, from impulsive and immature needs to be spontaneous and egocentric and arise from feelings of criticism and the judgment that our patients don't deserve our help. Or perhaps they grow out of unrecognized fears, such as not knowing the right thing to do. Perhaps they stem from not having clarified the values underlying a therapeutic presence.

VALUES THAT REINFORCE HEALING

Essential to a therapeutic use of self is the capacity to feel compassion for those who need our help. Compassion is quite different from pity, wherein I feel sorry for this poor person (and secretly feel smug and am thankful that this is not my problem). Compassion in a mature health care professional is a value that is fueled with imagination and the ability to envision what is possible from the other person's perspective. When we truly value our patients as human beings, we express behavior based on moral values that enhance healing, such as sincere and active listening and a desire to treat patients as adults, in charge of their own lives and capable of making wise and appropriate decisions for themselves. We treat what they say with confidence and respect, attend to them with interest, and obtain their informed consent for therapeutic procedures. We convey to them that their choice to come to us was well founded and that we will help within clearly set boundaries and expectations. In other words, we work to be able to feel sincere, genuine positive regard for all of our patients and relate to each with sensitivity to their uniqueness.

When we become professionals, we gain many things, but we also give up some things. One of the things we give up is the right to walk away from people we would rather not treat. What patient would be your most dreaded? Would it be the rapist? The child abuser? The alcoholic? The obese? The person who is HIV positive or who has AIDS? When we judge our patients, we cannot help but treat them as less than human. What is required is a sense of oneness with all human beings, regardless of the mistakes they may have made. Deciding that the mistakes **you** have made are far less evil only distances you from your patient.

As professionals, we also give up the right to say whatever we feel at any moment. We give up the right to speak and act impulsively and take on the responsibility to act in accordance with core values and the code of ethics or, in similar terms, to act according to the moral values that facilitate healing. No longer may we claim the luxury of spontaneous outbursts or selfish indifference. No longer may we put our own needs before the needs of our patients. No longer may we be run by unclear values or fears that have not yet been examined and resolved.

Professional rehabilitative care requires problem solving that is proactive; based on scientific data; and demonstrates a consistent, conscious value of choosing behavior that is conducive to healing. As a health care professional, you must become an informed reasoner. You must learn to value the systematic gathering of facts and compassionately relate to people who come to you for help. You must value taking the time to reflect on your behavior and choose to act in ways that reinforce healing. Central to this process is the courage to carefully examine your values and the values of healing and to make a commitment to change behaviors that interfere with effective and compassionate care. Feedback from others is important, but at this point in the text, you are asked to focus on self-examination.

DEVELOPMENT OF AN ETHICAL CONSCIOUSNESS

We are not born knowing the right thing to do; we develop the ability to solve moral problems in conjunction with cognition. There are 3 common approaches to teaching children the right thing to do[2]: *objectivism*, or *legalism*; *ethical subjectivism*, or *values clarification*; and *ethical relativism*. The most common is *objectivism*, or *legalism*, which asserts that to do the right thing is to obey the rules. The rightness of the value is within the value itself; therefore, it is always right, for example, to love people and to act justly, honestly, and with compassion. Organized religion teaches this approach to values education. To do the right thing, one should obey the higher authority, do as the Bible says, follow the Torah, the Qur'an, The Ten Commandments, etc. But objectivism offers little help in reconciling the contradictions that can be found in the Bible or resolving the dilemma, for example, between honoring your parents and following your own conscience in developing your career when your choice and the choice your parents would have you make are at odds. Likewise, objectivism fosters the development of a moral belief system based on outside authority. For these reasons, it does not adequately serve the purpose of dilemma resolution in health care.

The second approach, *ethical subjectivism*, or *values clarification*, offers an alternative that approaches ethical relativism.[10] The third approach, *ethical relativism*, is the view that each person's values should be considered equally valid. Subjectivism suggests that one examine the conflicting values to make sure that each is, indeed, a value. If a belief or idea does not meet true value status, it is relegated to a position of less importance than a true value. To satisfy the definition

TABLE 3-1
RATHS' 7 REQUIREMENTS FOR A VALUE
CHOOSING ONE'S BELIEFS AND BEHAVIORS 1. Choosing freely 2. Choosing from among alternatives 3. Choosing after considering consequences of choice
PRIZING ONE'S BELIEFS AND BEHAVIORS 4. Prizing and cherishing 5. Publicly affirming when appropriate
ACTING ON ONE'S BELIEFS AND BEHAVIORS 6. Acting 7. Acting repeatedly, showing consistency
Adapted from Raths LE, Harmin M, Simon S. *Values and Teaching.* Columbus, OH: Charles E. Merrill; 1966.

of value, Raths et al[10] suggested a value must satisfy the 7 criteria listed in Table 3-1. The content of a value, so important in objectivism, becomes secondary to the process of determining whether something is, indeed, a value.[10]

How well does subjectivism assist us in making value-based decisions? It probably does not make that much difference if one begins treating patients at 8:00 AM or 7:30 AM. People will (and often do) argue the importance of their priorities, but nonmoral values, or value preferences, are just that—relative preferences. Moral values present a different story. Moral relativism renders an ethical code meaningless.[6]

Thus, in a moral or ethical dilemma, in which one must choose between doing the loving thing and following the rules, it does little good to use a subjectivist approach, clarifying whether both compassion and justice fit the criteria of a value. What is needed is a way of weighing the relative goodness of each value **in the situation**. Thus, subjectivism and objectivism both fall short of informing us clearly how to decide between 2 conflicting values.

Gilligan[11] and Kohlberg[12] developed theories that assist us in our task. Their theories each fall under the category of *contextualism*, in which they assert that as people develop their ability to think, they also develop their ability to reason about the right or best thing to do **in a given situation**. This approach to dilemma resolution has been termed contextualism because the **context of the situation** provides the key information in deciding the right thing to do **in that situation**. Certain values are, as the objectivists suggest, always going to assume great importance, but the key to resolving the dilemma is to collect all the pertinent data about this particular situation and then weigh alternatives for the best thing to do according to the best and most mature debate. How do we discover the most adequate reasoning, the most mature debate? Developmental psychology and philosophy inform us here.

MORAL DECISION MAKING: DEVELOPMENTAL ASPECTS

In general, developmentalists assert that as people grow and change, they pass through predictable stages in which new behaviors are formed and stabilized. The maturation process consists of a progression through a series of passages or stages, which reflects the increasingly sophisticated changes occurring in a person's nervous system. Thus, children are not little adults and should not be treated as such, nor should they be asked to act like adults before they know what that means.

Perhaps the most famous developmentalist, Jean Piaget,[13] suggested that as cognitive abilities develop, the ability to know the right thing to do also develops. Piaget[13] suggested 4 stages of development of a moral conscience (Table 3-2): amoral (ages 0 to 2 years), egocentric (ages 2 to 7 years), heteronomous (ages 7 to 12 years), and autonomous (age 12 years and older). Kohlberg[12] based his work on that of Piaget[13] and further refined the stages, based on research conducted around the world. Kohlberg[12] suggested 6 stages that men and boys go through in developing a mature moral consciousness (Table 3-3). Earliest and most immature is the punishment and obedience stage, in which that which is wrong is that for which I get punished. Tables 3-2 and 3-3 illustrate the progression of stages through to stage 6, an autonomous stage of knowing the right thing based on a decision of conscience in accord with self-chosen, well-thought-out ethical principles appealing to logical comprehensiveness, universality, and consistence and that flow from the basic principle of justice.[12]

TABLE 3-2				
DEVELOPMENTAL MODEL COMPARISON				
PIAGET'S MORAL DEVELOPMENT MODEL	**KOHLBERG'S MORAL DEVELOPMENTAL COMPARISON**			
	Level	*Orientation Stage*	*Characterized by*	*Personally Stated as*
Amoral stage (ages 0 to 2)				
Egocentric stage (ages 2 to 7): Lacks morality, bends rules, and reacts instinctively to environment	Pre-conventional	1. Punishment and obedience orientation 2. Instrumental relativist orientation	Satisfying one's own needs	I must obey the authority figure or else...
Heteronomous stage (ages 7 to 12): Based on total acceptance of a morality imposed by others	Conventional	3. Good boy–nice girl orientation 4. Law and order orientation	○ Conformity to social conventions and expectations ○ Respect for authority and society's laws	○ I probably should because everyone expects me to ○ I ought to because of duty to obey the rules
Autonomous stage (ages 12 and older): Based on an internalized morality of cooperation	Post-conventional or autonomous	5. Social contract orientation 6. Universal-ethical principle orientation	○ Conformity to the ever-changing values and demands of society ○ My conscience holds me responsible for doing what is right	○ I may because of my role in society, but I often question the relative values of society ○ I will because I know it is the right thing to do

Reprinted with permission from Piaget J, Kohlberg L. Comparison of the stages in two models of moral development. In: Francoeur RT. *Becoming a Sexual Person.* New York, NY: John Wiley and Sons; 1982:673.

When faced with dilemmas, Kohlberg[12] observed that people did not just work out the right answer for themselves by guessing or by trial and error. Rather, depending on their age and maturity, they appealed to a category of reasons outlined in the stages in Table 3-3. Kohlberg[12] and Piaget[13] believed that children progress from a total abdication to an outside authority to an autonomous stage, wherein they make their own choices.

Gilligan,[11] also a contextualist and student of Kohlberg,[12] reacted to the fact that Kohlberg only studied men and boys and then generalized his theory to girls and women. Kohlberg[12] stated that girls and women get stuck in stage 3, good boy–nice girl orientation, which reveals conformity to social expectation because girls are socialized to stay at home and tend the house, yielding to the decisions of the man in the house. Right is that which pleases others. This is changing in today's contemporary society, yet many still hold these values.

Gilligan's[11] work challenged the rigidity of this assumption. In her studies of how girls, college women, and housewives perceive the same set of moral problems outlined by Kohlberg,[12] she revealed that women "appear to frame moral problems in terms of conflicting personal responsibilities, rather than conflicting rights and the concept of justice." Thus, as a function of social conditioning, adolescent boys may well focus first on achievement and self-identity and much later focus on developing a value of intimacy and friendship, whereas girls do just the opposite. Both genders have the same ability to mature to higher stages of moral conscience; girls and women do not simply stop maturing morally at stage 3. However, girls and women seem to mature not linearly as Kohlberg's scale illustrates, but horizontally, in a net-like fashion, favoring the higher importance of relationships over abstract goals such as social justice and achievement. As we mature and enter relationships, we may also tend to demonstrate these value scales, whereas "men are motivated when they feel needed, while women are motivated when they feel cherished."[14]

TABLE 3-3
KOHLBERG'S STAGES OF MORAL DEVELOPMENT

1. PRECONVENTIONAL LEVEL

Child is responsive to cultural rules and labels of good and bad or right and wrong as they relate to physical consequence of action (reward of punishment).

Stage 1: Punishment and obedience orientation. Avoidance of punishment and unquestioning deference to power valued in their own right, not in terms of respect for underlying moral order supported by punishment and authority (stage 4).

Stage 2: Instrumental relativist orientation. Right actions are those that satisfy one's own needs. Reciprocity is not a matter of loyalty or justice but of "You scratch my back and I'll scratch yours."

2. CONVENTIONAL LEVEL

Maintaining the expectations of the individual's family, group, or nation is valuable in its own right, regardless of consequences.

Stage 3: Interpersonal concordance or good boy–nice girl orientation. Good behavior is that which pleases others and is approved by them. Behavior is often judged by intention. One earns approval by being nice.

Stage 4: Law and order orientation. Right behavior consists of showing respect for authority, following the rules, doing one's duty, and maintaining the given social order for its own sake.

3. POSTCONVENTIONAL, AUTONOMOUS, PRINCIPLED LEVEL

Clear effort to define moral values and principles that have validity and application apart from authority of groups or other persons holding these principles.

Stage 5: Social contract, legalistic orientation. Right actions are defined as those that have been critically examined and agreed upon by the whole society. Emphasis placed on procedural rules for reaching consensus in the face of relativism. Aside from what is constitutionally and democratically agreed upon, what is right is a matter of personal values and opinion. It is possible to change the law when it is to the benefit of society. Outside the law, free agreement and contract are the binding elements of obligation (the "official" morality of the United States government and Constitution).

Stage 6: Universal-ethical principle orientation. Right is defined by the decision of conscience in accord with self-chosen ethical principles appealing to logical comprehensiveness, universality, and consistency. The basic universal principles are those of justice, the reciprocity and equality of human rights, and respect for the dignity of human beings as individual persons, no matter which nationality, race, color, or creed.

Adapted from Kohlberg L. The cognitive development approach to moral education. *Phi Delta Kappa.* 1975;June:670-677.

MORAL AWARENESS VERSUS MORAL CONSCIOUSNESS

To be morally aware is to know what the dictionary says about, for example, compassion, and to be somewhat aware of whether your behavior fits that description at any given time. To be morally conscious, however, is to examine how compassion weaves its way through your behavior, how it influences you in your various decisions, and how you feel about compassion with regard to justice, for example, in a moral dilemma. Thus, moral consciousness represents a deeper way of knowing and thus a firmer commitment to consistency in moral behavior or the way we interact with other human beings. The goal of this text is, at the least, to confirm your moral awareness and, ideally, to help stimulate a moral consciousness that is consistent with quality and compassionate health care. Knowing the right thing to do does not guarantee doing the right thing, but it is a major first step. Pellegrino[15] suggested that quick self-examination on the effectiveness of one's therapeutic presence might be accomplished by answering these 3 questions **truthfully**:

1. **Do I listen and not only respond to but satisfy the fundamental questions each person who is ill and anxious brings to me?**

2. **Can I accept the patient for what he or she is, not for what I think he or she should be?**

3. **Can I handle my authority in a humane way that respects the life and values of the patient?**

To be able to answer yes to any of these questions requires that we continue to grow as persons as we become health care professionals. It behooves us to revisit Pellegrino's[15] self-examination questions as a reminder of the values of therapeutic presence, not only as we develop, but as we mature as empathic health care professionals and self-monitor our values over the course of our careers and assure we do not need to change direction. Hopefully, you can find a mentor and/or good colleagues with whom you can debrief when needed. The value of a lifelong commitment to growth and increasing moral consciousness ensures a meaningful and peaceful professional as well as personal life.[15]

AWARENESS THROUGH ACTIVITY

Most health care professions are adversely affected by lack of acculturation to the values of the health care disciplines.[16-20] In a retrospective study, Papadakis et al[16] reported that 95% of the disciplinary actions taken by the state medical boards were linked with unprofessionalism exhibited in medical school. Hence, problem behaviors in medical school were directly associated with subsequent future disciplinary action by the state. In a subsequent study of 3 medical schools from 1990 to 2003, Papadakis et al[19] found that 235 graduates were disciplined by medical state license boards. The disciplinary action was strongly associated with prior unprofessional behavior while in medical school. The most strongly linked unprofessional behaviors were severe irresponsibility, followed by diminished capacity for self-improvement; the practicing medical school graduates who were disciplined also demonstrated low scores on the admissions tests and poor grades in the first 2 years of medical school. Wynia et al[17] stated that lists of desirable professional attributes and characteristics are highly important for education and to begin to understand the implications of values within the health professions that are needed for real-world practice, yet they are not by themselves sufficient. Even in the early phase of health professions education, the respect that is provided with a human cadaver is the opportunity to begin to demonstrate appropriate values and professionalism.[20]

In her Linda Crane Memorial Lecture entitled "Integrity: At the Heart of Our Profession," Ethel Frese, PT, DPT, MHS, CCS,[21] focused on integrity related to professionalism, ethics and core values, and associated professional responsibilities. Frese[21] described our calling today for developing health care professionals:

> *Students are growing up in a society with declining ethical values, and we cannot expect students to have strongly developed moral behaviors. Unfortunately, students may see dishonest, unethical behavior in the world, as a normal part of life. Evidence supports a high correlation between academic cheating and deviant behavior in the workplace ... our professional responsibility has increased even more with the growth of autonomous practice and the increased complexity of ethical situations ... physical therapists must adhere to the rules and regulations of state and federal institutions, insurance companies, and employers, but they also are expected to deliver high-quality, patient-centered care. The emphasis on productivity, can conflict with quality, but it can also challenge the moral behavior of a therapist. With integrity being 'at the heart of our profession' we must emphasize integrity in our professional education, and in our professional socialization. We cannot separate who we are from what we do.*

As future health care professionals, we must first examine our own personal values before we can begin to ascribe to the values of our profession. It remains relevant that we are able to adjust to the values of our health care discipline so as to avoid the potentials for disciplinary actions that might range from loss of your professional license to fines and reprimands that may require restitution and, once again, supervised practice. We must also recognize the problematic behaviors in others and assist in their professional socialization.[22] We may also need to reconcile our own personal values, such as embracing computerized technologies[23] and social media platforms[24] and/or the use of assistive technology,[25] with those that vary from the culture of the clinical practice arena and the values of our patients/clients, which may or may not be accepting of new technologies or cutting-edge research or accessibility to assistive technologies.[25] Reconciling our personal values, professional values, and the patients'/clients' values and beliefs, along with considerations of aspects of social justice, are paramount to the patients' experiences.[25] Many decisions we must make as health care professionals are not value neutral,[25] and first knowing your own values is key so you can best determine how to interface with the profession, the cultural values of the systems we work within, colleagues, and the people who are to be your patients and clients, each of whom comes with his or her own values and belief systems and who looks to you to provide appropriate clinical reasoning to affect a positive change in his or her preferred life.[21,24-30]

Hopefully you are now motivated to examine your own values, self-assess, and realize the importance of professionalism and the implications of values for true reflective practice.[26] We will further examine the concepts of self-assessment and reflective practice in Chapter 9. The exercises at the end of Chapter 3 are designed to help you further analyze important personal values you currently hold and to help you learn which of your values you value most or what your highest order value is today. A visit to a clinic or patient care area (or reflection upon these) where you will be asked to make careful observations of behavior and to comment on the values that seem to underlie it will help sensitize you to the stresses of patient care and will illustrate various kinds of interactions that take place with patients. Finally, a forced-choice exercise will pull out some introjected values that you may not even be aware that you hold.

References

1. Rogers CR, Stevens B. *Person to Person: The Problem of Being Human*. Lafayette, CA: Real People Press; 1967.
2. Morrill RL. *Teaching Values in College*. San Francisco, CA: Jossey-Bass; 1980.
3. Maslow A. *Motivation and Personality*. New York, NY: Harper and Row; 1954.
4. Beck C. A philosophical view of values and value education. In: Hennessy T, ed. *Values and Moral Development*. New York, NY: Paulist Press; 1976:13-23.
5. Davis CM. Influence of values on patient care: foundation for decision making. In: O'Sullivan S, Schmitz T, eds. *Foundations of Rehabilitation*. 2nd ed. Philadelphia, PA: FA Davis; 1988:31-37.
6. Wehlage G, Lockwood AL. Moral relativism and values education. In: Purpel D, Ryan K, eds. *Moral Education…It Comes With the Territory*. Berkeley, CA: McCutchen; 1976:334-335.
7. Hensel WA, Dickey NW. Teaching professionalism: passing the torch. *Acad Med*. 1998;73(8):865-870.
8. American Physical Therapy Association. Professionalism: physical therapy core values. http://www.apta.org/Professionalism/. Accessed June 1, 2015.
9. Peterson C, Seligman MEP. *Character Strengths and Virtues: A Handbook and Classification*. Washington, DC: American Psychological Association; 2004.
10. Raths LE, Harmin M, Simon S. *Values and Teaching*. Columbus, OH: Charles E. Merrill; 1966.
11. Gilligan C. *In a Different Voice*. Cambridge, MA: Harvard University Press; 2009.
12. Kohlberg L. The cognitive development approach to moral education. *Phi Delta Kappa*. 1975;June:670-677.
13. Piaget J. *The Construction of Reality in a Child*. New York, NY: Basic Books; 1954.
14. Gray J. *Men Are From Mars, Women Are From Venus*. New York, NY: Harper Collins Publishers; 1992.
15. Pellegrino ED. Educating the humanist physician—an ancient ideal reconsidered. *JAMA*. 1974;227(11):1288-1294.
16. Papadakis MA, Hodgson CS, Teherani A, Kohatsu ND. Unprofessional behavior in medical school is associated with subsequent disciplinary action by a state medical board. *Acad Med*. 2004;79(3)224-229.
17. Wynia MK, Papadakis MA, Sullivan WM, Hafferty FW. More than a list of values and desired behaviors: a foundational understanding of medical professionalism. *Acad Med*. 2014;89(5):712-714.
18. Papadakis MA, Osborn EH, Cooke M, Healy K. A strategy for the detection and evaluation of unprofessional behavior in medical students. University of California, San Francisco School of Medicine Clinical Clerkships Operation Committee. *Acad Med*. 1999;74(9):980-990.
19. Papadakis MA, Teherani A, Banach MA, et al. Disciplinary action by medical boards and prior behavior in medical school. *N Engl J Med*. 2005;353(25):2673-2682.
20. Talarico EF Jr. A change in paradigm: giving back identity to donors in the anatomy laboratory. *Clin Anat*. 2013;26(2):161-172.
21. Frese E. Integrity: at the heart of our profession. Paper presented at: APTA Combined Sections Meeting; February 5, 2015; Indianapolis, IN.
22. Lowe DL, Gabard DL. Physical therapist student experiences with ethical and legal violations during clinical rotations: reporting and barriers to reporting. *J Phys Ther Educ*. 2014;28(3):98-111.
23. Foreman KB, Morton DA, Musolino GM, Albertine KH. Design and utility of a web-based computer-assisted instructional tool for neuroanatomy self-study and review for physical and occupational therapy graduate students. *Anat Rec B New Anat*. 2005;285(1):26-31.
24. Gagnon K, Sabus C. Professionalism in a digital age: opportunities and considerations for using social media in health care. *Phys Ther*. 2015;95(3):406-414.
25. Greenfield B, Musolino GM. Technology in rehabilitation: ethical and curricular implications for physical therapist education. *J Phys Ther Educ*. 2012;26(2):81-90.
26. Musolino GM. Fostering reflective practice: self-assessment abilities of physical therapy students and entry-level graduates. *J Allied Health*. 2006;35(1):30-42.
27. Rindflesch A, Hoverstien K, Patterson B, Thomas L, Dunfee H. Students' description of factors contributing to a meaningful clinical experience in entry-level physical therapist professional education. *Work*. 2013;44(3):265-274.
28. Wong CK, Driscoll M. A modified jigsaw method: an active learning strategy to develop the cognitive and affective domains through curricular review. *J Phys Ther Educ*. 2008;22(1):15-23.
29. Noteboom JT, Allison SC, Cleland JA, Whitman JM. A primer on selected aspects of evidence-based practice relating to questions of treatment. Part 2: interpreting results, application to clinical practice, and self-evaluation. *J Orthop Sports Phys Ther*. 2008;38(8):485-501.
30. Simoneau GG, Allison SC. Physical therapists as evidence-based diagnosticians. *J Orthop Sports Phys Ther*. 2010;10(40):603-605.

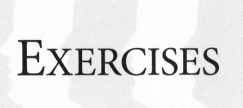

EXERCISES

<u>EXERCISE 1: VALUES PRIORITY</u>

This exercise takes place in 4 parts:

1. First, with each of the values listed in Step 1, indicate its degree of importance to you.
2. Then, list your 5 least and 5 most important values from this list.
3. Then, complete the Five-Sort Value Inventory.
4. Then, transfer the numbers from the Five-Sort Value Inventory to the Value Inventory Rating Summary.

Step 1

Read through the entire list. This is not a semantics test, so feel free to cross out the definition and add your own if you wish. Then, circle each item's level of importance to you.

Achievement (accomplishment; results brought by resolve, persistence, or endeavor)

Not very important   Important   Very important

Aesthetics (appreciation and enjoyment of beauty for beauty's sake, in both arts and nature)

Not very important   Important   Very important

Altruism (regard for or devotion to the interest of others; service to others)

Not very important   Important   Very important

Autonomy (ability to be a self-determining individual; personal freedom; making own choices)

Not very important   Important   Very important

Creativity (developing new ideas and designs; being innovative)

Not very important   Important   Very important

Emotional well-being (peace of mind, inner security; ability to recognize and handle inner conflicts)

Not very important   Important   Very important

Health (the condition of being sound in body)

Not very important   Important   Very important

Honesty (being frank and genuinely yourself with everyone)

Not very important   Important   Very important

Justice (treating others fairly or impartially; conforming to fact, truth, or reason)

    Not very important   Important   Very important

Knowledge (seeking truth, information, or principles for the satisfaction of curiosity)

    Not very important   Important   Very important

Love (want, caring; unselfish devotion that freely accepts another in loyalty and seeks the other's good)

    Not very important   Important   Very important

Loyalty (maintaining allegiance to a person, group, or institution)

    Not very important   Important   Very important

Morality (believing and keeping ethical standards; personal honor, integrity)

    Not very important   Important   Very important

Physical appearance (concern for one's attractiveness; being neat, clean, well-groomed)

    Not very important   Important   Very important

Pleasure (satisfaction, gratification, fun, joy)

    Not very important   Important   Very important

Power (possession of control, authority of influence over others)

    Not very important   Important   Very important

Recognition (being important, well-liked, accepted)

    Not very important   Important   Very important

Religious faith (having a religious belief; being in a relationship with God)

    Not very important   Important   Very important

Skill (being able to use one's knowledge effectively; being good at doing something important to me/others)

    Not very important   Important   Very important

Wealth (having many possessions and plenty of money to do anything desired)

    Not very important   Important   Very important

Wisdom (having mature understanding, insight, good sense, and judgment)

    Not very important   Important   Very important

Step 2

After completing Step 1, pick out and list in the spaces provided the 5 items that you feel are the most important to you and the 5 items that are the least important.

Five Most Important:
1.
2.
3.
4.
5.

Five Least Important:
1.
2.
3.
4.
5.

Step 3—Five-Sort Value Inventory

The following are 21 sets of 5 values each. Within each set, rank the values from 1 (favorite value of the set) to 5 (least favorite value of the set).

1. ( ) Achievement
   ( ) Altruism
   ( ) Justice
   ( ) Religious faith
   ( ) Wealth

2. ( ) Altruism
   ( ) Autonomy
   ( ) Loyalty
   ( ) Power
   ( ) Recognition

3. ( ) Creativity
   ( ) Love
   ( ) Pleasure
   ( ) Recognition
   ( ) Wealth

4. ( ) Aesthetics
   ( ) Justice
   ( ) Pleasure
   ( ) Power
   ( ) Wisdom

5. ( ) Altruism
   ( ) Honesty
   ( ) Love
   ( ) Physical appearance
   ( ) Wisdom

6. ( ) Achievement
   ( ) Aesthetics
   ( ) Health
   ( ) Honesty
   ( ) Recognition

7. ( ) Achievement
   ( ) Autonomy
   ( ) Physical appearance
   ( ) Pleasure
   ( ) Skill

8. ( ) Autonomy
   ( ) Emotional well-being
   ( ) Health
   ( ) Wealth
   ( ) Wisdom

9. ( ) Honesty
   ( ) Knowledge
   ( ) Power
   ( ) Skill
   ( ) Wealth

10. ( ) Achievement
    ( ) Emotional well-being
    ( ) Love
    ( ) Morality
    ( ) Power

11. ( ) Aesthetics
    ( ) Autonomy
    ( ) Knowledge
    ( ) Love
    ( ) Religious faith

12. ( ) Aesthetics
    ( ) Loyalty
    ( ) Morality
    ( ) Physical appearance
    ( ) Wealth

13. ( ) Creativity
    ( ) Health
    ( ) Physical appearance
    ( ) Power
    ( ) Religious faith

14. ( ) Health
    ( ) Justice
    ( ) Love
    ( ) Loyalty
    ( ) Skill

15. ( ) Aesthetics
    ( ) Altruism
    ( ) Creativity
    ( ) Emotional well-being
    ( ) Skill

16. ( ) Emotional well-being
    ( ) Justice
    ( ) Knowledge
    ( ) Physical appearance
    ( ) Recognition

17. ( ) Altruism
    ( ) Health
    ( ) Knowledge
    ( ) Morality
    ( ) Pleasure

18. ( ) Morality
    ( ) Recognition
    ( ) Religious faith
    ( ) Skill
    ( ) Wisdom

19. ( ) Emotional well-being
    ( ) Honesty
    ( ) Loyalty
    ( ) Pleasure
    ( ) Religious faith

20. ( ) Achievement
    ( ) Creativity
    ( ) Knowledge
    ( ) Loyalty
    ( ) Wisdom

21. ( ) Autonomy
    ( ) Creativity
    ( ) Honesty
    ( ) Justice
    ( ) Morality

Step 4—Value Inventory Rating Summary

To summarize the results in Step 3, begin entering the numbers you recorded for the first set of 5 values in the first box of each of those values below. Each value occurs 5 times, so when you are through recording all 21 sets of 5 values, you will have 5 entries for each value. Add those 5 numbers across. The Totals column will then give you some ideas of the respective weights you give to the values involved. Remember, the lower the number in the Totals column, the higher that value ranks in your priorities.

						TOTALS
Achievement						
Aesthetics						
Altruism						
Autonomy						
Creativity						
Emotional well-being						
Health						
Honesty						
Justice						
Knowledge						
Love						
Loyalty						
Morality						
Physical appearance						
Pleasure						
Power						
Recognition						
Religious faith						
Skill						
Wealth						
Wisdom						

Top 3 values:

1.

2.

3.

Are you surprised? If yes, why? If no, why not?

EXERCISE 2: ENVIRONMENTAL CRISIS

This is another exercise designed to help you learn more about the values you learned at home, some of which you may not have given much thought but accept as true and often believe that everyone accepts them as true.

The Situation

You are a young health care professional in a moderately sized metropolitan hospital that has an entire unit devoted to the care of patients with kidney disease. The kidney unit can accommodate 5 people at a time on dialysis and is the only unit within a 500-mile radius that has dialysis capability. At times, there are scheduling difficulties, at which time a committee is called together to help resolve decisions of priority. The committee is made up of health personnel from the hospital and community and of laypeople from the community. You are on that committee.

The community in which you live and work has had a crisis. A toxin has leaked into the water supply for the city and has made more than half of the citizens terribly ill. Those most vulnerable to the toxin are people with kidney disease. Ten people are near death (within 1 hour) unless their blood is dialyzed. There are only 5 machines.

The committee has been called together to decide who should receive priority. It is impossible to save the lives of all of the victims, but you must make the decision of which 5 will be saved.

Your group has only minimal chart information about the 10 people and 30 minutes to make the decision. Your group realizes that there is no alternative to making this choice if 5 people are to be saved. With no decision, all 10 people will die.

Here is what you know about the 10 people:

1. Bookkeeper, 31-year-old man
2. Bookkeeper's wife, 30 years old, 6 months pregnant
3. Second-year medical student, man, African American
4. Famous historian and author, 41-year-old woman
5. Hollywood actress, 50 years old
6. Biochemist, 35-year-old woman
7. Rabbi, 54-year-old man
8. Olympic athlete, shot put, 19-year-old man
9. College student majoring in health profession other than medicine, woman
10. Owner of a topless bar, 56-year-old man, prison record

Instructions

1. Read the situation carefully.
2. Working alone, decide which 5 people are to go on dialysis. You have 10 minutes to make your personal decision.
3. At the instructor's signal, join with 3 others in the room and, working as a group of 4, decide on the 5 people to receive dialysis. You have only 20 minutes to make your decision. Argue strongly for your ideas and opinions. The future of these people's lives depends on your group decision. Make sure that your group is satisfied with the final list. Agree with other group members only if they truly convince you that their idea is better than yours.
4. Decisions by majority vote are not permitted. Every member of your group must agree with, and be committed to, the decision.
5. Group discussion: At the end of 30 minutes, one member of each group comes forward and places a mark in the data summary box on the board in the front of the room. Discuss as a group.

GROUP	1	2	3	4	5	6	7	TOTAL
Bookkeeper								
Bookkeeper's wife								
Medical student								
Historian/ author								
Hollywood actress								
Biochemist								
Rabbi								
Olympic athlete								
Health profession student								
Topless bar owner								

a. Why did you decide on each person? What were the assumptions you made that convinced you and others of the worth of each person's life?

b. What process did you go through to decide? Once you accepted the responsibility for the decision, was it difficult to decide on the final 5? Who in the group was most convincing? How vocal were you in arguing for what you felt was right?

c. What values emerged as you decided on the worth of a person's life and the opportunity for that person to continue living? Where did those values come from? When your decision was challenged, were you surprised that someone placed a different value higher than yours? Or did you assume that most everyone would agree with you?

d. After reflecting for a few minutes, comment on this exercise and what it teaches us about the nature of stereotype, labeling, and prejudice. How might this affect our decisions as clinicians?

e. Did everyone agree that every life has equal value and therefore suggest a lottery? How do you feel about that idea?

Journal about what you felt as you completed the exercise and what you learned about yourself with regard to what you believe is true and worthwhile and what you learned about your style of arguing for what you believe in. What are you feeling?

EXERCISE 3: CLINICAL FIELD TRIP

This is an exercise designed to deepen your understanding of the nature of health care behavior and, specifically, of patient-practitioner interaction. Read over the questions below carefully and then visit a facility where patients are being treated by health care professionals from the profession you have chosen. Visit as an observer only, and carefully make observations from which you will respond to the questions asked. Once the questions are answered, journal about what you learned and felt with this experience.

1. What pleased you about what you saw?

2. What bothered you?

3. How did this experience impact on your choice to be a health care professional?

Clinical Interaction Observation

1. Observe the environment. Describe how things are ordered and how things appear, and comment on possible underlying values.

2. Is efficiency a value? How do the health care professionals perform or function in relation to wise use of time?

The patient-practitioner relationship is one of the major factors that affects the success of treatment. This relationship is based on the establishment of sound, professional judgment. No 2 practitioners approach the patient in exactly the same manner. With experience, you will develop your own personal style of rapport. By observing interactions between experienced health care professionals and their patients, you will be better prepared to form your own approach to patient-practitioner interaction.

Use the following questions as a guide to direct your attention to specific aspects of patient treatment. You will be concerned primarily with the verbal and nonverbal communication that exists between practitioner and patient.

Attending Skills

1. What did the practitioner do to attend to the patient's personal needs and/or comfort before, during, and after treatment?

2. How did the practitioner maintain the patient's dignity during treatment?

3. Did the practitioner seem to really listen to the patient's description of his or her illness/disability as it is lived by that person?

Communication Skills

NONVERBAL BEHAVIOR

1. Did the practitioner exhibit any personal mannerisms/behavior that might have added to or detracted from gaining the patient's confidence?

2. Could you explain why any additional behaviors might have been effective?

3. Was the practitioner a good listener? What behaviors make you say that?

4. Did the practitioner maintain eye contact while talking with the patient? If not, did it seem to detract?

5. Were practitioner and patient at the same eye level for most of the time? Comment.

VERBAL BEHAVIOR

1. Describe and comment on the practitioner's voice quality as he or she communicated with the patient (soft-spoken, brusque, rapid, etc).

2. How did the practitioner seem to motivate the patient? Was the method effective?

Summary

1. What impressed you most about your visit?

2. What impressed you least?

3. What did you learn that you didn't know before?

(Adapted from material developed by Marilyn DeMont Philips, MS, PT, at that time Assistant Professor, Sargent College, Boston University and retired, following 20 years as Director of Professional Development, American Physical Therapy Association. She currently serves on the Parkinson's Disease Foundation [PDF] Advisory Council as a research advocate and volunteer ensuring PDF grants meet patient needs.)

**The exercises at the end of this chapter are also available online.
Please refer to the sticker in the front of the book and enter the access code provided.**

IDENTIFYING AND RESOLVING MORAL DILEMMAS

*Carol M. Davis, DPT, EdD, MS, FAPTA and
Gina Maria Musolino, PT, MSEd, EdD*

"It is curious that physical courage should be so common in the world, and moral courage so rare." –Mark Twain

"You are what you repeatedly do. Excellence is not an event—it is a habit." –Aristotle

OBJECTIVES

- To describe professional ethics and to distinguish among ethical situations, ethical problems, moral temptation, and true ethical dilemmas.
- To compare manners and etiquette with ethics and distinguish the continuum between moral obligations and nonmoral obligations as health care professionals (HCPs).
- To examine contemporary research that explores ethical and moral decision making in developing and licensed health care professionals in everyday practice.
- To describe the various factors to consider in making sound ethical decisions.
- To compare discursive or principled ethical reasoning processes with nondiscursive aspects of ethical reasoning.
- To outline the difficulties inherent in using the principles and rules of traditional biomedical, ethical reasoning alone in resolving dilemmas.
- To offer the Realm–Individual Process–Situation (RIPS) model and Applied Ethics Model: Active Engagement for ethical problem solving in order to incorporate traditional discursive ethical reasoning with nondiscursive elements, such as story, virtue, discernment, and meta-beliefs, and to apply these to individual, organizational, and societal dilemmas.

Ethics is the study of morality or the study of moral behavior. *Moral decisions* are decisions about what is right and wrong or better and best to do in a situation. *Descriptive ethics* discusses the moral systems of a group or culture; *normative ethics* deals with establishing a moral system that people can use to make moral decisions, and *meta-ethics* is the study of the meanings of ethical terms.[1] *Bioethics*, or *biomedical ethics*, is the application of ethics to health care.

Why should health care professionals have to consider the ethical? Practitioners are faced with many decisions each day. Most health care professionals place great importance on making sound clinical or therapeutic decisions in their practice.

Davis CM, Musolino GM. *Patient Practitioner Interaction: An Experiential
Manual for Developing the Art of Health Care, Sixth Edition* (pp 49-72).
© 2016 SLACK Incorporated.

At times, the legal ramifications of a clinical decision become apparent, but less seldom do practitioners consider the ethical or moral implications of their decisions unless they come face-to-face with a difficult moral dilemma that is not easy to resolve with confidence.

ETHICAL DECISIONS APPERTAIN TO CLINICAL DECISION MAKING

Whereas clinical decisions are based on weighing and considering facts (eg, given these laboratory values and these symptoms, the diagnosis is likely to be X), moral decisions are based on weighing and considering values, so there is no such thing as a true or false moral decision. However, just as it is highly important for health care professionals to make the right clinical decision, it is assumed that practitioners would rather act ethically than not, choosing the highest or best moral alternative in a value-laden dilemma.

Clinical decisions, no matter how purely factual they seem, still deal with people making decisions about what is best and true for other people. Few clinical decisions, especially those that deal with integrative or alternative treatment choices, are void of a moral component because most clinical decisions necessitate weighing the value of various outcomes. Different people may place different importance on the values aspects of any decisions.[2] Value-laden ethical decisions, like factual clinical decisions, are better made if they are made thoughtfully and rationally, not based solely on intuition or the emotion of the moment.

MANNERS ARE MINOR MORAL BEHAVIORS

The value-laden decisions we make at any one moment in the clinical setting can be analyzed as stemming from 2 main circumstances. Genuinely moral situations, which we discussed in Chapter 3, are those situations pertaining to how we interact with fellow human beings vs nonmoral choices or value preferences, which relate more to social convention and personal predilection.

But the social and cultural rules that can be observed in patient care settings often have grown up around moral choices while working with patients and colleagues. A common example would be the rules around dress and appearance that can be directly associated on a continuum of individual preference to responses to one's attire that lead to trust, comfort, and confidence (or its opposite). For example, students who push the dress code regulations by wearing attire more suited to leisure will risk losing patients' respect and trust.

Mueller[3] made the excellent point that "[m]any times the lines between etiquette, laws, and ethics are difficult to distinguish, leaving the individual to decide the best course of action." Proper behavior in the professional cultural setting often must be learned in much the same way that we learned manners and rules in our families (Chapter 2). Many of the habitual behaviors of Millennials will be in direct conflict in the patient care setting, and some could be determined to be unethical or immoral (eg, accepting a large gift from a grateful patient without realizing the ethical ramifications of this, texting one's friends or family while supervising a patient carrying out an exercise program, or leaving a patient abruptly because it's 5 o'clock and you put in your 8 hours).

The professions mandate moral behaviors in a way that occupations do not. A clinical decision that results in **not** putting the patient first—or, in moral language, not showing *beneficence*—must be able to be justified only on the grounds that there is a higher competing value. Let's examine the various ethical situations that call for decisions by health care professionals.

ETHICAL SITUATIONS, PROBLEMS, AND DILEMMAS

There are 3 major kinds of ethical decision-making opportunities in clinical practice: ethical situations, ethical problems, and ethical dilemmas. *Ethical situations* contain important values or duties but require no problem solving or difficult decision making, but ethical action may be part of the situation. Many ethical decisions are simple to solve. In the same or similar situation, the majority of people would do the same thing, say, in deciding between good and evil (eg, refusing to assist—or trying to prevent—a depressed person from taking his or her own life). Or perhaps you are with a group discussing an ethical situation but you need not act to resolve it.

Then there are *ethical problems*. *Ethical temptations* fall in this category, where we know what we should do but do not want to do it, often because we stand to profit or self-interest takes precedence over doing good for others (or beneficence). Another kind of ethical problem is *ethical distress*, where we know what we would like to do but are prohibited or constrained from doing it by organizational policies and procedures (eg, you want to have your patient seen on a Sunday before discharge, but institutional policy does not allow patient care on Sundays) or societal laws or rules (eg, you would like to be able to treat your Medicare patients, but you are prohibited from seeing them and charge for providing services because you do not have a Centers for Medicare and Medicaid Services provider number).

Ethical dilemmas, more difficult ethical decisions, deal with which is better and which is worse—do I continue to treat (and bill) this terminally ill patient even when my treatment is of little benefit but my visit seems to make a big difference in the quality of his or her day-to-day existence? This example might be seen to be a struggle between the ethical principles of beneficence (contribute to the good of each patient) and *distributive justice* (just distribution of limited resources to those who would benefit most).

The choice of the right thing to do is not only very unclear, but acting on one moral conviction can mean breaking another.[1] For example, as a physical therapist, if I act on behalf of my patient recovering from a stroke but in a plateau stage and document in the medical record that he is still progressing with physical therapy, I am not telling the truth because he has gone into a stage in which progress is not obvious each day. However, if I tell the truth, the best interests of my patient are compromised because the third-party reimbursement will likely be withdrawn, and he will not be able to pay for therapy and then, in my professional opinion, he will regress. This illustrates a dilemma where beneficence—acting in the best interest of my patient—means breaking a moral conviction to tell the truth. Which is the higher moral alternative? How do I decide?

Some would say that the most difficult of all moral decisions in health care have to do with allocation of scarce resources. Who deserves to receive help, and on what do we base our decision?[2] The above situation may illustrate the third-party payer's reply to the question of distributive justice; that is, only those who are showing regular change—improvement or decline—should be reimbursed for physical therapy services.

WHAT DO WE DO WHEN FACED WITH NOT KNOWING WHAT TO DO?

When faced with an ethical decision, what choices do we have? We could ignore it, follow our ideas or perceptions of current custom (what everyone else would do in this situation), ask our superior what to do, search for a policy that speaks to our problem or a rule to follow, do what feels emotionally best or right, follow our perception of the dictates of our religion, follow our perception of the dictates of our family rules, or apply traditional methods of ethical dilemma resolution in the search for the best moral alternative.[2] (This last suggestion is advocated in bioethics, but, unfortunately, many health care professionals choose one of the former alternatives and hope for the best.[4])

Ethical dilemma resolution has not received the attention in professional curricula that clinical decision making has received. Many health professions educators feel uncomfortable teaching students how to decide the best moral alternative because there is no one principle that binds us, and there is no absolute dictum against which we can measure the adequacy of our moral choice as being best.

BIOMEDICAL ETHICS VERSUS EVERYDAY ETHICS

What issues come to your mind when we speak of biomedical ethics or health care ethical decisions? The media favors reporting life-and-death moral dilemmas that deal with issues that reflect the increasing impact of high technology on health care (eg, organ transplants, fetal tissue research, euthanasia, and abortion). Granted, these ethical dilemmas are important, and we all benefit from studying the ethical treatment given these issues from ethicists who help direct us in our own decision making. Our task is to read the various arguments and decide which argument and conclusion seem to match our own evaluation of the best alternative in terms of logical soundness and consistency and what we feel in our hearts is the highest moral alternative.

Many bioethicists would tell us that our hearts should have nothing to do with this problem solving because our hearts contaminate our reasoning with subjectivity that cannot be substantiated with logic.[5] This would seem more acceptable if we were robots dealing with robots. Because we are people—health care professionals dealing with the everyday issues of deciding the best thing to do with people who are our patients, as well as their families—it is impossible for many of us to find comfort solely in the **rationalistic discursive resolving of dilemmas according to principles alone**. The compelling facts of each situation, our own personal priorities, our personal knowledge of the individuals and situation involved, and our own personal integrity developed over time by making decisions and weighing the consequences will all come into play to help us decide which is the best decision in this particular situation with the limited information we have in this moment.

Rarely do we deal with life-and-death ethical problems of euthanasia day-to-day. The ethical dilemmas we face day-to-day have to do with trying to do the best thing for our patients within the organization or institution of health care delivery, created mainly to meet the needs of great numbers of people, not necessarily individuals. These dilemmas often have to do with maintaining or improving the quality of a single patient's life. In discussing quality of life in the nursing home, Kane and Caplan[6] said it this way:

> *In one sense the disproportion of time and energy spent discussing transplants, artificial hearts, and other issues of high technology, acute care medicine, is appropriate. Matters of when and whether life should be maintained are of fundamental ethical importance, but the seemingly small stakes involved in the nursing home context—setting mealtimes and bedtimes, use of the phone, the right to keep personal property in one's nightstand—should not lull anyone into thinking that daily life in a nursing home lacks either ethical content or importance.*

The content of ethical concerns in health care parallels shifting cultural mores and values. A 1980 survey of the most common ethical issues faced by physical therapists in New England listed issues such as which patients should be treated, the obligations entailed by that decision, who should pay for treatment, and what duties are incumbent on physical therapists as they relate to physicians and other professionals.[7]

In 1996, Triezenberg[8] published data that indicated that there was a shift in most common ethical issues toward concerns about overutilization, supervision of support personnel, informed consent, protection of patients' rights to confidentiality, justification of appropriate fees, truth in advertising, preventing sexual misconduct and abuse, maintaining clinical competence, and ethical guidelines for the use of human subjects in research, and inappropriate endorsement of equipment and products by physical therapists. A panel of experts listed what they felt would be future ethical issues within the next 10 years (1995 to 2005). That list included responses of physical therapists to environmental issues of pollutants and health hazards associated with specific treatment modalities (eg, fluoromethane sprays effect on the ozone layer), employment discrimination, duty of physical therapists to report misconduct in colleagues, defining the limits of personal relationships in physical therapy, encroachment on practice, use of treatments not validated by research, use of advertising, and sexual and physical abuse of patients by physical therapists and those whom they supervise.[8]

The actual retrospective data analysis of physical therapist professional liability claims was elucidated by a claims study[9] examining the time period from December 1993 to March 31, 2006. Claims were made in all practice settings, most frequently in hospitals and patient homes, followed by nursing homes, schools, and outpatient service areas. The most frequently cited injury claims were trauma, including fractures; burns; delayed recovery; not providing additional needed procedures; injury; loss of limb use; abrasions/lacerations; emotional distress; bruises/contusions; and sprains and strains. The most frequently claimed (7% to 15%) primary allegations included during the time period were failure to supervise treatments and procedures, injury during manipulation, improper techniques, injury due to heat therapies, and injury during stretching or exercise. Less frequently (4% to 5%) cited primary allegations were failure to monitor the patient; improper management of the course of treatment; injury during electrotherapy; and inappropriate behavior by the clinician, including physical, sexual or emotional abuse/misconduct. These were followed by even less frequent (<2% to 3%) primary allegations claimed of improper use of equipment, equipment malfunction or failure, improper performance of a test, injury during passive range of motion, and improper positioning. Even less frequently cited (<1% to 2%) were primary allegations of failure to refer/seek consultation, injury from cold therapies, manipulation or massage, failure to report patient's changed condition(s), and injury during traction. Even less frequently cited (<1%), yet no less relevant to point out, were primary allegations of various issues, such as failure to maintain proper infection control, failure to follow established policy, failure to diagnose, breach of confidentiality/privacy, inadequate record keeping/documentation, failure to treat, lack of informed consent, and failure to respond to the patient.[9] Health care professionals are encouraged to be mindful of the primary claim concerns as a matter of ethical obligation and safety for the patients/clients to **first do no harm**.

Because the provision of health care remains a hands-on profession, the need to continue to seek informed consent, not just initially, and educate your patients/clients as therapeutic touch evolves in the course of care is continually reemphasized based on the prior claims alleged and in the suggested self-assessment for risk management. We must not forgo high touch with the high tech merely due to fear of litigation. Establishing an appropriate therapeutic presence in our patient-practitioner interaction (PPI) remains paramount, and effective communication is important for diminishing risk. We shall cover these topics related to communication and therapeutic presence more in-depth in subsequent chapters.

Physical therapy was further studied from 2001 to 2010, with the liability underwriter[10] retrospectively examining closed liability claims for the designated time period. As a result of the study, physical therapists were "encouraged to examine their own practice and policies to discern areas of possible improvement and dedicate themselves to maximizing patient safety and minimizing risk."[10] Similar outcomes studies[9,10] have been completed for nurses, nurse practitioners, pharmacists, counselors, and other health care professionals. The physical therapy study[10] results from 2001 to 2010 demonstrated that the highest average paid claims were in a hospital setting, yet the highest total paid claims were in offices or clinics. The most common allegations were improper performance using therapeutic exercise, improper performance using a physical agent, and failure to supervise or monitor. The highest claim indemnity was due to failure to properly test or treat the patient, but this specific claim was low in the overall percentage of closed claims. Many of the recommendations to decrease risk are related to components of PPIs. To minimize risk, the Healthcare Providers Service Organization recommended a Risk Control Self-Assessment Checklist for Physical Therapists and the following risk management overview[10]:

- Communicate effectively with patients, families, and colleagues.

- Delegate patient therapy services only to the appropriate level of staff.

- Provide appropriate supervision for all delegated patient services.

- Adopt an informed consent process that includes discussion and demonstrates that the patient understands all the risks associated with treatment.

- Ensure that clinical documentation practices comply with the standards promulgated by physical therapist professional associations, state practice acts, and facility protocols.

- Avoid documentation errors that may weaken legal defense efforts in the event of litigation.

- Maintain clinical competencies specific to the relevant patient population.

- Be vigilant about protecting patients from the most common types of injuries.

- Recognize patients' medical conditions and comorbidities that may affect therapy.

- Know and comply with state laws regarding scope of practice.

Licensing board outcomes, as a result of the claims, ranged anywhere from license probation, stipulations, reprimands, and/or suspension, and/or fines, to prescribed continuing education. Everyday ethics can have far-reaching impacts, and it remains in the health care professional's best interest to complete self-assessment activities to ensure currency and management of risk related to PPIs while considering ethical and legal implications of decision making related to patient care. It is recommended that you visit the claims website (http://www.hpso.com/resources/claim-studies.jsp?refID=ptclaimreport2011) and review the various health care professional risk-control self-assessment checklists to gain additional insights now, as a developing health care professional, and as you prepare to enter practice for clinical or fieldwork experiences and/or your first career position. Revisiting as an early career health care professional and keeping current in this area is appropriate and essential for all health care professionals.

Health professions students in educational settings in classroom and clinical education environments are not without ethical challenges in terms of environmental influences and practice exposures. Remarkably, in terms of toxins in the environment related to physical therapy education, Cope et al[11] and Cope[12] discovered and confirmed the hazards of air quality in anatomy laboratories used by students and faculty in relation to formaldehyde exposure, and pleaded for the removal of the health hazard. The ethical decision making relates to the cost benefits of an exposure to a known carcinogen compared with alternate forms of instruction combined with availability of anatomical structures with less exposures and/or decreasing the exposure risk with improved air quality management. Efforts to monitor the risk of exposures are significant in anatomical laboratories. Perhaps as 3- and 4-dimensional and haptic technologies continue to improve, the need for exposures shall be lessened, with alternative educational instructional formats.

In addition, Lowe and Gabard[13] gained insight into students' experiences with ethical and legal violations during clinical education with reporting and barriers to reporting. The survey included many of the commonly claimed areas, such as inappropriate use of resources, improper supervision, lack of truth telling, sexual harassment, blatant wrongdoing, and medical billing fraud. They surveyed 70 clinical students who noted violations but who oftentimes failed to report due to "low hierarchical position, fear of not being a team player, that they did not recognize as an issue, and personal consequences."[13] The researchers recommended that all students complete a mandatory competency test on the state practice act prior to clinical affiliations and that coursework also include instruction in moral reasoning, options, and outcomes for reporting, with process steps, to diminish barriers.[13]

Now that we have piqued your ethical interest from a personal, professional, and everyday standpoint, let's look more closely at the need for approaches aimed at ethical action, as well as components of moral decision making.

FOUR COMPONENTS OF ETHICAL ACTION

The ability to make a mature moral or ethical decision requires 4 behaviors that are often viewed as progressing developmentally: *moral sensitivity, moral judgment, moral motivation,* and *moral character.*[14]

Table 4-1 illustrates why simply knowing the best or right thing to do does not ensure that a person will do it. Most difficult of all of the components is moral character or moral courage. Moral sensitivity, judgment, and motivation can be encouraged and taught, but standing up for what you believe in in the face of adversity requires self-discipline, impulse control, and resistance to the fear of rejection and losing one's position.

TABLE 4-1
FOUR COMPONENTS OF MORAL ACTION
MORAL SENSITIVITY ○ Ability to interpret a situation correctly and appropriately ○ Awareness of how our actions will affect others ○ Awareness of all possible lines of action and their effects on others and self ○ Ability to imagine various scenarios with limited facts ○ Ability to role play and take the other's part
MORAL JUDGMENT ○ Judging which action is right or best, wrong or worst ○ Judging which line of action is more morally justified given the facts ○ Grasping the importance of the context of the situation that will point to the higher, more caring, more morally justified value
MORAL MOTIVATION ○ Prioritizing moral values over personal values ○ Wanting to do the caring or beneficent thing over self-interest
MORAL CHARACTER OR MORAL COURAGE ○ Having the strength of your convictions, courage, and persistence in overcoming distractions, pressures, and obstacles, no matter how large ○ Having implementation skills, focus, and ego strength: "Here I stand. I can do no other." (Martin Luther, 1483-1546) ○ Resisting fatigue, the morality of the day, the morality of expedience ○ Having self-discipline, impulse control, and skill to act according to one's highest goals ○ Resisting the need to be approved of and liked
Adapted from Rest JR. Background: theory and research. In: Rest JR, Narvaez D, eds. *Moral Development in Professions*. Hillsdale, NJ: Lawrence Erlbaum Associates; 1994:1-26.

INGREDIENTS OF A MORAL DECISION

A moral statement says that, in situation X, person Y should do Z. Thus, a moral statement includes what should be done (Z), who is to do it (Y), and the conditions under which the statement is applicable (X).[2] Most decisions made each day in health care are working decisions based on the facts of the situation. The decision is subject to modification or reversal when more facts become known. Decisions have to be provisional when each day brings new facts to bear. This is the reality of day-to-day health care. "Our task then," according to Francoeur,[15] "is to collect as much information as possible and then refer to the principles involved and choose the highest or best moral alternative in light of the situation at hand."

Let's take a look at discursive or principled ethical reasoning and see how it can guide us in deciding the highest or best alternative and then look at nondiscursive methods that will help us discover our own meta-beliefs that underlie and influence our final decisions about what is truly right and best in each situation.

TRADITIONAL BIOMEDICAL ETHICS

Traditional discursive or principled ethical reasoning requires adherence to 4 levels of thinking: (1) the particular ethical decision will be made by (2) favoring an ethical rule that (3) sits within an ethical principle that (4) evolves out of an ethical system. Ethical systems grow out of how we tend to view the world or how we "set our lenses." We try on and adopt points of view about right and wrong as we are growing up and following the dictates of higher authorities, such as our parents and church authorities.

Two ethical systems predominate: (1) ends- or results-oriented systems that say that the best way to decide the right thing to do is to act to bring about the best result or the maximum good (teleological systems) and (2) duty- or principle-oriented systems or deontological systems that say that the proper decision should not simply be decided by the results. The highest moral alternative should be situated in principles or rules known to be right whether or not they serve good ends.[2] In sum, in deciding the best thing to do, does the end (commonly the greatest good) most of the time justify the means, or do the means need to be carefully weighed without primary concern for the outcome?

An example of a principle that stems from a teleological or consequential way of looking at an ethical problem (ends are the most important) would be to act so that the greatest good can be brought about for the greatest number. That which is best is that which benefits everyone. Individuals come second to the good of the group. Hospital and nursing home administrators often make decisions based on this principle (eg, when all patients are required to go to bed at a certain time for the convenience of the staff). Another question that could be asked to weigh the good of an action from this perspective would be, "Would I be satisfied with the consequence of this action if it were done to me?"

However, duty-oriented ethicists would look to ethical principles that are those general and foundational truths, laws, or doctrines used by deontological ethicists to generate ethical rules about how to act in certain situations, regardless of the consequences. Many principles exist, and in each situation, we appeal to the most relevant and appropriate principle to generate the highest moral action.[16] Previously, we described ethical dilemmas that seemed to be related to the principles of beneficence, truth telling, and distributive justice. We had to decide whether telling the truth or loyalty to the patient was the highest moral alternative in the context of the situation.

MORAL PRINCIPLES AND RULES OF PROFESSIONAL CODES OF ETHICS

Four moral principles and 3 rules that stem from those principles make up the foundational ethical framework for the professions (law, theology, and medicine), each one of which provides service to the community.[15,17] A scan of most code of ethics documents will reveal ethical standards based on the following principles and rules:

1. **Autonomy:** Do that which enables the patient's or client's right to choose for one's life and to voice that choice for as long as possible. Informed consent, or the freedom to act on one's own behalf and to implement one's free decision, is a right situated in the principle of autonomy.

2. **Beneficence:** Do that which is best for your patient or client. Professionals are obliged to act in the best interests of the patient when the benefit to the patient outweighs harm it may cause the professional. At first glance, it may seem as if beneficence and nonmaleficence are the same, but they are not.

3. **Nonmaleficence:** Above all, do no harm. Do not do anything that may cause injury to, disable, or kill a person or undermine the person's reputation, property, privacy, or liability. In all cases, prevent any harm from happening. This principle is often the one that is cited as the higher alternative to not allowing a patient to die because removing life support is seen as causing harm rather than allowing a natural event to occur (allowing death to take place rather than stopping it). The key question to be answered is, "By your action, are you preventing harm (an untimely death) or preventing death from taking place when it is inevitable and no semblance of meaningful life is probable?"

4. **Justice:** Act with fairness to all.

   a. *Distributive* justice: Equal distribution of goods (attention, service) to all members of a group. (All qualified drivers with disabilities receive the same sticker to be used on their cars for parking privileges.)

   b. *Compensatory* justice: Act to make up for past injustice (affirmative action).

   c. *Procedural* justice: First come–first served or alphabetical order are the most common procedures used to be fair to several.

The 3 ethical rules that follow from these 4 principles include the following:

1. **Veracity** (from autonomy and beneficence): Tell the truth; do not lie. Most often, this rule is challenged with the question of just how much of the truth the patient should hear and when.

2. **Confidentiality, privacy** (from beneficence): Moral obligation to keep confidential all information concerning patients/clients **even if not specifically requested by the patient or client**, except when doing so would bring harm to innocent people or to the patient or client personally. In addition, patients or clients have the right to keep private information not relevant to care.

3. **Fidelity** (from beneficence): Actions should at all times be faithful not only to one's patient or client but to one's fellow colleagues. Criticizing the opinion of a colleague to a patient or family members undermines the whole of health care. When you disagree with a colleague, you can simply say that you have formed a different opinion.[15,18]

In sum, these principles and rules serve as a beacon to all health care professionals when confronted with a moral dilemma. Due to the nature of the professions (bound in service), these values turn out to be the higher ones in principled decision making. At times, we are confronted with a patient who requests one thing (autonomy) and we feel that it is not in his or her best interest to comply (beneficence). Then we must guard against paternalism or choosing for the patient what is best because we think we know better. Instead we must strive to inform the patient so that he or she can make the best decision for him- or herself. Then, we must do what we can to ensure our patient's right to choose for him- or herself, even if we disagree.

Unfortunately, most often the common dilemma is between autonomy or beneficence and self-interest (ie, moral temptation that becomes disguised or rationalized).[16] For example, the physical therapist may say that 10 or more treatments are necessary to meet the functional goals set for the patient to ensure the income from those visits, whereas if the patient had been placed on an adequate home program, those visits may not have been necessary. The extra income is a self-interest decision that would be rationalized as necessary treatment for quality care. This decision was far more common a decade ago than it is today and, in part, poor judgments such as this (multiplied by millions) are what helped push the pendulum of reimbursement to the other, highly unfair extreme, where in this century it is the exception rather than the rule to be reimbursed fully by third-party payers for care that is given. Today there are more serious concerns with professional integrity related to fraud, abuse, and waste in health care, which we will address further in subsequent chapters.

Principle Utilization: Advantages and Challenges

When one has to decide what the highest moral action to take is in any given situation, it helps to be freed up from the intensity and confusion of spontaneous feelings. This is true whether we're deciding a true biomedical dilemma, such as distributive justice (ie, who should be treated and who should not) or a day-to-day dilemma, such as the head nurse who has to decide whether the dying patient on the unit can have a visit from his grandchildren from out of town who arrived after visiting hours were over.

Using a reflective, problem-solving process that takes into account all of the given facts and uncovers all of the principles and rules that might apply is a way to rise above the subjective moment in an attempt to articulate an objective and defensible rationale for your decision. Trying to discern the *best* rule or principle or the *highest* moral action is often the most difficult decision, especially when you have limited information and must act right away.

We have stated that a teleologist will adopt the point of view that the facts should be weighed and the action that is best would be the action that benefits the greatest number. (The head nurse decides that the visit of young grandchildren might be disruptive to other patients—the greatest number—and decides not to allow it.) Meanwhile, the duty-oriented person will refer to a list of principles and pull out all of those that seem to bear on the case and, weighing the facts, decide which principle is the highest in this situation. (The head nurse decides that beneficence, contributing to the good of the patient, is more important than worrying about future decisions; if all patients ask for this privilege, chaos might result [justice].)

The Difficulties of Principled Decision Making

Well-known medical ethicists Pellegrino and Thomasma[18] asked, "Is there a set of obligations which bind all who practice medicine? Is there one rule, or set of rules, that health care professionals will find almost always is the highest moral alternative in health care?" This task of deciding would be made simpler if there were; put simply, adherence to principles does not always work because people disagree about which principles are most acceptable. Gilligan[19] posits, "The way people define moral problems, the situations they construe as moral conflicts in their lives, and the values they use in resolving them are all a function of their social conditioning." Thus, even recognizing a problem as having an ethical aspect to it has a lot to do with how we were brought up, how we view the world, and how our lenses are set.

Nondiscursive Approach to Ethical Dilemma Resolution

"While acknowledging the power of such rational systems, nondiscursive ethicists … challenge the narrowness of a strictly applied, formal system of ethical reasoning."[17] Nondiscursive ethicists do not claim that discursive ethics is too theoretical or difficult to perform. Rather, their complaint is that theories, principles, and rules alone promote a formalized, purely objective, cognitive way of thinking that is excessively rational and unbalanced. Principles are too often in conflict. Nondiscursive ethicists attempt to balance the process of dilemma resolution by incorporating such aspects of thought as imagination, virtue, character, role, power, discernment, and liberation in their search for an adequate method to decide the highest moral alternative.[17]

The Importance of a Person's Story

The final ethical choice, even the decision of which theory seems more compelling, ends vs means, derives from within a personal moral narrative developed over time that we all inherit. Nash[17] believed that to restrict ethical decisions to rules and principles alone "sends out the false message that a person's story is irrelevant to (or worse, destructive of) the 'proper' formation of a moral self." A person's story is a "moral necessity because it provides one with the ethical skills to form one's life truthfully, committedly, and courageously. … Objective discursive systems allow for rational, step-by-step deliberation and decision-making. **But the individual's moral intentions and motives originate in, and are formed by, significant people and events in the individual's life**" (bold added).

The key perspective in discussing the nondiscursive aspect of dilemma resolution is to make clear that a choice of the highest moral alternative can be seen to be seated in a rather consistent system of values that can be uncovered by proving one's moral convictions in a deliberate fashion or by writing a personal ethical autobiography. Once this story is better understood, important questions of character and virtue (What kind of a person am I? What kind of a person should I be as a health care professional?) can be asked. Health care professionals must be helped to recognize the way they've set their lenses so that they can adjust to a more professional perspective. For example, if what emerges on self-examination is a preoccupation with self-interest or a fear-laden perspective that takes precedence over autonomy, nonmaleficence, or beneficence, which are critical to professional health care value decisions, the health care professional must realize that decisions he or she makes very often will not be with highest concern for the welfare of the patient.

Deontology and teleology *presume* personal integrity. Principled ethicists believe that one develops moral character and integrity by making rule-based decisions, justified by ethical principles. Nondiscursive ethicists insist that moral character and integrity consist of more. To be moral requires constant training as a child and young person, and that training is more than applied ethics. "Integrity is the lifelong outcome of actions that shape particular kinds of character… And the character that develops is like the narrative of a good novel: it gives coherence to ethical decisions, and forces individuals to claim their actions as their own."[17]

As we learned in the previous chapter, cognitive developmental psychologists, such as Kohlberg,[20] favor a type of training to be moral, maintaining that children are only able to learn how to make higher or more adequate ethical decisions as they develop their cognitive reasoning skills. Moral developmentalists advocate teaching children how to reason morally by teaching them how to solve moral problems. The best moral decisions, according to Kohlberg,[20] are those that are logically consistent and admit to fewer exceptions, respect the dignity of all persons, and aim toward just treatment of all people, regardless of the law or of the person's race, creed, color, gender, or sexual orientation. Finally, cognitive developmentalists[14,20] offer methods of testing the developmental level of moral consciousness of a person by asking him or her to comment on the moral aspects of a dilemma that he or she identifies as being most relevant. In this way, subjects reveal whether they have progressed in their reasoning to an understanding of moral principles or remain stuck in simply obeying the law or doing that which is socially appropriate.[21]

VIRTUE ETHICS: THE DEVELOPMENT OF INTEGRITY OR CONSISTENT MORAL BEHAVIOR

What kind of a person should I be? Integrity is built from a continuum of choices, some important enough to be remembered, some almost habitual and unreflective. Each time a student cheats in class or a citizen cheats on reporting income for tax purposes, that choice to behave unethically, no matter what the rationale, wears away at the development of integrity. Choice is not only about what to do in a given situation; choice in making moral decisions is about **who I want to become**. The key question in self-examination is, "How does a truthful examination of my moral actions fit my moral image of myself?" Do I claim to be a person of virtue and integrity but choose to participate in gossip, judge others with prejudice, lose my temper, break my promises if I believe they're stupid promises, hurt people under the guise of trying to help by being honest, or lie when it is expedient to my goals? Answering truthfully requires our lenses to be set to listen carefully to the essential self; the ego must be still. The ego, the pragmatic goal seeker, will act to get ahead and rationalize that action so that it sounds acceptable and even clever.

How does this detrimental pattern of choice make sense? It makes sense if in my autobiography I remember the moral axioms of a parent who repeated such phrases to me as, "Get them before they get you." "If you don't look out for yourself, no one else will." "People get what they deserve." "The only thing that matters is who wins." "The winner is the one with the largest or most possessions or salary." "Life is hell and then you die and they throw dirt in your face." This pattern of negative choices also makes more sense today in light of commonly reported ethical lapses by our national- and state-elected and appointed leaders who most often publicly claim to be highly moral. The moral dictum of "do and say whatever you think will get you reelected" is the behavior we read about continually. Our country seems to have slipped into a period of the morality of personal gain and expediency, with the emphasis on not being caught. Only now are we waking up to the fact that one result is that we are destroying the planet we live on in the name of personal gain and technological progress.

Fear-based axioms, such as "Get them before they get you," are often behind this behavior, and, over time and with repeated exposure, this negativity will seat itself in one's conscience. Feelings of guilt and shame will then surface when you feel that someone is out ahead of you or is better than you are in class, or when you feel as if you've acted naïvely or allowed yourself to be taken advantage of in life.

In a conflict over altruism or beneficence vs self-interest or personal gain, it will be difficult to act for the good of your patient when doing so makes you feel as if you have been taken advantage of in the situation. Very often, day-to-day ethical decisions are made by deferring to policies and procedures as a way to assuage guilt. For example, a day-to-day decision of what to do about a walker, paid for by the patient but left behind after her discharge to a nursing home, may not be seen as an ethical decision, if one refuses to deal with this mistake because she's "too busy with more important things." "It's just too bad that the walker was left behind. Thanks for the donation to the department. I don't have time to chase down discharged patients. They're not our concern once they've left this facility." This treatment of a decision ignores the ethical aspect entirely. Selfish concern over the value of one's time vs concern over returning property to its rightful owner and then "passing the buck" by claiming that it's not your fault or problem are attempts to brush away the inadequacy of this mistaken choice. Or, following repeated patient falls, a health care professional who defends herself based on the system that these patients are expected to fall because it's a dementia unit rather than proactively working to prevent falls on the unit is blaming the system rather than taking accountability and responsibility to provide best practice for a culture of falls prevention.

Thus, one's character, built up over the years by listening to important moral statements and making little decisions day after day, will dictate whether a clinical decision has a moral component to it. If a value-laden decision is not recognized, the process of solving the dilemma for the highest good will never begin.

In other words, being moral means (1) being able to identify the moral aspect of a problem as well as (2) being a certain kind of person who wants to be able to reason adequately, and, finally, (3) doing the right thing. Virtue ethicists claim that virtues such as compassion, generosity, fidelity, graciousness, justice, and prudence should be cultivated in people so that doing the right thing becomes consistent with one's character.[22] A person will choose one's ethical behaviors more wisely if he or she chooses in accordance with commonly held virtues.[23] Virtue ethicists argue about which are the most important virtues. Lebaqcz[24] argued that the virtues of fidelity and prudence should be central to the professions. Fidelity to clients includes trustworthiness, promise keeping, honesty, and confidentiality; prudence has to do with "an accurate and deliberate perception that enables professionals to perceive realistically what is required in any situation."[24]

DISCERNMENT AS A VIRTUE

The common criticism of virtue theory is that cultivating virtue in one's being does not dictate that one will act virtuously in all instances. One might argue that a virtuous person, by definition, would tend to act in a virtuous way, but character traits alone are not enough to ensure the highest moral action.[23] But, if one has reflected on one's values, paid attention to moral choices, and developed integrity and compassion over time, it becomes easier to act with moral consistency, and inconsistencies serve to stir one's conscience in a way not as available to the morally unaware.[25] As Table 4-1 suggests, moral character or courage is more assured following components of moral actions, through moral sensitivity, judgment, and motivation.

The concept of *discernment* is integral to the development of character because discernment is the ability to assert that there is more than objective rationality to moral decision making. Thus, by introducing the whole topic of nondiscursive aspects of moral dilemma resolution in this chapter, I am acting on the quality within me of discernment. I believe that the best truth to be found is found within the human decision maker, within the essential self, and that every moral decision should combine the best of logic and rational methods with attention to the various impulses and movements that occur within a deliberative consciousness.

What is required in day-to-day ethics is a balance of heart and head, founded in a virtuous moral character that places the good of our patients foremost. Ethical decision making should never be reduced to subjectivity and feelings or intuition alone. The nondiscursive aspects of moral decision making are not meant to replace the discursive, but to add to it, to approach a balance with head and heart. Attention to the nondiscursive elements in a moral decision helps one to gain a personal understanding of the moral life. It is in paying attention to this aspect of moral reasoning that one can decide, for example, "when one is willing to make or break a promise, when to tell only the truth, to decide what one is willing to die for."[17] To learn to live the consistent and good moral life is one reason we believe we are all here on this earth.

THE ETHIC OF CARE

The ethic of care suggests that we do what is most important to preserve the integrity of the therapist-patient relationship.[16] To care for the patient is to have regard for his or her views, interests, and cultural mores and to hold warm acceptance and trust for the other, rather than doing good simply because beneficence dictates it. Sensitivity to the deepest values and concerns of the patient in the context of his or her life situation is what drives the decision making. To follow an ethic of care requires moral sensitivity and judgment, discernment, and excellent interpersonal skills. Health care professionals must listen carefully to the initial history and the patient's description of the problem and the meaning that this has in the person's life. The current economic pressures of the health care system commonly place restrictions on the ability of the health care professional to engage with patients in such a way as the ethic of care requires. The institutional constraints on caring have to be confronted as an ethical situation for health care professionals to be able to practice without feelings of conflict or doubt. Once this is done, the quality of one's practice can be anticipated to improve.

ETHICS AND THE LAW

As a general rule, ethics provide higher standards of the best or right thing to do than do state laws. Laws are created to protect the citizens of the state from unsafe practice; ethics bind a health care professional to the highest form of care.

With regard to the laws of health care practice, each jurisdiction in the United States has statutes called *practice acts* that guide the limits of professional obligation and responsibility for health care professionals in that state alone. The statute itself is accompanied by a document, usually referred to as the rules, that further clarifies the statute. The rules can be clarified and changed more easily than the statute itself, which was created by the lawmakers of that jurisdiction for its citizens.

Changes in health care management are occurring so rapidly that health care professionals constantly have to refer to their practice acts to ascertain what is within and what lies outside the scope of their practice, as well as the scope of practice for paraprofessionals, such as physical and occupational therapist assistants. For example, as of 2015, 29 jurisdictions required jurisprudence exams for new licensees on the laws and rules of practice for physical therapy, and 27 for the physical therapist assistant.

In the past, when no specific law existed to cover an action that ended up in the courts, the court (the judge) ruled according to interpretation of the facts of the case and his or her interpretation of the practice act. However, in recent years, courts have been holding health care professionals to a higher standard than the state practice act dictates.[26] For example, despite the fact that not all physical therapists are members of the American Physical Therapy Association, which binds its members to a code of ethics for proper practice, the court is starting to accumulate case law decisions that all physical therapists are professionals who should be held to this code of ethics standard. Many state practice acts today incorporate the code of ethics and standards of practice espoused by the professional associations and, therefore, hold nonmembers to the same standards and ethical obligations from a legal standpoint. Students and licensed health care professionals must comply with jurisdictional laws and rules; hence, it would behoove you to begin to become familiar with your state practice act and/or the jurisdiction in which you are going to train or practice. The Federation of State Boards of your profession of practice provides extensive information and links to guide licensees, those applying for license, jurisprudence and information for the public (eg, the Federation of State Boards of Physical Therapy [https://www.fsbpt.org/], with a mission to promote safety and competence).

The Federation works closely with the professional association and is currently collaborating on efforts to have a Licensure Compact to develop an interstate license; yet, state legislators must also be willing to adopt these changes. So, you can see the need for advocacy with the legislative body, which we will address in Chapter 10.

MODELS OF CARE

Corporate health care, managed competition, capitation, and prepaid health organizations in many cases have been limiting patient access to physical and occupational therapists and limiting therapists' choice of and duration of reimbursed treatments. Under managed care, physical therapists have professional obligations to patients and may have contractual obligations to managed care organizations (MCOs). It is important that health care professionals be able to carefully analyze their patients' needs and use sound moral reasoning and ethical dilemma resolution skills to decide on the appropriate actions for the good of the patient and for justice or appropriate fairness when there is a shortage of professional care available.

Until recently, MCOs had no moral obligations to their clients, the patients. Managed care is a business only. In the eyes of the law, MCOs do not practice health care. The primary duty of the health care professional is always to the patient and secondarily to the business contract. This can result in ethical distress when you know the best thing to do but are prohibited from doing it by the organization within which you practice. For example, if, under capitation agreement, the MCO provides coverage for only 6 visits and the goals set for the patient at the initial evaluation cannot be met in such a short time, the health care professional can be held liable for abandonment if his or her response is to discharge the patient short of the agreed-upon goals with the comment, "Your MCO told me I had to stop care." Business cannot dictate to a health care professional when to discontinue treatment.[26] Health care professionals are obligated to provide needed care. Likewise, health care professionals have the right to maintain an adequate financial base of practice and thus should seek private or other reimbursement from the patient.

Case law now indicates that the court's expectations are for the health care professional to carry out the duty to continue to serve the patient pro bono or without compensation. Thus, each practice needs to develop a policy or guide outlining how it will determine the incidence and limits of pro bono care and, beyond that, the care of the patient who cannot pay but requires treatment should be transferred to colleagues who have pro bono capacity at that time.[26]

When health care as a service is managed only as if it were a business, where profit is the primary reason for its existence, a conflict is bound to emerge. We have seen the concept of facilitating the healing of the whole patient or client all but disappear from health care. Business executives, with their eyes on the bottom line and dictating to health care professionals who they can treat, for how long, and what is reasonable to charge strip health care professionals of their ethical foundations. The definition of a profession's autonomy requires that health care professionals are the only ones who can make those judgments, and they are morally obliged to make them not with profit in mind but with service for those in need.[16]

It is important that you, as an early career health care professional, stay current with local, state, and federal guidelines on health care practice and reimbursement and learn how to resolve the ethical dilemmas that result in these unstable times. Your professional association assists health care professionals in timely updates regarding these matters, yet individual health care professionals are responsible, as professionals, to stay current. Only time will tell just how the Affordable Care Act (ACA), which refers to 2 separate pieces of legislation—the Patient Protection and Affordable Care Act (P.L.111-148) and the Health Care and Education Reconciliation Act of 2010 (P.L. 111-152)—will affect all these issues. Some predict that the negative impact of business on health care will become more restrictive to providing quality care before improvements begin. The ACA was challenged to the US Supreme Court and upheld in June 2012 as an exercise of Congress' taxing power; however, states may not be forced to participate in the ACA Medicaid expansion, leading to some state contentions and potential fallout of the ACA. This aspect of ACA has led to many state and federal battles and political divides. Some benefits have occurred as a result of this shift toward managed care. Some providers have also further boycotted the ACA and set up boutique-type health care where providers are placed on robust annual retainers and you may use the service at any time, whereas others have implemented cash-only services, leading to additional ethical conundrums. In terms of the ACA, although the patient/client savings in health care costs are far less than were predicted, the current trend has resulted in isolated areas of cost containment, as well as a greater shift of the burden of care to patients and their families, some of whom are experiencing greater expenses. This results in more responsibility on the part of patients for their health and for prevention and maintenance of their own care. We will discuss the challenges of health behavior change for health care professionals in Chapter 15. Once again, the value of health care as a right vs a privilege in the United States is changing and evolving, and it remains important that we monitor and advocate for our patients, which we will also discuss more in Chapter 10.

Above and beyond all trends and reimbursement mechanisms, when the interests of the patient and the health care professional collide, always remember that beneficence and autonomy ethically must outweigh self-interest.[16] If health care professionals were engaged only in business, there would be no dilemma. But health care professionals are bound by codes of ethics of service, not profit, that mandate advocacy for our patients who come to us because we have the education and the commitment to help them.

REALM—INDIVIDUAL PROCESS—SITUATION CONCEPTUAL ANALYSIS MODEL

Professional behavior requires fulfilling a role in society in relationship to individual patients or clients, the institutions and organizations in which we practice, and society as a whole. In the past, resolving ethical dilemmas concentrated on one aspect of this complicated relationship alone—the relationship with individual patients or colleagues. Although all ethics are interpersonal, the most compelling dilemmas we deal with in the 21st century often concern our relationship with our organizations and institutions and with society. To be ethically competent, we must be able to resolve all kinds of ethical situations, taking into consideration the context of the situation (the realm), the individual process involved (moral sensitivity, judgment, motivation, and courage), and the kind of ethical situation that is before us (an issue, problem, temptation, or dilemma).

In 2004, a theoretical model of analysis[27] was developed that combines the prior work of Glaser[28] in the realm arena, Rest[14] in the individual process arena, and Purtilo[29] in the ethical situation arena. Glaser[28] first developed a model in 1994 for exploring beneficence in 3 realms: individual, institutional, and societal. Glaser[28] posited that within the individual realm, a question might be, "May I deliberately and actively end my own life?" At the societal level, the appropriate question might be, "Does patient autonomy include the right to medically assisted death?" Once we determine the level or realms involved, we have a starting point for ethically based reasoning. The 3 realms are interdependent and help guide ethical decision making by providing guidelines or a partial map of ethics. The collective works of ethicists Glaser,[28,30] Rest,[14,31] Purtilo,[1] and Kidder[32] are combined in the conceptual model, termed the *RIPS conceptual model of analysis.*[27] The ethical rules of veracity or informed consent or confidentiality are well worked out at the individual level, but when it comes to the systems, policies, and procedures of organizations and institutions or the cultural dictates of society, it becomes less clear how to act. Each of the realms, at best, tries to promote the good and encourages moral behavior, but each realm will differ on definitions, priorities, authority, and what data are meaningful in coming to the decision of what is best and right in a given situation.[27] In other words, ethics becomes more complicated as you move beyond the concerns of individuals, and it is believed that you cannot resolve organizational and societal ethical distress and dilemmas with purely individual modes of action. For example, the inability of a person in a wheelchair to access an entrance to a public building is, in part, an issue of justice (individual), but it requires policy changes beyond simply changing the rules (organizational and societal). Likewise, the unwillingness of Medicare to reimburse for treatment based on faulty research or inaccurate reimbursement formulas goes beyond veracity. Policies and procedures, authority, laws, and bureaucratic customs all converge on decisions of federal reimbursement, and "organizational and social problems demand strategies and solutions appropriate to that realm."[27] For example, there are times when the best thing we can do to feel as if we have acted in good conscience is to email, phone, and/or meet with members of Congress and their staffers to advocate on behalf of our patients or make phone calls to request payments for our patients from third-party payers and follow-up with appropriate appeals and evidence-based justification letters for care.

SOLVING ETHICAL PROBLEMS: SUGGESTED PROCESS

Ethical issues, problems, and dilemmas occur frequently and require different problem analyses and solutions. The most difficult problem to resolve is a dilemma—when 2 or more ethical principles conflict with each other in a given situation and it is unclear what the best or highest moral action would be in this case or instance. The following problem-solving process method is suggested for application to solving ethical situations, including ethical dilemmas. It incorporates rule-based method (deontology) with consideration of the consequences (teleology) and attends to nondiscursive elements (virtue theory and the ethic of care). The suggested method is a combined adaptation of the work of Seedhouse and Lovett[33] and the RIPS conceptual model of analysis.[27]

1. Gather all the facts that can be known about this situation.

2. Decide which realm is primary: individual, organizational, or societal (Table 4-2).

3. Then, decide the process that seems to be called for: sensitivity, judgment, motivation, or character (see Tables 4-1 and 4-2)

4. Decide what level of ethical situation is involved: issue, problem, temptation, distress, or dilemma (see Table 4-2).

5. If the situation is within the realm of individual, organizational, or societal, efforts for resolution should focus on identifying needed policy and systems changes. Suggest the values that are involved and the policies and procedures that contribute to the ethical problem. Tackle the problem at the individual process level required—sensitivity, judgment, motivation, or courage (see example that follows).

6. If the situation is a true ethical dilemma at the individual level, proceed to decide which ethical principles are involved (eg, beneficence, nonmaleficence, justice, autonomy, confidentiality, veracity, and/or fidelity).

7. Clarify your professional duties in this situation (eg, do no harm, tell the truth, keep promises, be faithful to colleagues, etc. Duties such as these are often outlined in one's code of ethics.).

TABLE 4-2
RIPS CONCEPTUAL MODEL: FRAMEWORK

REALMS	INDIVIDUAL PROCESS	SITUATION
Individual	Moral sensitivity	Issue
Organizational	Moral judgment	Problem
Societal	Moral motivation	Dilemma
	Moral courage	Distress
		Temptation

Adapted from Swisher LL. Realm-individual process-situation (RIPS) ethical analysis model. In: Arslanian LE, Davis CM, Swisher LL. *Ethics From the Trenches: Everyday Ethics and the Real World.* Presented at: APTA Combined Sections meeting; February 2004; Nashville, TN.

8. Describe the general nature of the outcome desired or the consequences. Which seems most important in this case—an outcome that is most beneficial for the patient, the family, or your colleagues?

9. Describe pertinent practical features of this situation—one or more of the following: disputed facts, the law, the wishes of the others, resources available, effectiveness and efficiency of action, the risk, your code of ethics and standards of practice, the degree of certainty of the facts on which you base your decision, and the predominant values of the others involved (which may or may not coincide with predominant values in US health care).

When all of the pertinent aspects that go into this particular decision are laid out before you, you must use your discernment to decide which action is the highest moral alternative. You should be able to justify your decision by explaining your ethical reasoning process and your conscious weighing of one value over another in this situation based on what you know about your moral character; the virtues, traditions, and beliefs that frame your choices in life; and your professional ethical mandates.

APPLICATION OF THE SUGGESTED PROBLEM-SOLVING PROCESS

Let's take an example first of an ethical situation that involves the expectation of a kickback or gift in exchange for referring patients.

An occupational therapist certified in hand therapy visits a local orthopedic hand surgery practice with information about her skills and her practice in hopes of educating the physicians and office staff about the benefits of referring their patients to her for rehabilitation. She is told by the receptionist that unless she was prepared to offer regular golf outings at the local country club, she could not compete with the local physical therapist who got there before she did, although he was not board certified.

This surely is an ethical problem. Let's apply the problem-solving process to the case. The facts are that a highly qualified hand therapist would like to receive referrals from an orthopedic surgery practice, but she is told she must give a kickback, or pay for the referrals, in competition with another therapist who at face value seems less qualified to help the patients than she is based on advanced certification. Another fact is that kickbacks are against the law. But, unlike pharmaceutical manufacturers and medicine, exactly what constitutes a kickback and what constitutes an expense associated with promoting one's business has not been clearly delineated by physical or occupational therapy organizations.

Going to Table 4-2, we decide that the principal realm involved here is organizational. The ethical situation is between the occupational therapist and the orthopedic practice or the organization. The individual process required is one of moral courage or implementation. The occupational therapist is motivated to want to work for change but will need the courage to report this infraction and still remain in her mind a viable therapist in the community. The situation would be one of distress. She may be tempted to just look away and not make waves and thus protect her business, but she knows that what is going on currently is unethical, illegal, and not good for patients. She knows what she must do, but she has to work up the courage to take the appropriate course of action. She has to report the physical therapist and the orthopedists to their state boards of practice. So, this is not an ethical dilemma at all, but an uncomfortable ethical distress.

Now, let's illustrate how this process is used to solve a dilemma. One rather common ethical problem that occurs in spinal cord rehabilitation facilities is the ethical dilemma of what to do when a mentally competent patient refuses beneficial treatment. (We already know that this is at the realm of the individual.) But first, the facts:

Alex is a 23-year-old patient with a cervical fracture and spinal cord lesion at the level of C6-C7. He has had a surgical fusion, is medically stable, and is ready to begin rehabilitation, but he refuses to allow others to transfer him from bed to begin the process of tolerating sitting. Testing has revealed normal intelligence and a suspected level of grief and depression following this accident. No active motion has yet been seen below the level of the lesion. The nurses have had problems with his refusal to eat, the physical and occupational therapists have been unable to get him out of bed, and the social worker has been unable to engage him in discussion about his depression. He lies in bed with the covers over his head and says, "Leave me alone. I want to die." The physician on the case refuses to take Alex's desires seriously but also shows little compassion or sensitivity and commands the orderly to bodily remove Alex from the bed and wheel him to physical therapy. The other members of the team, although not wanting simply to yield indefinitely to Alex's depression, believe that the physician's order is inappropriate and are struggling with what to do next. They feel a strong pull of loyalty to other members of the team, including the physician, but resist the command to force Alex to comply. They feel a loyalty to their patient but believe that his depression blocks him from making the best decisions for himself at this time.

APPLICATION OF THE PROBLEM-SOLVING METHOD

1. Gather all of the facts.

   a. Cervical lesion, complete, at C6-C7.

   b. Young man, 23 years old. No committed relationship to a partner. Family (ie, father, mother, sister) supporting and visit regularly.

   c. Completed 2 years of college, proven intelligence, taking a year off to "find himself," risk taker, athlete.

   d. Accident occurred showing off by diving into shallow water of friend's pool at a party late at night.

   e. From family history, suspected addiction to alcohol, history of risk-taking behaviors.

   f. Family has excellent health insurance.

   g. Friendly, bright personality, strong previous desire to contribute to society, active in Big Brothers and Boy Scouts.

   h. Without conferring with the team, the physician has ordered that they act in a way that seems to many to be abusive and insensitive to the patient's (hopefully) temporary feelings of depression and hopelessness.

2. Decide which realm—individual—between the team, the patient, and the physician.

3. Decide which process is required. It's not moral sensitivity. The team understands and recognizes the problem. But they do not know the best thing to do, so this requires a process of moral judgment.

4. Decide which situation is present. There is no moral temptation, really. The team genuinely does not know what is best to do. This is a problem that seems to come to the level of a dilemma. To act in fidelity to the physician who believes that he is doing the best for the patient will be going against what the team believes is beneficent for the patient.

5. Organizational or societal issues at work here are not primary, so we go to the following.

6. Ethical principles involved: Decision to allow the patient to have his freedom to act in his own interest (autonomy) vs acting in a way to convince the patient to get motivated to begin rehabilitation (beneficence) contributing to the overall benefit of the patient. But the other factor is, what is the action that is most beneficial? The doctor's demand to bodily force the patient to comply with a rehab plan may be the end desired, but the means do not seem to be justified. Above all, do no harm (nonbeneficence) is an issue, and a logical question would be what harm might result from physically forcing the patient to comply. Fidelity to one's professional colleague seems to be less important than do no harm.

7. Clarify your duties in the situation: If I am the physical therapist, I have a different specific duty than if I were the social worker, occupational therapist, recreation therapist, or nurse. But each of us has the duty to act in such a way that the patient is supported in overcoming his natural depression and becoming invested in hope for a new life. Once Alex gets beyond his depression and understands, at the deepest levels, what his choices will be living with quadriplegia, then his decision to live or die will be his to make, free of interference. Right now, he doesn't have all of the facts, and his depression keeps him from even considering what those facts might be and how important they are to his decision. In other words, his depression renders him mentally incapable of deciding adequately in his own best interest. My duty as a health care professional is to contribute to the team's individual and collective effort to support Alex through his depression and to help him learn what he can expect from life living with quadriplegia.

   I am also obliged to be faithful to my colleagues so that we are united in our approach and work together for a good outcome, but I cannot be faithful to a plan that might cause the patient harm. The physician's order is not one that I can readily follow, so the desire to do no harm and the patient's beneficence seem more important than fidelity to my colleague, the physician.

8. Describe the general nature of the outcome desired: I want Alex to become involved in rehabilitation and to learn what it is like to be as independent as possible with his quadriplegia without having to go through the humiliation of being bodily forced to participate in rehabilitation.

9. Describe pertinent practical features of the situation.

   a. Disputed facts: (1) It is permissible to insist that patients not yield to depression by bodily forcing them to go to rehab. The end justifies the means. This fact can be disputed. (2) Alex is taking up someone else's bed who wants to be involved in rehab, and someone else deserves the bed more.

   b. Wishes of others: (1) Family wants everything done for Alex as soon as possible. (2) Mother has little tolerance for her son's depression. Concurs with physician's order. Father asks for patience and perseverance, plus treatment of depression.

   c. Resources available: Rehab beds are in demand, but money is not an issue for the family.

   d. Risk: Forcing Alex to be involved in rehab could cause injury to body or emotions. Also, it may backfire, causing more resistance.

   e. Degree of certainty of facts: The most uncertain of the facts concerns the nature of the cervical lesion. What will Alex's physical and emotional deficit look like in 6 months? In 1 year? How debilitated will Alex be, and how independent can we hope he can become? How successful will he be in reforming his core self-worth and values so that he might live a fulfilled life as a patient with a disability? Likewise, we are uncertain just how long Alex's depression will last. Even with the uncertainty of the future, the fact now is that he is physically ready to participate in rehab. Also certain is the fact that rehab cannot take place successfully without Alex's cooperation.

Decision

1. Meet with the team physician to discuss unwillingness to carry out the order to force Alex to go to rehab.

2. Confer with the psychologist, physician, nurse, and/or social worker and agree on a plan to systematically confront Alex's depression in a supportive way, with the goal of helping him through it in as timely a way as possible. Commit as a team to giving him the time he needs.

3. Once rehab has begun, practice beneficence and guarded paternalism while Alex is gaining a sense of himself with his new identity, and then be careful to relinquish any paternalism as Alex becomes able to cognitively and emotionally make decisions for himself, even if the health care team and/or family disagree with those decisions.

Two things seem obvious at this point. Moral decision making takes time and practice, and we may not have considered aspects of this situation that seem quite apparent to you. What if the physician becomes enraged that the team has not followed his instructions and threatens to have each one fired? Sometimes moral stances come to this level of confrontation, but not often. When one's integrity is challenged, moral temptation seems to become more compelling. It helps to have systematically thought through your decision to avoid this lapse in moral judgment.

Hopefully, the case application of the problem-solving approach has assisted you in further understanding the value of ethics in clinical decision making. The relevance of the impact of not considering ethical aspects of clinical decision making could lead to not only the incorrect decisions, but sometimes more harmful or hurtful ones. Research studies of physical therapy students in ethics content demonstrate that students who consider case-based, ethical applications with

	TABLE 4-3
	ACTIVE ENGAGEMENT MODEL: STEPS AND QUESTIONS
STEPS	**FACILITATING QUESTIONS**
Step 1: Active listening	○ How has the patient and health care team member cast their story? ○ Within the story, how do they portray themselves? ○ Why are they telling the story in this way? ○ Whose voice in the story is dominant? ○ Whose voice in the story is not being heard? ○ How else might this story have been told? ○ What is ethically at stake in this story? ○ What are the ethically important moments in the story?
Step 2: Reflexive thinking	○ What goals and values do I, as the physical therapist, personally bring to a given treatment? ○ What goals and values are inherent within the physical therapy treatment that I offer? ○ What influence do my language and my treatment methods have on the patient and others? ○ How do others (patients, colleagues, managers) know what they know? ○ What shapes and has shaped their world view? ○ How do they perceive me and why? ○ How do I perceive them? ○ How do they make sense of what I give them? ○ What perspectives do they bring to the findings I offer?
Step 3: Critical reasoning	***Realm of Patient and Therapist Relationship*** ○ What values and goals do I bring to the therapeutic relationship? ○ How do my professional and personal values and goals differ from the patient's? ***Organizational Realm*** ○ What is my relationship with the health care organization? ○ How does this relationship influence the clinical encounter? ○ How do institutional systems and structures affect the patient's ability to receive treatment? ***Societal Realm*** ○ What are the health care structures, resources, and economic policies that influence the goals and provision of physical therapy?

Reprinted from *Phys Ther.* 2010;90:1068-1078, with permission of the American Physical Therapy Association. © 2010 American Physical Therapy Association.

ethical problem-solving processes in the classroom find that the material is easier to integrate with real-world practical applications and have improved critical thinking with respect to clinical practice scenarios encountered.[34,35]

Delany et al[35] shared that "as moral agents, physical therapists are required to make autonomous clinical and ethical decisions based on connections and relationships with their patients, other health care team members, and health institutions and policies." Their perspective study also proposed an applied ethics model termed the *active engagement model* to further integrate clinical and ethical dimensions of practice. The active engagement model includes "3 practical steps: (1) to listen actively, (2) to think reflexively, and (3) to reason critically."[35] The active engagement model is further expanded on in Table 4-3, with steps and questions; and step 3, critical reasoning, incorporates the components of realms in PPIs, organizations, and society. The model suggests within each of the 3 steps specific facilitating questions (or sideways questions[36]) to support the process. The questions attempt to go deeper and facilitate active engagement for the broader aspects of care. You may wish to revisit the prior case and/or consider a case of your own once you are in fieldwork or clinical experiences to apply these deeper and expanded steps of the active engagement model for ethics in professional practice.[35]

CONCLUSION

We hope you see that the systematic processes to examine ethical encounters works to raise the decision-making process up out of the murky waters of intuition and subjectivity alone, and one could defend the decision as the best or highest decision one could make at the time with the facts provided. To go back on ethical decisions because of a threat would weaken one's integrity. We hope that the situations would not come to that end, but if they did, we would be confident in one's discernment and, one would hope, remain committed to one's decision.

Never forget that this process of deciding the highest moral choice must always be reflective of the needs of the patient and the patient's family. The real-live person before you with whom you are interacting is who you are accountable to and responsible for in health care. As Greenfield and Jensen[37] so eloquently put it, "We are not well served by a rationale, principlist approach to ethical issues that excludes the possibility of contextual understanding from the perspectives of our patients." The starting point for all of the processes of ethical clinical decision making must be the patient's own story if we are truly in service to meet the needs of society as partners in health care.[37,38]

The exercises that follow will give you a chance to discover more clearly the qualities of your discernment by asking you to write your moral autobiography and will give you the opportunity to practice ethical dilemma resolution using the suggested processes. Remember, you have been making personal moral decisions all of your life. Now, what is asked of you is to search for the values, beliefs, stories, myths, and parables that have informed those choices in a consistent way. How well will that way serve you now as a health care professional? What changes must you make, if any, to remain true to a commitment to therapeutic presence and healing? Don't forget to journal about your discoveries.

REFERENCES

1. Purtilo RB, Cassel C. *Ethical Dimensions in the Health Professions*. Philadelphia, PA: Elsevier Health Sciences; 2010.
2. Brody H. *Ethical Decisions in Medicine*. 2nd ed. Boston, MA: Little, Brown and Co; 1981.
3. Mueller K. *Communication From the Inside Out*. Philadelphia, PA: FA Davis; 2010.
4. Nalette E. Constrained physical therapist practice: an ethical case analysis of recommending discharge placement from the acute care setting. *Phys Ther*. 2010;90(6):939-952.
5. Callahan S. The role of emotion in ethical decision making. *Hastings Cent Rep*. 1988;18(3):9-14.
6. Kane RA, Caplan AL. *Everyday Ethics: Resolving Dilemmas in Nursing Home Life*. New York, NY: Springer Publishing Co; 1990.
7. Guccione AA. Ethical issues in physical therapy practice. A survey of physical therapists in New England. *Phys Ther*. 1980;60(10):1264-1272.
8. Triezenberg HL. The identification of ethical issues in physical therapy practice. *Phys Ther*. 1996;76(10):1097-1107.
9. CNA/Health Providers Service Organization. Physical Therapy Claims Study, 1993-2006. CNA HealthPro. www.cna.com. Accessed June 1, 2015.
10. CNA/Health Providers Service Organization. Physical Therapy Liability 2001-2010. CNA. http://www.hpso.com/Documents/pdfs/CNA_CLS_PTreport_final_011312.pdf. Accessed June 1, 2015.
11. Cope JM, Sanders E, Holt SM, Pappas K, Thomas KJ, Kernick E. Comparison of personal formaldehyde levels in the anatomy laboratories of 5 physical therapy education program. *J Phys Ther Educ*. 2011;25(3):21-29.
12. Cope JM. Comparison of two formaldehyde exposure assessment devices in a physical therapy education program anatomy laboratory. *J Phys Ther Educ*. 2014;28(3):15-20.
13. Lowe DL, Gabard DL. Physical therapist student experiences with ethical and legal violations during clinical rotations: reporting and barriers to reporting. *J Phys Ther Educ*. 2014;28(3):98-111.
14. Rest JR. Background: theory and research. In: Rest JR, Narvaez D, eds. *Moral Development in Professions*. Hillsdale, NJ: Lawrence Erlbaum Associates; 1994:1-26.
15. Francoeur RT. *Biomedical Ethics: A Guide to Decision Making*. New York, NY: John Wiley & Sons; 1983.
16. Pellegrino ED. Altruism, self-interest, and medical ethics. *JAMA*. 1987;258(14):1939-1940.
17. Nash RJ. Applied ethics and moral imagination: issues for educators. *J Thought*. 1987;22(3):68-77.
18. Pellegrino ED, Thomasma DC. *A Philosophical Basis of Medical Practice: Toward a Philosophy and Ethic of the Healing Professions*. New York, NY: Oxford University Press; 1981.
19. Gilligan C. *In a Different Voice: Psychological Theory and Women's Development*. Cambridge, MA: Harvard University Press; 1993.
20. Kohlberg L. The cognitive development approach to moral education. *Phi Delta Kappa*. 1975;56(10):670-677.
21. Munsey B. *Moral Development, Moral Education and Kohlberg*. Birmingham, AL: Religious Education Press; 1980.
22. Noddings N. *Caring: A Feminine Approach to Ethics and Moral Education*. 2nd ed. Berkeley, CA: University of California Press; 2003.
23. Pence GE. *Ethical Options in Medicine*. Oradell, NJ: Medical Economics Co; 1980.
24. Lebaqcz K. *Professional Ethics: Power and Paradox*. Nashville, TN: Abingdon Press; 1985.
25. Purtilo RB, Haddad A, Doherty R. *Health Professional/Patient Interaction*. 8th ed. Philadelphia, PA: Elsevier Health Sciences; 2014.

26. Scott R. *Legal, Ethical, and Practical Aspects of Patient Care Documentation: A Guide for Rehabilitation Professionals*. 4th ed. Burlington, MA: Jones & Bartlett Learning; 2013.

27. Swisher LL, Arslanian LE, Davis CM. Realm-individual process-situation (RIPS) model of ethical analysis decision-making. *HPA Resource*. 2005;(3):1, 3-8.

28. Glaser J. *Three Realms of Ethics: Individual, Institutional, Societal: Theoretical Model and Case Studies*. New York, NY: Rowman & Littlefield Publishers; 1994.

29. Purtilo RB. A time to harvest, a time to sow: ethics for a shifting landscape. *Phys Ther*. 2000;80(11):1112-1119.

30. Glaser JW. Three realms of ethics: an integrative map of ethics for the future. In: Purtilo RB, Jensen GM, Brasic-Royeen C, eds. *Educating for Moral Action: A Sourcebook in Health and Rehabilitation Ethics*. Philadelphia, PA: FA Davis; 2005:169-184.

31. Rest JR, Narvaez D, Bebeau MJ, Thoma SJ. *Postconventional Moral Thinking: A Neo-Kohlbergian Approach*. Mahwah, NJ: Lawrence Erlbaum Associates; 1999.

32. Kidder RM. *How Good People Make Tough Choices: Resolving the Dilemmas of Ethical Living*. New York, NY: Fireside; 1995.

33. Seedhouse D, Lovett L. *Practical Medical Ethics*. New York, NY: John Wiley & Sons; 1992.

34. Venglar M, Theall M. Case-based ethics education in physical therapy. *J School Teach Learn*. 2007;7(1):64-76.

35. Delany CM, Edwards I, Jensen GM, Skinner E. Closing the gap between ethics knowledge and practice through active engagement: an applied model of physical therapy ethics. *Phys Ther*. 2010;90(7):1068-1078.

36. Guillemin M, Gilliam L. *Telling Moments: Everyday Ethics in Health Care*. Melbourne, Australia: IP Communications; 2006.

37. Greenfield BH, Jensen GM. Understanding the lived experiences of patients: application of a phenomenological approach to ethics. *Phys Ther*. 2010;90(8):1185-1197.

38. Sullivan KJ, Wallace JG Jr, O'Neil ME, et al. A vision for society: physical therapy as partners in the national health agenda. *Phys Ther*. 2011;91(11):1664-1672.

39. Christ C. *Diving Deep and Surfacing*. Boston, MA: Beacon Press; 1995.

SUGGESTED READINGS

American Physical Therapy Association. Ethics in practice articles. http://www.apta.org/Ethics/Tools/Articles/. Accessed May 25, 2015.

Banja JD. Ethics, outcomes, and reimbursement. *Rehab Manag*. 1994;7(1):61-65.

Clancy CM, Brody H. Managed care. Jekyll or Hyde? *JAMA*. 1995;273(4):338-339.

Curtin LL. Why good people do bad things. *Nursing Manage*. 1996;27(7):63-65.

DeGrazia D, Mappes TA, Ballard J, eds. *Biomedical Ethics*. 7th ed. New York, NY: McGraw Hill Higher Education; 2010.

Federation of State Boards of Physical Therapy Practice. www.fsbpt.org.

Gawande A. *Being Mortal: Medicine and What Matters in the End*. New York, NY: Metropolitan Books; 2014.

Gawande A. Overkill: an avalanche of unnecessary medical care is harming patients physically and financially. What can we do about it? *The New Yorker*. May 11, 2015.

Gawande A. The cost conundrum redux. *The New Yorker*. June 25, 2009.

Grimaldi PL. Protection for patients or providers? *Nursing Manage*. 1996;27(7):12-17.

Hiepler MO. *Managed Care: A Revolution in Progress: Lawsuits Against HMOs/Gatekeeper Physicians*. Berkeley, CA: Conference Recording Service; 1996:Publication HFM96-3.

Page CG. *Management in Physical Therapy Practices*. 2nd ed. Philadelphia, PA: F.A. Davis; 2015.

Palermo BJ. Capitation on trial. *Calif Med*. 1996;7:25-29.

Rawal PH. *The Affordable Care Act: Examining the Facts*. Santa Barbara, CA: ABC-CLIO; 2015.

Rodwin MA. *Medicine, Money and Morals*. New York, NY: Oxford University Press; 1993.

Salladay SA. Rehabilitation, ethics and managed care. *Rehab Manag*. 1996;9(6):38-42.

Stahl DA. Risk shifting in subacute care. *Nurs Manage*. 1996;27(7):20,22.

Steinbock B, London AJ, Arras J. *Ethical Issues in Modern Medicine: Contemporary Readings in Bioethics*. 8th ed. New York, NY: McGraw-Hill College; 2013.

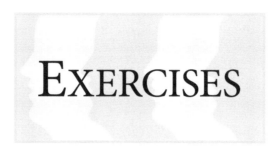

EXERCISES

EXERCISE 1: WRITE YOUR MORAL AUTOBIOGRAPHY

People reveal themselves in telling stories. We all have stories to tell about ourselves, our lives growing up, the choices we had to make, close calls we've had, funny incidents where we were caught off guard, a great (or terrible) date, a wonderful concert or movie, and a great time with an old friend.

Carol Christ wrote in *Diving Deep and Surfacing*[39]:

> *When meeting new friends or lovers, people reenact the ritual of telling stories. Why? Because they sense the meaning of their lives is revealed in the stories they tell, in their perception of the forces they contended with, in the choices they made, in their feelings about what they did or did not do. In telling their stories, people speak of parents, lovers, ecstasy, and death—of moments when life's meaning seemed clear or unfathomable.*

One of the most important aspects of your story is your perception of how, growing up, the values of your family provided a sense of orientation for you that perhaps became a taken-for-granted set of boundaries against which you played out your life, against which you had to contend, the currents in which you learned to swim, and the forces that helped you to define yourself. In this way, those values provided a sense of meaning. They grounded you in powers of being that enabled you to challenge the obstacles of the world to become who you are now.

Think back to when you were a child. You may want to interview parents and grandparents for more information.

1. What were the rules of the family? Where did those rules seem to come from? The Bible? The church? From ancient wisdom passed down?

2. What do you remember being punished for? What were your siblings punished for? Were you punished, or would you say you were "disciplined"? What is the difference to you?

3. What were you praised for? What were you encouraged to do? How did that make you feel?

4. Were there certain favorite virtues that were emphasized? For example, always refer to older people as Mr. or Mrs., always do your best, always tell the truth, get good grades, and go out for sports?

5.   What were the family rules for making decisions, or did that remain a mystery?

6.   What do you remember being most emotional about? Did you have a favorite cause? Have you ever participated in a march for a cause or in any actions of civil disobedience? Would you if you were challenged to? Why or why not?

Recount any major moral decisions you remember making. Write a story of the development of your moral consciousness. What values do you see as most important, and how, from your story, do you know this? Does this have implications for your choice of profession?

EXERCISE 2: EXAMINE YOUR CODE OF ETHICS AND PRACTICE ACT

Locate a copy of your profession's code of ethics. Analyze the code statements to determine the values and ethical principles that are most esteemed by your profession. Next, examine the code and its accompanying rules for what seems to be missing. What would you wish the code and rules would speak to that is not present? Are the directions for moral action specific enough for your guidance? Why not?

Locate a copy of your licensing authority's practice act for your profession and its accompanying rules. Outline the scope of practice allowed by the act. What are you able to do, and what are you prohibited from doing? What guidelines are given with regard to delegation of care to aides and assistants? What might you be asked to do by an uninformed superior that would not be legal? What might you be asked to do that is legal but would not be ethical? How would you respond?

EXERCISE 3: ETHICAL DILEMMA RESOLUTION

Below are several day-to-day ethical situations faced by health care professionals. Choose one. Go through the process to solve it as illustrated in this chapter.

1. A physical therapist colleague in private practice admits that he charges less money for patients who pay with cash because he never records his income for tax purposes. You have been working for this therapist for 6 months, and in order to keep your job, he is asking you to adopt the same system and offers you a cash bonus of $5000 at Christmas because you deserve the money more than the Internal Revenue Service. Personal circumstances make this the only place where you can practice and still fulfill your family responsibilities. You are the only person in your family employed at this time, and you are supporting 2 children and an elderly mother.

    a. Look at Table 4-2. Is this an individual, organizational, or societal problem?

    b. What kind of ethical situation is described here—an issue, problem, dilemma, distress, or temptation?

    c. Finally, what kind of process is required on the part of the physical therapist—moral sensitivity, judgment, motivation, or courage?

    d. What should this physical therapist do? Why?

    e. Consider the queries for active listening, reflective thinking, and critical reasoning in Table 4-3 applying the active engagement model.

2. You have agreed to fill in for a home care therapist for 2 weeks. At 4 of the 5 patients' homes in 1 day, as you evaluated and treated according to your standards, the patients have made comments that the other therapist never did any of this kind of therapy. It becomes apparent to you that the therapist you are filling in for is giving no professional care. You are scheduled to move out of this town to another state as soon as this 2-week time period ends. If you report this person, you would need to return to the state to testify, but the state would pay your expenses to do so.

    a. Look at Table 4-2. Is this an individual, organizational, or societal problem?

    b. What kind of ethical situation is described here—an issue, problem, dilemma, distress, or temptation?

    c. Finally, what kind of process is required on the part of the physical therapist—moral sensitivity, judgment, motivation, or courage?

    d. What should this physical therapist do? Why?

    e. Consider the queries for active listening, reflective thinking, and critical reasoning in Table 4-3 applying the active engagement model.

3. At 4:45 PM, a woman in severe pain walks into the physical therapy department with a referral from her physician to be evaluated and treated for severe low back pain. The physical therapist in charge (and the only one present) had stayed late to see patients well after the usual closing time of 5 o'clock for the past week. Furthermore, the day care center had called just before the woman walked in, stating that the therapist's 6-month-old daughter was very sick with severe vomiting and diarrhea, and they were very worried about her. The therapist's wife is out of town. The therapist tells the patient, "I'm sorry, we're closed for the day and I must leave. You'll have to come back in the morning." The woman bursts into tears and says she doesn't even know if she can make it home, she is in such pain.

    a. Look at Table 4-2. Is this an individual, organizational, or societal problem?

    b. What kind of ethical situation is described here—an issue, problem, dilemma, distress, or temptation?

    c. Finally, what kind of process is required on the part of the physical therapist—moral sensitivity, judgment, motivation, or courage?

    d. What should this physical therapist do? Why?

    e. Consider the queries for active listening, reflective thinking, and critical reasoning in Table 4-3 applying the active engagement model.

4. You are treating a woman who recently had a stroke. Her insurance allows for payment for only 10 treatments. What ethical implications are there when you cannot achieve agreed-upon functional goals in 10 treatments?

    a. What is your professional responsibility? What is your legal responsibility? What would you do to resolve this problem short of refusing care?

    b. How might you go about working to change this organizational limitation from the insurance company? Would you do it? Why or why not?

    c. Consider the queries for critical reasoning in Table 4-3 applying the active engagement model.

The exercises at the end of this chapter are also available online.
Please refer to the sticker in the front of the book and enter the access code provided.

STRESS MANAGEMENT

*Carol M. Davis, DPT, EdD, MS, FAPTA and
Gina Maria Musolino, PT, MSEd, EdD*

"We don't stop playing because we grow old; we grow old because we stop playing." –George Bernard Shaw

OBJECTIVES

- To define burnout and explore personal sources of stress.
- To explore the effects of stress on the body and on our perceptions of situations.
- To discuss the negative effects of stress in health care organizations on quality of care and provider stress.
- To discuss the stress development model and related screening tools.
- To describe external and internal factors that contribute to the buildup of stress in professional helpers.
- To emphasize the importance of one's thoughts on the quality of life.
- To explore mechanisms that interfere with stress buildup and thus help control the negative effects.

One of the most powerful rewards of the healing professions is the tremendous job satisfaction they bring. Most people enter the helping professions to work with people who need help in overcoming illness or disability or to help well people stay well and fit. The expectation is a career in which one assumes that each day will be interesting and rewarding, with the expectation of a great deal of personal satisfaction and meaning in helping others. Few people ever anticipate or prepare for the tremendous amount of stress that is inherent in the helping professions. Despite the deepest feelings of caring and altruism, caring for people who need help can bring with it great emotional and physical exhaustion to those who do not prepare for it.

STRESS

Let's take a closer look at stress in general. *Stress* is a value-neutral word; that is, it need not indicate something negative. In fact, stress is simply a response to being alive, and the human organism requires certain stress to have something to respond to in order to live.

Davis CM, Musolino GM. *Patient Practitioner Interaction: An Experiential Manual for Developing the Art of Health Care, Sixth Edition* (pp 73-89).
© 2016 SLACK Incorporated.

What we perceive as negative stress results from our inability to solve a problem or to reach a goal that is believed (or feared) to be unattainable. We feel out of control, and tension arises from attempts to figure out how to get back in control and reach our goals.[1] This is similar to standing at the bottom of a huge mountain and not knowing how in the world we will ever manage to get to the top. This kind of stress has effects on our perspective of the situation, and it has effects on our bodies. Sometimes, even positive stress or having lots of opportunities and options may be more stressful than negative stress. Due to the fact that many good options are presented with choices or careers/career opportunities, the stress arises from making the best choice(s), which unfortunately can often be paralyzing, leading to no choice, forced choices, or, worse yet, an unrelenting feeling of being overwhelmed, leading to paralysis by analysis.

When we feel the anxiety of negative stress, we tend to misread the situation at hand, blow things out of proportion, take on unrealistic guilt, or internalize and personalize thoughts that have little to do with us. For example, let's say you feel under the stress of seeing 5 more patients in the next 12 minutes (an unattainable goal), and a colleague comes into your office and is noticeably upset about something. There's a high likelihood that one of your immediate responses to your colleague would be, "Oh great! What did I do now?"

The fact is that you are often not the cause of another person's anger or frustration, and you increase your stress by making that erroneous assumption. Under stress, you have simply distorted a situation and, depending on the energy of your paranoia, blew it all out of proportion. Stress distorts our ability to see the world as it truly is, and this distortion then increases our stress, causing a positive progression or escalation of our anxiety. The greater the existing stress, the more likely the addition of more stress. In other words, a positive feedback loop is established.

Many aspects of day-to-day life, positive and negative, cause some minor stress (eg, change in sleeping habits, church, social activities, new school, vacation, and personal achievement). Many life events are sources of major stress (eg, death, divorce, separation, injury, illness, change in health [self or family member], sexual difficulties, changing jobs, and relocation).

Stressors Commonly Experienced by Health Care Professionals

The health care profession underwent massive change in the past 3 decades and continues to reflect those changes. The impact of managed care on the quality of care of patients has received mixed reviews, but, for the most part, patients now report more depersonalized care; are disappointed with the quality of the care they are receiving, particularly the lack of individual time spent with their providers; and resent the increasing cost of health insurance.[2,3] Today, more access to care is available, but with varying quality and proximity. Less comprehensive coverage is available, but more preventive coverage is generally attainable. Catastrophic care is still problematic for those without private insurance, and federal and state governments continue to offer a range of plans. The burden is now on the public, more than in the past, to select a plan. Limited consultation is available to assist the public in selecting insurance coverage, and choices are now mandated. Just making a choice about health care has now become a point of stress for the untrained public, and many have no idea how to examine a policy to learn how different aspects of care, such as rehabilitation therapies, will or will not be covered. Often, the coding and billing staff in your practice setting may help to offer advisement, and you may be asked to provide guidance as a health care professional (HCP). As policies change, health care professionals are stressed to keep up with current payment models and a plethora of insurance types while staying current in evidence-based practice and striving for excellence in patient-practitioner interactions. Health care is not for the faint of heart. Health care professionals are being challenged to do more for less. Different payment models and systems continue to be studied and considered, causing even greater stress on health care professionals to provide accurate documentation to support the payment systems. Health care professionals must select appropriate codes and provide standardized measures to support progressions of care. Ensuring compliance with federal regulations (eg, Medicare [www.medicare.gov], third-party payers, federal civil rights laws, and the Health Insurance Portability and Accountability Act Privacy Rule [www.hhs.gov/ocr/office]) may be a source of stress in everyday practice. We will discuss some key legislation affecting patients and health care professionals in Chapter 16.

Assessing risk for fraud and abuse and doing the right thing is part of practice management for all health care professionals. If one does not manage these practice demands on a daily basis, they can become an escalated, negative, and unnecessary stress and potentially lead to devastating fines and criminal charges or behaviors. Together, the American Physical Therapy Association (APTA), American Occupational Therapy Association (AOTA), and American Speech-Language-Hearing Association (ASHA) have issued a consensus statement related to clinical judgment in health care settings regarding ethical service delivery, the need to know rules and regulations, evaluation, treatment, documentation, and upholding clinical integrity. The statement also provides information on the Office of Inspector General hotline for reporting fraud anonymously. You may access the joint statement via http://www.apta.org/NationalIssues/FraudAbuse/, as well as many other compliance tips and educational opportunities to assist in integrity in practice. Each professional association's website offers additional information with related links provided in the consensus statement.

Knowledge is certainly a way to combat stress and reassures that you are doing the right or best things in practice and conscientiously choosing to make the wisest possible decision. Staying active in your professional associations helps to keep you abreast of changing practice needs on national and state levels. Although the rewards of the profession in assisting another human being accomplish therapeutic goals is paramount, the stress of care management in an ever-changing health care world demands that health care professionals manage their stressors daily. One cannot be like an ostrich and stick his or her head in the sand when it comes to managing stress in health care practice arenas.

Select research studies have explored issues of stress in health care professional practice. A study examining the impact of the changing health care environment on fieldwork education in occupational therapy revealed that stress was increased by increased productivity expectations, number of hours worked, and time spent in documentation, with a decrease in job security, time for continuing education, and quality of patient care.[4] In a study of primary care physician practices, patients reported a lower rating on the quality of care from physicians in managed care practices.[5] Some of the most common sources of workplace stress for nurses included more intense workload, conflicts with leadership/management style, professional conflicts in general, and the emotional cost of caring.[5]

It remains a sign of the times that the environment of health care has changed significantly to become more stressful for health care professionals and their patients, and it will take a quantum shift for health care to once again be characterized by healing and less by business practices. When patients become a means to an end for profit, the stress on health care professionals who want to serve those in need becomes enormous when they are forced by organizations to pay more attention to the bottom line.[6]

Stressors Commonly Experienced by Students

Purtilo et al[1] discussed ongoing anxieties commonly related to student life. Remember that negative stress is experienced in the presence of a fear that a goal that we have set is unattainable. They reported that students respond most dramatically to 3 anxiety-provoking questions throughout their education[1]:

1. **Am I good enough?** This is not only troublesome just before exams, but it is also an ongoing fear related to questions of moral and intellectual competence—in other words, this is an issue of self-esteem and can be fueled by constant comparison of oneself with "more talented" classmates and professionals.

2. **Do I have what it takes?** Similar to question 1, this relates to perceptions of and fears about one's physical and emotional limits. This anxiety rears its ugly head the first time a student feels faint while in a hospital or experiences the exhaustion of long hours of work without breaks.

3. **Can I pay?** The cost of tuition is steadily rising with little concurrent increase in financial aid. The anxiety of having to take out another loan, take on an override loan, pay for temporary housing, take on another job, or quit weighs on students and often affects their performance in classes and clinics.

A review of the literature by Dyrbye et al[7] examining students' difficulties with stressors in medical school described sources of stress for medical students, varying by year in training:

- First-year stressors
  - Challenges of being uprooted from family and friends
  - Adapting to a demanding new learning environment
  - Human cadaver dissection
  - Substantially increased scholastic workload
  - Concern for academic performance
- Preclinical years
  - Attempting to master a large volume of information
  - Peer groups of equal motivation and intelligence, particularly for those who struggle academically
  - High-stakes examinations, such as the part I examination of the National Board of Medical Examiners
  - Tests that must be passed before academic advancement
- Clinical years
  - Separation from their peer support group
  - Frequent rotations to new work environments at different hospitals requiring a unique medical knowledge base and skill set, which tends to highlight students' deficiencies rather than their progress
  - An unstructured learning environment

- ○ Lack of time for recreation
- ○ Concerns about financial issues
- ○ Long on-duty assignments
- ○ Student abuse
- ○ Exposure to human suffering

Life issues go on while students are in school, and as the age of students entering the professions increases, life issues become more complex, with families and partners to be concerned about during professional school training (eg, illnesses, pregnancies, having to move, marriage, divorce, disconnecting from social networks, and marital and/or parent problems do not automatically disappear while the student finishes his or her education). The anxieties feed into the base level of life stress and can markedly affect students' abilities to learn and focus. Professional students are encouraged to use their student support services to assist in their educational endeavors when encountering stress management concerns. Individual and group counseling support services are available to assist learners with the notable stresses of life and with being a professional student in training. Part of becoming a professional means being able to effectively cope and manage your stress. Taking advantage of available resources is not a sign of weakness; it is a sign of **courage** and **strength** and is critical to you becoming the best health care professional. Not only will you learn coping skills for yourself, but you can also gain insights into patient stress management as you travel your personal and professional development journeys. Do not be afraid to seek support; rather, embrace the learning and growth opportunity and often-needed support during an important time for your ability to be devoted to the necessary learning and capabilities as a health care professional in training. A little help goes a long way with those willing and interested to effect change.

Physical Effects of Stress

Stress takes its toll physically as well. Now that medicine has made great strides in eradicating infectious diseases, most illnesses are of a more chronic nature, and most chronic diseases have been found to be greatly influenced by stress. When we perceive stress, the endocrine system goes into action. This was quite useful when we depended on the sympathetic nervous system for our survival in the jungle. Fight or flight was, at one time, our only alternative in stressful situations, most of which were life threatening. However, it seems as if our nervous system has not kept up with our progress as a civilized society. Few wild animals threaten our survival, but in some situations, we respond as if that were exactly the case.[8] This outpouring of adrenaline and other neuropeptides acts as a stressor on our bodies.[9] Individuals' physical responses differ. Some suffer from headaches, diarrhea, nausea, or cardiac palpitations. Over time, organ systems break down under constant stress, and the result might be diabetes mellitus, high blood pressure, ulcers, colitis, arthritis, or chronic fatigue. Again, maintaining your mental and physical health as a health care professional remains critical to your success. Do not skip your annual physical and dental exams and screens, and seek medical care when needed. Do not be your own worst patient; seek the expertise of those who can provide any required care needed. This way, you shall also serve as a role model for your patient by maintaining your own optimal health status.

Stress Development Model

The key to understanding stress and preventing negative effects lies in understanding a continuum model:

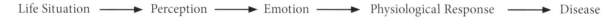

Life Situation ⟶ Perception ⟶ Emotion ⟶ Physiological Response ⟶ Disease

The life situation is **not** the key component in this model; it is the **perception** I have that this life situation is a tiger that is going to eat me unless I get out of here fast or fight like crazy for my survival. Some people live all day, every day as if there were a tiger just around the corner. They have learned a world view that life is a hostile place and one must always be on guard.[8] (Remember that Chapter 2 gives us insights into how people learn this world view.) Others simply periodically find themselves in situations where they realize that their stress is too high, that the world view has been distorted, and that it is time to get a grip on things and time to do what they must to get back in control of their lives.

How Misperceptions Develop

When there is a misperception of the current situation, it is most often a result of the influence of past experience. We become programmed in a sense, based on unfortunate things that have happened to us in the past, and thus we misperceive what is happening right now and fear the unknown of the future. As a result, we allow history or old data to distort the present, and our anxiety mounts. Thought is at the heart of all stress. Our thoughts create our reality in the largest sense. When you think of it, there are 4 kinds of thoughts. Only one kind of thought is truly beneficial to the quality of our lives—**positive** thoughts. Thoughts that are focused on optimism, possibility, connection with others and the world, gratitude, appreciation, and love are thoughts that will develop a feeling of oneness, confidence, and hopefulness. However, too often we are consumed by negative thoughts, wasted thoughts (*If only I had…*), and neutral thoughts (thoughts needed to get through the day). Thoughts lead to feelings, which lead to attitudes, which lead to actions and behavior, which lead to habits, and which lead to destiny.

The key to changing the negative effects of stress is to carefully examine the nature of our thoughts and misperceptions. Negative thoughts and beliefs (thoughts we just keep telling ourselves over and over) leave us feeling exhausted, worried, frustrated, drained, combative, and angry. Positive thoughts leave us feeling hopeful, appreciative, optimistic, and caring. We have an internal mechanism that can help us recognize immediately whether our thoughts are helpful or stressful. If we can interrupt the stress buildup by changing what we think and what we believe about what is happening, then the emotion will be more realistic and the sympathetic nervous system need not be overstimulated.[10] By reaching for the positive thought or even just a more neutral thought, we can interrupt the sympathetic response and choose a more life-nurturing activity. We then can make the best of a situation; we can transform our day from stressful to uplifting, but this takes practice.

Learning to stay in the present is a place to start. As soon as we begin to feel anxious, we should take a deep breath and simply say to ourselves, "Stay in the now. Do not be influenced by the past that is gone forever, or the future that has yet to happen. Listen carefully to what is going on now. Do not personalize or react. Listen."[11] This is not an easy thing to do because our reactions are firmly set in place by years of habitual ways of thinking. To interrupt these ingrained habits takes conscious practice and commitment to change. According to Tolle[11] and Kabat-Zinn,[12] the skill of staying in the now is best learned by purposefully quieting your mind. This can be done by learning meditation techniques, such as transcendental meditation,[9] or by practicing tracking your breath for 10 to 30 minutes every day.

Sit quietly and practice focusing 100% of your concentration on the breath as it flows in and out of your nostrils. Quiet the "monkey chatter" in your brain, let all thoughts float away in imaginary bubbles, and simply breathe. Soon, your body will relax, and your parasympathetic nervous system will help you to slow down and feel more centered and peaceful. Be patient with yourself. When you find yourself thinking thoughts, just say to yourself "Thinking," and then gently return your awareness to your breathing.[12]

BURNOUT

Burnout is a term that has been popularized to indicate a state of emotional and physical exhaustion that results from intense and long-standing professional stress. Maslach[13] first described burnout in 1976. The subjects in her investigation were human service personnel, or people helpers. When we agree to help people, there are always professional demands that seem impossible to meet, and this creates stress and tension that builds over time. This professional stress and tension has been termed burnout, and it is a dynamic process that is fed by a negative self-concept and negative job attitudes, which result in a loss of concern for people, a withdrawal from interaction, and alienation from the work environment.[14]

Signs and Symptoms of Burnout

Health care professionals enter the professions with enthusiasm and optimism and often soon realize that the demands of the work far exceed their expectations. The common response is to double the effort, with little change in productivity.[5] Soon, fatigue and discouragement set in. The stress of the intense emotional demands of health care interaction builds, and a common coping mechanism is to distance oneself or become emotionally detached from work.[14] Detachment is often unconscious and can take the form of actual physical withdrawal, spending shorter time with people, or emotional withdrawal, objectifying people (eg, by labeling them). A patient with back pain becomes "the low back in 343."

Other signs of burnout are the drawing of crisp boundaries between work and home; compartmentalizing one's life sharply; and demonstrating less creativity in treatment, offering more rigid, by-the-book responses to problems, lowering the risk of making a mistake. Feelings of personal inadequacy from not achieving (often unrealistic) goals can result in self-dissatisfaction, which results in projected anger and frustration. People tend to stay away from you because of your short fuse.

At-home burnout can contribute to marital tension. There is a tendency to engage in compulsive behavior (addictions) to numb oneself from stress, so use of food, drugs, sex, and alcohol may increase. Physical signs, such as headaches, stomach ailments, or problems with elimination, begin to appear. Sleep may be disturbed. By this time, one is well on the way to increased absenteeism and begins to job hunt or seriously consider applying to graduate school, often believing that finding the right place to work, or be, will solve all of these problems.

	TABLE 5-1			
	BURNOUT MANIFESTATIONS IN OCCUPATIONAL THERAPISTS			
COMPONENTS	STAGE 1: ENTHUSIASM	STAGE 2: STAGNATION	STAGE 3: FRUSTRATION	STAGE 4: APATHY
Personal characteristics	Do I invest my whole self in my work? Do I set extremely high goals for myself?	Am I beginning to question whether I like my job and whether it meets my personal needs? Am I beginning to see that there are limitations in my work environment?	Am I not only questioning the value of my job but also the value of the entire profession? Do I blame myself when a patient does not improve or return to treatment?	Am I feeling totally disinterested in my job? Do I avoid work by using all of my sick time? Am I disinterested in patient progress?
Modality use	Do I work to increase my repertoire of activities and/or attempt to create new program ideas? Do I verbally discuss with my patients the purpose of an activity and observed progress?	Do I find myself using the same activities over and over again? Do I focus with the patient on only 1 or 2 aspects of their performance?	Is my stress so great that I no longer feel creative? Do I look at product vs process?	Do I always let the patients choose their activity, even when another modality may be more therapeutic? Am I disinterested in my patient's response to the modality selected?
Use of theoretical	Am I interested in learning about new theories and applying them to my practice?	Do I prefer to use the theory base with which I am most comfortable? Do I attempt to use new concepts after discussion with peers and supervisors?	Do I find new theories to be a waste of time and more professional jargon?	Do I find myself using no theoretical base at all?
				(continued)

Table 5-1 illustrates that the symptoms of burnout permeate several areas of our lives and build over time and, as they escalate, they can be seen to fall into 4 stages.[15] Stage 1, enthusiasm, characterizes the symptoms of early burnout. Without appropriate intervention, a person inevitably progresses to stage 4, which carries many of the symptoms of a full-scale depression.[10] Stage 4 burnout is a serious condition, and professional help is very often needed to free oneself from this situation.

Physical Stress Symptom Scale

In most families, people react to stress in similar ways. The data are inconclusive as to whether this is primarily due to genetic weakness or learned behavior, but it is common to see several people in a family respond to stress with similar symptoms. Refer to the Physical Stress Symptom Scale (Table 5-2).[16] Which of your organs or systems are most vulnerable to stress? You may want to compare your results with those of other members of your family.

TABLE 5-1 (CONTINUED)				
BURNOUT MANIFESTATIONS IN OCCUPATIONAL THERAPISTS				
COMPONENTS	STAGE 1: ENTHUSIASM	STAGE 2: STAGNATION	STAGE 3: FRUSTRATION	STAGE 4: APATHY
Interprofessional relationships	Do I attempt to engage other disciplines in the activity process? Do I work to increase communication among team members and to effectively resolve conflicts?	Do I get annoyed when people from other professions ask to observe my groups? Do I feel that my domain is being stepped on by other team members?	Do I feel competitive with team members and avoid talking to them outside required meetings? Do I find myself expressing my anger about the team to the other therapists in my department?	Do I feel there is no need to deal with my team about unresolved issues because nothing helps?
Education	Do I enjoy the opportunity to educate others about what I do as an occupational therapist?	Do I get tired of always having to explain my practice?	Am I beginning to resent the need to always educate others, especially team members?	Do I avoid having to explain what to do?
Budget	Do I find it easy to adapt to a low budget by finding creative ways to use limited supplies?	Am I becoming tired of the constant need to adapt my programs to supply and budget constraints?	Do I find myself frequently complaining to my coworkers and supervisor about our limited budget and supplies?	Have I given in to our low budget by limiting my program to only those supplies that are readily available?
Response to supervision and increased responsibilities	Do I look forward to supervision and the opportunity to improve my job performance?	Do I become anxious when my supervisor suggests a change or that I take on additional responsibilities?	Do I resent changes implemented within the department and frequently discuss my resentment with peers?	Do I avoid work because of what will happen next?
Professional development	Do I actively pursue workshops, seminars, and courses to improve my skills? Do I put a lot of energy into my professional organizations?	Do I find that outside of work I always choose to pursue activities other than continuing education? Am I questioning the value of the profession and its organization?	Do I find suggestions to pursue continuing education to be an imposition? Will I pursue these activities only on work time?	Am I disinterested in professional activities and continuing education?

TABLE 5-2

PHYSICAL STRESS SYMPTOM SCALE

In the space provided, indicate how often each of the following effects happens to you either when you are experiencing stress or following exposures to a significant stressor. Respond to each item with a number between 0 and 5, using the following scale: 0 = never, 1 = once or twice a year, 2 = every few months, 3 = every few weeks, 4 = once or more each week, 5 = daily.

Cardiovascular Symptoms

_____ Heart pounding

_____ Heart racing or beating erratically

_____ Cold, sweaty hands

_____ Headache (throbbing pain)

_____ **Subtotal**

Respiratory Symptoms

_____ Rapid, erratic, or shallow breathing

_____ Shortness of breath

_____ Asthma attack

_____ Difficulty in speaking because of poor breathing control

_____ **Subtotal**

Gastrointestinal Symptoms

_____ Upset stomach, nausea, or vomiting

_____ Constipation

_____ Diarrhea

_____ Sharp abdominal pains

_____ **Subtotal**

Muscular Symptoms

_____ Headaches (steady pain)

_____ Back or shoulder pain

_____ Muscle tremors or hand shaking

_____ Arthritis

_____ **Subtotal**

Skin Symptoms

_____ Acne

_____ Dandruff

_____ Perspiration

_____ Excessive dryness of skin or hair

_____ **Subtotal**

Immunity Symptoms

_____ Allergy flare-up

_____ Catching colds

_____ Catching the flu

_____ Skin rash

_____ **Subtotal**

Metabolic Symptoms

_____ Increased appetite

_____ Increased craving for tobacco or sweets

_____ Thoughts racing or difficulty sleeping

_____ Feelings of crawling anxiety or nervousness

_____ **Subtotal**

_____ **Overall Symptoms Total (add all 7 subtotals)**

Physical Stress Symptom Scale:

0 to 5: No predisposition in that symptom

6 to 13: Slightly higher risk of disease in that symptom

14+: Likely to experience psychosomatic disease in that symptom

Adapted from Allen R. *Progressive Neuromuscular Relaxation.* College Park, MD: Autumn Wind Press; 1979.

Causes of Burnout

Factors that lead to burnout can be grouped into internal and external causes.[14] External causes include conditions in the workplace that make it virtually impossible to experience consistent success, such as the following[14]:

- Work overload
  - Understaffed conditions
  - Overload of too many of one type of patient or one type of activity; not enough variety
  - Inability to use professional skills and creativity due to lack of time
- Role ambiguity
  - Less-than-clear guidelines of boundaries of responsibility
  - Nebulous expectations not communicated clearly
- Role conflict
  - Several health care professionals perceive they are responsible for achieving the same goal; especially apparent in multidisciplinary team situations in which there is inadequate communication
  - Physicians make all decisions with no regard for input from other health care professionals

Internal causes of burnout are more difficult to identify and often are more challenging to influence. They include the following[14]:

- Health care professional's self-esteem. How individuals view themselves personally and professionally has an impact on their work. Low self-esteem facilitates imagined feelings of failure.
- Inability to set clear boundaries between personal and professional needs. Unclear ideas about the motives for wanting to help people (ie, the desire to fix it for people rather than encouraging autonomy) result in inadvertently contributing to patients' neediness and dependence on health care workers, which results in a feeling of becoming too close or trapped in a relationship with a patient.
- The establishment of unrealistically optimistic goals for patients and the failure to meet them, which lowers self-image, a common event for overachieving new graduates. Intervention and guidance is required from mentors or supervisors.

In a study of burnout in practicing physical therapists in rehabilitation hospitals, the Maslach Burnout Inventory scores indicated that 46% of the respondents scored high on the emotional exhaustion subscale, 20% scored high on the depersonalization subscale, and 60% scored low on the personal accomplishments subscale.[17] As a whole, 52% of the 250 therapists responded to the questionnaire, and the respondent sample presented with moderate burnout. Several factors were considered as contributing most, including communication and connectedness, achievement, time constraints, variability in depersonalization, and personal accomplishment. The majority of the physical therapists in this study were in practice for less than 4 years. Continuing to work toward recognition of burnout by health care professionals and how to address to change the burnout syndrome remains crucial. Health care professionals should watch for signs and symptoms of burnout, not only in themselves, but to help coworkers and patients, in recognition of burnout components, with appropriate referrals.

INTERVENTION

Previously, we discussed the importance of perception in handling stress. Cultivating an ability to stay present or stay in the now and resisting the habit of interpreting present, ongoing events from past history or fear of the future will greatly assist one in remaining clear and realistic from moment to moment.[11,12] Asking clarification questions and using active listening skills will reduce the tendency to personalize and take undue responsibility for others' problems. Learning to inventory one's thoughts by checking on how you feel is critical to replacing negative thoughts with more energetic and hopeful thoughts that feel better.

However, the next step in reducing the problem of burnout is recognition that it is occurring, that it is happening right now to you, and choosing to believe that you have the power to stop its escalation. Because burnout has internal and external antecedents, intervention must take place in both areas.[14]

Externally or organizationally, lowering staff-to-patient ratios is critical, as is allowing for time away from contact with patients. Doing less stressful tasks—such as record keeping; reading journal articles; and planning patient research, student education, or quality assurance activities—is an effective way to lower the stress exacerbated by intense interaction with people.[13] Required use of vacation time also helps those who tend to overwork and deny the presence of burnout.[15] Mixing of patient loads and scheduling of regular staff rotations also helps to reduce the stress of seeing too many of any one type of patient.[15] Organizationally sanctioned support groups are also an effective way to help reduce stress.[18] In these sessions, discussion of feelings is more important than discussion of patient problems. Many health care professionals keep fears and feelings of personal failure to themselves, but most will welcome the opportunity to discuss frustrations concerning patients, especially if the organization encourages this opportunity for all its members.[18]

In rehabilitation, we must maintain a constant awareness that strict adherence to the medical model of diagnose-treat-discharge "cured" very often does not apply to our patients. Most patients we see have multiple chronic illnesses, and we must learn how to expect an appropriate amount of effort from them, maintaining a somewhat more realistic goal than a hope for a cure. Patients' values and hopes must be clearly delineated and integrated into any plan of care.[19]

Studying burnout and its prevention while still in school gives you an added advantage before you get caught up in the confusing situations that your first position offers. You may also wish to become familiar with some of the scales and tools to screen for burnout, stress, and work addiction (eg, the Dutch Work Addiction Scale,[20] Holmes-Rahe Life Stress Inventory,[21] and Workplace Stress Survey[22]). Self-monitoring and being able to screen for stress is important professionally, with our patients/clients, for ourselves, and often for colleagues. Internally or personally, health care professionals must develop a realistic view of helping and learn effective ways to handle repeated, intense, emotional interactions with people.[14] Regular exercise is critical in reducing stress. A lunch break that is taken away from the patient care milieu and that includes a brisk walk, bike ride, or swim has immediate and long-term positive benefits. Sufficient sleep and a nutritional diet also serve to keep one's internal stress low.

The logical, systematic left brain is the seat of the anxiety that leads to burnout. It is the left brain that can't seem to figure out how to get the goal met. The right brain, however, is the source of relief from this pressure. The right brain functions by way of pictures, symbols, colors, and dreams. Meditation and activities that balance left and right brain activity and engage the right brain in activities, such as daydreaming or imagery for relaxation, during breaks in the workday also help. Tracking your breath, as described previously, is one such activity.[12]

Above and beyond all is the importance of each health care professional carefully examining his or her own needs in becoming a health care professional to identify and curtail the tendency to overwork that is so common among us.[10] Work is just as addictive as alcohol, food, and drugs. We engage in compulsive behavior to keep from dealing with our problems or from feeling the pain of normal growth and development. When work is used to keep us from growing, everyone suffers. Unfortunately, unlike drugs and alcohol, which do not carry public sanction, workaholics are often praised for their dedication and allow themselves to be taken advantage of by others.

Eventually, workaholics come to the realization that they are receiving from their efforts far less than they are contributing, and this awareness often leads to a temporary decrease in activity. Unless the original pain and need for personal growth are examined and confronted at this time, a new addictive behavior will move in rapidly to fill the void. Chapter 2 focuses on the need to not only confront compulsive behavior, but to locate and communicate with the abandoned child within all of us to begin the healing process before real change can be experienced.

PREVENTION

Because stress occurs from the perception of the inability to successfully achieve goals, one way to prevent this from occurring is to set goals that are predictably attainable. Stewart[18] wrote, "Unless the goals of therapy are agreed upon in the beginning, the therapist and the patient can be forced to work together over a long period of time attempting to achieve goals which are not shared by both." When working with patients, Stewart[18] suggested the following steps to help lower stress:

- Establish a clear contract with the patient. This should contain an explicit description of the goals and responsibilities of both parties, should take into account the patient's values and priorities.

- Do not promise more than you are prepared to deliver to the patient, the family, or the referring practitioner.

- Be aware of the patient's feelings of dependency, loneliness, and fears of abandonment. Deal with feelings with active listening, encouraging open discussion. Give plenty of advance notice before taking time off or separating from patients in any way.

Another skill that is useful in helping to keep control over the work environment is assertiveness training for those who lack the skills needed to communicate ideas for change. Learning how to speak up from a position of personal confidence can help revitalize an entire work setting.[23] Chapter 8 will assist you in developing these skills.

TABLE 5-3
STRESS RELIEF: BALANCING THE 4 QUADRANTS OF CARE

PHYSICAL	**EMOTIONAL**
○ Eat breakfast, eat nutritious food	○ Find and keep a confidant, and talk often
○ Drink plenty of water	○ Join a group
○ Don't smoke, don't do drugs	○ Be a good listener who does not judge
○ Exercise regularly but moderately	○ Cherish a pet of your own
○ Sleep at least 8 hours a night	○ Make use of the counseling center on campus
○ If you drink alcohol, drink moderately	○ Journal
○ Alternate work with rest and play	
INTELLECTUAL	**SPIRITUAL**
○ Read material that adds energy to your life	○ Establish a regular meditation practice
○ Listen to good music	○ Attend religious services
○ Crossword puzzles, chess, bridge	○ Read inspiring literature
○ Design and build, write	○ Get out into nature regularly
○ Learn another language	○ Listen to inspiring music
○ Learn to play a musical instrument	

CONCLUSION

Health care professionals are responsible for clearly understanding patients' problems and, perhaps most important and most stressful, for teaching them how to avoid future problems; we are responsible for helping people take responsibility for themselves and their health. This can be the most demanding of our obligations to those we serve. We must learn to handle situations that fail to respond to our interventions. We must learn to set realistic limits as to what we are willing and able to do to facilitate change. We must learn to face the inevitability of terminal illness and death. Each of these realities in health care, if perceived as failure, will cause stress because the ideal, hoped-for goal of cure and wellness is unattainable. We set ourselves up to experience burnout if curing is our only goal in health care.

When one enters the health professions, there must be an early commitment to taking care of oneself to prevent the negative effects of inevitable stress. We suggest that people can be seen to be composed of 4 quadrants: the physical, the intellectual, the emotional, and the spiritual. To avoid stress, one must keep a healthy balance of activity and growth in all 4 quadrants (Table 5-3). This would include a commitment to eat well, get enough rest and sleep, get regular exercise, take time away from people, seek emotional confirmation and support, and dedicate time to play and fun.

Some of us who become health care professionals who grew up in troubled homes have had to be serious from the very start, and we lack the ability for spontaneous play. If that is true, we must find others to help us. Our healthy survival depends on a true dedication to play and fun. Unfortunately, according to a national study of more than 2000 individuals, findings suggest that people are not receiving what they need from health care professionals to manage stress and address lifestyle changes to improve their health.[24] The American Psychological Association study found that only 17% of Americans are having needed conversations with their health care professionals about stress management.[24] The study clearly demonstrated that Americans are struggling with managing stress and that stress is on the increase. The Millennials (aged 18 to 33 years) were noted as having particular trouble managing stress, with their stress levels exceeding national averages compared with other generations.[24]

The exercises that follow are designed to help you identify the amount of stress you are currently experiencing and how that stress affects you physically. Please also consider completing some of the life stress inventories as a baseline for yourself as a developing health care professional. The final exercise addresses health care professionals' Integrity in Practice[25] and specifically fraud, abuse, and waste, which may arise from health care professional stress and burnout.

REFERENCES

1. Purtilo RB, Haddad A, Doherty R. *Health Professional and Patient Interaction*. 8th ed. St. Louis, MO: Elsevier Health Sciences; 2014.
2. Barr DA. The effects of organizational structure on primary care outcomes under managed care. *Ann Intern Med*. 1995;122(5):353-359.
3. Tu HT. More Americans willing to limit physician-hospital choice for lower medical costs. *Issue Brief Cent Stud Health Syst Change*. 2005;(94):1-5.
4. Casares GS, Bradley KP, Jaffe LE, Lee GP. Impact of the changing environment on fieldwork education: perceptions of occupational therapy educators. *J Allied Health*. 2003;32(4):246-251.
5. Grembowski DE, Patrick DL, Williams B, Diehr P, Martin DP. Managed care and patient-related quality of care from primary physicians. *Med Care Res Rev*. 2005;62(1):31-55.
6. Nalette E. Constrained physical therapist practice: an ethical case analysis of recommending discharge placement from the acute care setting. *Phys Ther*. 2010;90(6):939-952.
7. Dyrbye LN, Thomas MR, Shanafelt TD. Medical student distress: causes, consequences, and proposed solutions. *Mayo Clin Proc*. 2005;80(12):1613-1622.
8. Keyes K. *Handbook to Higher Consciousness*. Coos Bay, OR: Living Love Publications; 1975.
9. Chopra D. *Ageless Body, Timeless Mind: The Quantum Alternative to Growing Old*. New York, NY: Harmony Books; 1993.
10. Lipton BH. *The Biology of Belief*. Carlsbad, CA: Hay House; 2011.
11. Tolle E. *The Power of Now: A Guide to Spiritual Enlightenment*. Novato, CA: New World Library; 2004
12. Kabat-Zinn J. *Coming to Our Senses: Healing Ourselves and the World Through Mindfulness*. New York, NY: Hyperion; 2005.
13. Maslach C. Burned-out. *Human Behav*. 1976;9(5):16-22.
14. Wolfe GA. Burnout of therapists: inevitable or preventable? *Phys Ther*. 1981;61(7):1046-1050.
15. Apter LC, Kolodner EL. Professional burnout—are you a candidate? *Phys Ther Forum*. 1987;6:6-10.
16. Allen R. *Progressive Neuromuscular Relaxation*. College Park, MD: Autumn Wind Press; 1979.
17. Donohoe E, Nawawi A, Wilker L, Schindler T, Jette DU. Factors associated with burnout of physical therapists in Massachusetts Rehabilitation Hospitals. *Phys Ther*. 1993;73(11):750-756.
18. Stewart TD. Psychotherapy and physical therapy common grounds. *Phys Ther*. 1977;57(3):279-283.
19. Pines A, Maslach C. Characteristics of staff burnout in mental health settings. *Hosp Community Psychiatry*. 1978;29(4):233-237.
20. Schaufeli WB, Taris TW. Dutch Work Addiction Scale. http://www.wilmarschaufeli.nl/publications/Schaufeli/Test%20Manuals/Scoring_DUWAS.pdf. Published 2004. Accessed April 30, 2015.
21. Rahe R. Holmes-Rahe Life Stress Inventory: The Social Readjustment Scale. http://www.stress.org/self-assessment/. Accessed April 30, 2015.
22. The American Institute of Stress. Workplace Stress Survey. http://www.stress.org/wp-content/uploads/2011/08/Workplace-Stress-Survey.pdf. Published 1998. Accessed April 30, 2015.
23. Davis CM. The "difficult" elderly patient: stressful effects on the therapist. *Top Geriatr Rehabil*. 1988;3(3):74-84.
24. American Psychological Association. Paying with our health. http://www.apa.org/news/press/releases/stress/index.aspx. Published February 4, 2015. Accessed May 3, 2015.
25. American Physical Therapy Association. Preventing Fraud, Abuse and Waste and the Choosing Wisely Campaign. http://integrity.apta.org/ChoosingWisely/. Accessed May 3, 2015.

EXERCISES

EXERCISE 1: RECOGNIZING PROFESSIONAL STRESS

1. I realize I am stressed when:

    Which makes me feel:

    And I react by:

    Afterwards, thinking about it calmly and quietly, I realize and tell myself next time I may choose to:

2. Signs and symptoms of burnout for me:
    a.

    b.

    c.

    d.

3. Coping mechanisms that I use now within my environment:
    a.

    b.

    c.

    d.

4. Three things I did last week to take care of myself:

  a.

  b.

  c.

EXERCISE 2: MAJOR SOURCES OF STRESS IN STUDENTS

Purtilo[1] mentioned that there are 3 major sources of anxiety for students:

1. Am I good enough? (basically)

2. Do I have what it takes? (physically, emotionally)

3. Can I pay?

First of all, do you agree that these are stressors for you? What would you add to that list? Are there life issues that cause you stress (eg, developing identity and finding a life partner)? Is the task of breaking away from your home and parents a major stress for you? Are you concerned that you may have chosen the wrong profession? Do you have a habit of procrastination that gets you into trouble rather consistently? Make a personal list of stressors and prioritize them. Assign relative stress points to each item.

Now, journal about how those stressors affect you each day physically, emotionally, mentally, and spiritually. For each stressor, list any actions you might be able and willing to take right now to minimize their negative influence and learn to put away anxiety about things you have no control over. Carrying a list of constant worries around in your mind or on your back makes it difficult to be present to the world and to people. Develop the habit of taking regular inventory of what you're worried about, what you can do about it right now, and what you must "offer up" and get off your mind. Make it a goal regularly to flush your mind and your heart of anxieties that are not appropriate or welcome. You will feel lighter if you do.

EXERCISE 3: HOW TO THINK IN A HEALTHIER WAY

Recognizing unhelpful negative thoughts is the first step to stopping them. The best way to change your thinking is to write negative thoughts down and come up with alternatives. The key is to recognize, through negative feelings, that you are thinking negative thoughts and then change those thoughts and reach for the better thought to pull you up on the emotional scale toward positivity.

Track your thoughts:

Situation: Late for class. Lost track of time. Traffic was unforgiving. No place to park.

FEELINGS/BODY RESPONSES	NEGATIVE THOUGHT	ALTERNATIVE THOUGHT
Sick to my stomach, down on myself, anxious that I will be embarrassed in front of the group.	I'm not good enough. I'll never be successful. I can't be trusted.	I'm under a lot of stress. I'm making too much of this one incident.

Now it's your turn. Track your thoughts:

Situation:

FEELINGS/BODY RESPONSES	NEGATIVE THOUGHT	ALTERNATIVE THOUGHT

Journal Reflections

As I reflect on my responses to the above questions, what did I learn about myself?

EXERCISE 4: INTEGRITY IN PRACTICE

Review the resources for the APTA Preventing Fraud, Abuse and Waste and the Choosing Wisely Campaign[25] (http://integrity.apta.org/ChoosingWisely/) and the American Board of Internal Medicine (ABIM), Advancing Medical Professionals to Improve Healthcare website (http://www.choosingwisely.org/). You may also wish to review the various "Choosing Wisely" suggestions provided through several other health professions via the ABIM site.

APTA student members may also complete the online course for Navigating the Regulatory Environment: Ensuring Compliance while Promoting Professional Integrity, through the APTA PT Learning Center (http://learningcenter.apta.org/Courses.aspx).[25]

Course instructors include Dr. Shantanu Agrawal, MD; Dr. Anthony Delitto, PT, PhD, FAPTA; Katherine Karker-Jennings, JD, MS; Ellen R. Strunk, PT, MS, GCS; and Becky Clearwater, PT, MS, DPT. This 2-part module provides expert guidance and strategies to prevent fraud and abuse in practice. Part 1 consists of a moderated audio roundtable covering laws and regulations related to health care fraud and abuse, the government's efforts to find and address fraud and abuse, and a discussion of a mock case scenario. Part 2 provides 5 case vignettes drawn from real-world situations that illustrate some of the types of fraud or abuse involving physical therapist services. Interactive questions and answers guide the learner through each situation. The modules are particularly helpful in distinguishing perceived gray areas in health care practice.

Be prepared to discuss your learning, insights, and feelings based on the campaign and learning modules for promoting professional integrity. Consider how, in each of the cases presented, **stress** may have contributed to the health care professional's lapse in judgment or practice.

The exercises at the end of this chapter are also available online.
Please refer to the sticker in the front of the book and enter the access code provided.

THE NATURE OF EFFECTIVE HELPING

EMPATHY AND SYMPATHY VERSUS PITY

*Carol M. Davis, DPT, EdD, MS, FAPTA and
Gina Maria Musolino, PT, MSEd, EdD*

"It is one of the beautiful compensations in this life that no one can sincerely try to help another without helping himself." –Ralph Waldo Emerson

OBJECTIVES

- To describe the ideal overall aim of helping.
- To explore the behaviors that interfere with effective helping.
- To distinguish among sympathy, pity, identification, self-transposal, and empathy.
- To describe the characteristics of helping communication.
- To reveal the characteristics of effective helpers.

When someone needs help, no matter what the nature of the help needed, we can assume that something's not right and that something is interfering with day-to-day function and growth. Those of us in the healing professions have devoted our lives, for the most part, to helping those who need help in understanding and overcoming illness or disability. However, some of us are more concerned with working with people who are essentially well but need help in becoming more fit or preventing illness or injury. Whatever the problem, health care professionals (HCPs) have devoted their professional lives to helping people overcome whatever is blocking them from living functionally useful and productive lives. Let's start by examining a case scenario:

Ariel, the supervisor in occupational therapy, was also the clinical instructor (field work coordinator/instructor) for Erin, a student in her last clinical before graduating. For the most part, Erin was independent in her patient care, but occasionally she would ask for Ariel's help in solving a clinical problem. At the end of one day, Erin asked Ariel for the answer to a question that Ariel felt Erin should know by now. She was tempted to tell her, "Go look that up! You should know the answer to that by now." But it was late in the day, and both of them were tired. Ariel gave in and told her the answer to her question, but then gave her a dirty look, as if to let her know she was not happy to be asked that question. Erin was confused about why she seemed unhappy.

Davis CM, Musolino GM. *Patient Practitioner Interaction: An Experiential
Manual for Developing the Art of Health Care, Sixth Edition* (pp 91-102).
© 2016 SLACK Incorporated.

What should the overall aim of helping be? When we were small and needed help, we searched out whomever we felt could fix the problem and make us feel better. As children, we lacked the skills to solve our own problems, and so we depended on our mothers and fathers or some other capable adult to take charge. Unlike children, adults require a different sort of helping because when someone constantly tries to "fix it," we often become resentful and angry and feel helpless and dependent. It is an important sign of maturity when we prefer to complete tasks and solve problems ourselves and take pride in our individual accomplishments.

There are times, however, when we feel particularly alone and helpless and we may appreciate that "fixing" kind of attention and help offered by a friend. Remember the comment from a previous chapter that greeting cards emphasize this common human need in phrases like "Before I even knew my own needs, you were there with a loving heart to respond." But this sentiment fails to acknowledge the more enduring need for adults to feel self-sufficient and capable of identifying and solving their own problems.

The overall aim of mature helping is always to make the helpee self-sufficient and to assist the helpee in achieving a more effective relationship between self and others and between self and the world.

We have discovered in previous chapters that our behavior is an expression of our values and our beliefs. Those who believe that they are called to help others, whether they want help or not, can become annoying at the least and obstructive to others' development at the worst. Not all help is helpful. Many of us have laughed at the turmoil that can occur when a well-meaning person tries to open a door for us and actually blocks our way. At the other end of the continuum, however, is the well-meaning friend or parent who takes great care in telling us what to do in a given situation and then abandons us with indifference, refusing to support us until we comply with the advice given: "You asked me. I told you. You did what you wanted. Now I will have nothing to do with you." Not very helpful.

As was pointed out in Chapter 2, helpers who had to develop parenting skills too early bring immature ideas about the nature of effective help into adulthood. A few familiar characteristics of unhelpful helpers include too much concern with matters that are none of their business, a need to be told how helpful—how irreplaceable—they are to the functioning of a group, and a need to have others depend on them as if their very self-worth revolved totally around their ability to fix problems for others. Sadly, often it does.

The important *truth* in this matter is that no person can take responsibility for another person. **We can only take responsibility for ourselves.** Exceptions exist, of course, with children and with people who, for whatever reason, have lost the ability to be adequately in charge of their own lives—those with certain mental illnesses or those with brain dysfunction. But for most of us, the world exists for us the way we see it, the way we think about it. No one outside of us can make us happy or unhappy unless we allow it. Circumstances exist the way they are, but we have a choice as to how we think about them.

Effective helping usually has, as a primary component, a problem identification and problem-solving process. As health care professionals, we learn important knowledge, skills, and values that we offer to assist those needing help, to understand the nature of their problem(s) and to act in ways so that the problem is solved and a return to normal function and quality living is facilitated. **Our goal must always be to help the helpee become self-sufficient once again.** We must provide the conditions for our patients to identify their own goals around their own health problems and provide the knowledge and skill to advise them on the wisdom of their desires and then help them get their needs met. Later in this textbook, we will discuss considerations of where one is in the ability to change (Chapter 15), but for now we shall stay focused on the nature of effective helping.

Patients may come to us with or without a diagnosis; however, contrary to common practice in most medical environments, the diagnosis serves as little more than a place to start in the helping process. The key questions remain: What are the problems from the **patient's or client's** perspective? What are the **patient's** goals in the healing process? Contemporary practice demands evidence-based practice (EBP), which first and foremost includes the patient's values, beliefs, and preferences. If these are not at the forefront, the therapeutic relationship will almost certainly fail. David Sackett, MD, clinical epidemiologist and pioneer in EBP, defined EBP as "the integration of best research evidence with clinical expertise and patient values."[1,2]

Effective helping includes not merely a provision of information and therapeutic procedures, but also helping the patient or client with the discovery of personal meaning. Otherwise, what good does illness or efforts toward optimal wellness serve?

THERAPEUTIC USE OF SELF

Central to this perspective on helping is therapeutic communication and the therapeutic use of one's self. How you view yourself will markedly affect your communication. Remember that the self-concept acts as a screen through which we view the world. Most of us have felt the discomfort of interacting with a person who continually apologizes for him- or herself, distorts what we say out of feelings of insecurity, or responds with negativity and self-contempt. Each of us holds many varied opinions and ideas about ourselves, but our essential self-worth forms the core around which those ideas merge, and negative self-worth is one of the most important factors that needs to be changed to communicate from a healing perspective.

Earlier chapters focused on the development of the ideas about the self and how our feelings of self-worth evolve. This chapter focuses on the nature of effective communication in the helping process.

THERAPEUTIC COMMUNICATION

Certain identifiable elements characterize therapeutic or healing communication. In the patient-practitioner interaction, the health care professional:

- **Speaks**—Communicates not just with an expression of ideas, but with the ability to *translate those ideas* from an inner conviction to an outer clarity. Self-awareness enables the speaker to voice articulately, and with sensitivity to the response of the other person, well-thought-out ideas regarding the role of the patient in the healing process.

- **Is fully present**—Is *totally* focused on the patient or client and his or her ideas about the problem. Does not get lost in memories of patients past or possible future problems. Allows the interaction with the patient to command his or her focused attention.

- **Listens**—Listens with the whole self, with the third ear, to ascertain the patient's meanings and goals. Clarifies interpretations of what is heard. Resists categorizing or projecting personal beliefs and values. Resists giving quick advice, telling the patient what to do (see Chapter 12).

- **Develops trust**—Resists trying to influence the patient; instead, asks questions only to ascertain the truth about the problem as the patient perceives the problem. Communicates that the patient is worth listening to, that he or she has important information to add to the process. Resists assuming a priestly or parental role that conveys that the patient is dumb and that he or she is smart. At the same time, however, conveys the values of expertise and confidentiality and never neglects the opportunity for *informed consent* so that the patient feels that trust has been appropriately placed.

- **Carefully considers**—The *patient's values, beliefs, and preferences* in the development of mutually agreeable therapeutic goals and expectations.[1,2]

Thus, the art of professional helping in the healing professions centers around the therapeutic use of oneself by way of a style of humanistic communication that places the patient in a position of informed, equal, and inevitably responsible for any positive outcomes in the helping process. Health care professionals do the following:

- Listen, clarify, ask, never assume or make quick judgments
- Identify problems with the patient, examine and evaluate
- Hypothesize causes
- Treat through therapeutic measures and education
- Reevaluate
- Readjust to new states and begin again until mutually agreed upon goals are reached

A CLOSER LOOK AT INTERPERSONAL INTERACTION PROCESSES

At the heart of listening with the third ear is the process of *self-transposal*, which is often confused with empathy.[3] *Empathy* (Figure 6-1) is often used interchangeably with several other interaction terms. Each term has a unique meaning, and it is helpful to understand and distinguish among them. The terms most commonly used interchangeably with empathy include *sympathy, pity, identification*, and *self-transposal*. Of these, pity and identification often are not appropriate to the healing process. Let's take a closer look at each of these interactive processes.

When I sympathize (Figure 6-2) with you, I feel similar feelings about something outside of us along with you. I can feel joyful about your success, or I can feel sadness about the bad news that my patient received today. This is sympathy, or "fellow feeling." It is commonly felt in health care, and it is totally appropriate in the healing relationship with patients.[3]

However, pity (see Figure 6-2) is rarely, if ever, appropriate. When I pity my patient, I feel sympathy **with condescension**. "You poor thing" conveys an inappropriate inequality between myself and the other person; I lift myself up to be better than the other, and in that process, I demean the personhood of the other. Granted, pity may draw us to help others, but to help with condescension gives the message to the patient that you are judging him or her to be pitiful.[3]

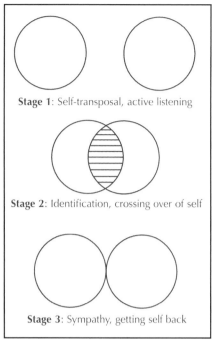

Figure 6-1. Three stages of empathy as described by Stein.

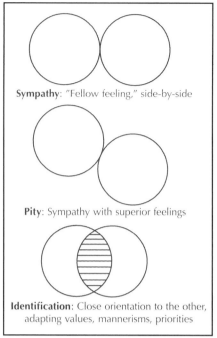

Figure 6-2. Graphic representation of 3 intersubjective processes.

Identification (see Figure 6-2) can interfere with healing communication as well. When I identify with my patient, I begin to feel at one with him or her, and in that process, I often lose sight of the differences between us. For example, just because we both have the same last name or we come from similar backgrounds, I may forget that he or she might have different values than I do. I may assume that my patient feels as I do about wanting to know everything there is to know about a disease or disorder, or I may project that my patient is at his or her best in the morning and schedule to treat him or her before noon. I forget to ask, to clarify. As a result, I confuse my meanings and values with those of my patient; I make assumptions and I project my values onto the patient and act in ways that make the patient less important or less relevant to the healing process. **The source of all conflicts is missed expectations.**

In addition, as I identify with or become one with the patient, I risk losing my own perspective, which weakens my therapeutic objectivity, and I often become subjective in the information I convey. Identification with patients often leads to being overly friendly with patients and an inappropriate sharing of personal information that can interfere with the therapeutic nature of the relationship. *Self-transposal* is a cognitive thinking of myself into the position of the other. It is the process most often confused with *empathy*, putting myself in the other's place or, more commonly, "walking a mile in another person's shoes." In his earlier writings, Carl Rogers[4] referred to this as empathy, but in truth, self-transposal merely sets the stage for empathy to occur. In self-transposal, I listen carefully and try to imagine what it must be like for the patient to be experiencing what he or she is describing.[5]

EMPATHY AS UNIQUE AMONG ALL INTERACTIVE PROCESSES

The process of empathy was first fully described by Edith Stein.[5] In her scholarly work published in the 1930s, Stein characterized empathy as absolutely unique from all other forms of interactions, distinguishable from other intersubjective processes, first by the fact that we never empathize; empathy happens **to** us. It catches us. It is given to us much like true forgiveness; when it finally comes, it seems to be given to us. We can want to forgive and try to forgive, but when the forgiveness finally comes, there is a sense that we have not done a thing except allowed it to happen.

Empathy takes place in 3 overlapping stages (see Figure 6-1). The first stage is the cognitive attending to the other, or self-transposal, as described previously. We listen carefully in an attempt to put ourselves in the place of the other. The second stage, following just a millisecond after, is by far the most significant; the crossing over stage, wherein we feel ourselves crossing over for a moment into the frame of reference or the lived world of the other person. We feel so at one with the other that we forget momentarily that we are 2 separate beings. This is the identification stage of empathy. The third stage resolves the temporary confusion as we come back into our own skin and feel a special alignment with the other after having experienced the crossing over.[5] The third stage resembles sympathy, or fellow feeling. Thus, empathy can be described as a momentary merging with another person in a unique moment of shared meaning.

When empathy occurs, health care professionals need not lose their therapeutic objectivity, as so many fear, in getting too close to their patients. Instead, what is experienced is a kind of holistic listening that can unite the therapist with the patient yet allows the patient and therapist to remain fully separate in the healing process. It is in identification alone that we lose our objectivity and become destructively fused with the patient, as described earlier. Thus, empathy is the intersubjective process that, among other things, empowers us to listen with the third ear, to communicate in a humanistic and therapeutic manner with patients, thus contributing to helpful helping.

SETTING APPROPRIATE BOUNDARIES WITH PATIENTS/CLIENTS

The challenge, then, is for health care professionals to be in therapeutic relationships with patients yet maintain the helper-helpee relationship. It is imperative that this relationship remain functional, always serving the purpose of healing. How does the clinician reveal just enough about him- or herself to maintain the trust and collegiality without allowing the relationship to change into a more involved friendship or intimate relationship? Revealing too much might confuse the patient by seeming to convey that you are willing to give more than is appropriate for the helping process. Powell[6] described 5 levels of communication that one can use as guidelines for communicating effectively without revealing too much about oneself. These levels lie on a continuum from near indifference to extreme intimacy.

- **Level 5: Clichéd conversation.** No genuine human sharing takes place. "How are you?" "It's nice to see you." Protects people from each other and prevents the likelihood of meaningful communication.

- **Level 4: Reporting facts.** Almost nothing personal is revealed. Some sharing takes place about information such as diagnostic data or the weather.

- **Level 3: Personal ideas and judgments.** Some information about oneself is shared, often in response to the patient's conversation. Topics talked about often relate to the patient's illness or the process the patient is going through, and if the patient looks bored or confused, conversation reverts back to level 4.

- **Level 2: Feelings and emotions.** A deep trust is required to share at this level, and if a person fears judgment, it will be impossible to relate at this level. True friendship and caring require this level of communication. Each person wants to be deeply known and accepted just as he or she is.

- **Level 1: Peak communication.** Mutual complete openness, honesty, respect, and love are required to communicate at this level. An all-encompassing intimacy is shared, often involving relating sexually. The minority of human interactions take place at this level.

In therapeutic communication with patients, it is important for health care professionals to have clear ideas about appropriate boundaries that will facilitate healing. Once crossed over, interaction beyond this boundary will confuse patients, and health care professionals will appear to be offering more of themselves to the relationship than is facilitative to the helper-helpee relationship. In most instances, interaction will take place at levels 5, 4, and 3, with an occasional interchange at level 2, but **never** at level 1.

New health care professionals often confuse the appropriate boundaries and find themselves caring too much, spending more time with one patient than is wise, or telling inappropriate stories or jokes in an attempt to make the patient feel at ease. The reverse often occurs when the patient feels compelled to help put the health care professional at ease. Patients don't need this added anxiety; they need to relax and trust that the health care professional has his or her best interests at heart and can manage the healing interaction free of awkwardness or threats to confidentiality and trust.

BELIEFS OF EFFECTIVE HELPERS

Combs and Gonzales[7] conducted research on the characteristics of effective helpers and concluded the following:

> *Good helpers are not born, nor are they made in the sense of being taught. … Becoming a helper is a time-consuming process. It is not simply a matter of learning methods or of acquiring gadgets and gimmicks. It is a deeply personal process of exploration and discovery, the growth of unique individuals learning over a period of time how to use themselves effectively for helping other people.*

Helpers were evaluated for their effectiveness, and the most effective responded to specific questions about their beliefs in 6 major categories. The summary of the beliefs of effective helpers are summarized in Table 6-1.[7]

TABLE 6-1

SUMMARY OF THE BELIEFS OF "EFFECTIVE" HELPERS

Combs describes commonly held beliefs and perceptions of effective helpers in 6 categories.

1. Subject or Discipline

One is committed to knowing one's discipline well, but mere knowledge is not enough. Knowledge about one's discipline is so personally integrated and meaningful as to have the quality of belief. Effective helpers are committed to discovering the personal meaning of knowledge and converting it to belief.

2. Helper's Frame of Reference

Effective helpers tend to favor an internal frame of reference emphasizing the importance of people's attitudes, feelings, and values that are uniquely human over an external frame of reference that emphasizes facts, things, organization, money, etc.

3. Beliefs About People

Effective helpers believe that people are essentially:

- Able to understand and deal with their own problems given sufficient time and information.
- Basically friendly and well-intentioned.
- Worthy and have great value; they possess dignity and integrity that must be maintained.
- Essentially internally motivated, maturing from within and striving to grow and help themselves.
- A source of satisfaction in professional work rather than a source of suspicion and frustration.

4. Helper's Self-Concept

Effective helpers must have a clear sense of self and their own personal boundaries before they enter into relationships with others. They feel basically fulfilled and adequate, so self-discipline is well practiced. Therapeutic presence for the other is made possible by a strong sense of self, of personal fulfillment, and of personal adequacy.

5. Helper's Purposes

Effective helpers believe that their purpose is to facilitate and assist rather than control people. They favor responding to the larger issues, the broader perspective, rather than the minute details in life. They tend to be willing to be themselves, to be self-revealing. Their purpose includes honesty, acknowledging personal inadequacies, and need for growth. Another purpose is to be involved and committed to the helping process. They are process oriented and committed to working out solutions rather than working toward preconceived goals or notions. They see themselves as altruistic, oriented toward assisting people rather than simply responding to selfish needs.

6. Beliefs About Appropriate Methods or Approaches to the Task

Effective helpers are more oriented toward people than toward rules and regulations or things. They are more concerned with people's perceptions than with the objective framework within which they practice. In helping people, the most effective approach is to discover how the world seems to that person. Self-concept is at the heart of the way one views the world, and so working with self-concept is imperative. Helpers have to be committed to gaining the trust of helpees so that self-control can be relearned in a positive way. The helping relationship makes this growth possible.

Adapted from Combs AW. *Florida Studies in the Helping Professions.* Gainesville, FL: University of Florida Press; 1969.

These beliefs are all developed in a growth process that is very much influenced by the way the lenses are set that we talked about in earlier chapters. The key to becoming an effective helper is to allow oneself to grow, mature, become more aware of feelings and thoughts, be able to identify those beliefs that lead to behaviors that facilitate healing, and grow beyond defensive behaviors that result in negativity and fragmentation.

Corey and Corey[8] outlined the picture of a helper who is making a significant difference, as follows:

- Is aware of personal strengths and weaknesses. Recognizes that "who you are as a person is the most important instrument you possess."
- Has a basic curiosity and openness to new learning.
- Possesses the interpersonal skills needed to establish good contact with others.
- Genuinely cares for people.
- Is willing and able to see the world through the eyes of the "helpee."
- Is able to challenge clients to dream. Is aware that you "cannot inspire clients to do in their lives what you are unwilling to do in your own."
- Is willing to use multiple resources to assist.
- Is willing to adapt approach and techniques to the client's situation.
- Respects differences in the client and does not expect him or her to fit into a preconceived mold.
- Takes care of self physically, mentally, emotionally, and spiritually.
- Deals with personal problems.
- Is willing to examine and challenge personal beliefs and values.
- Recognizes that your philosophy of life has been personally developed and not imposed on you.
- Is able to and has established meaningful relationships with at least a few others.
- Has a healthy sense of self-love and pride but is not self-absorbed.

THE PURPOSE OF HELPING

Health care professionals will act according to what they believe their purpose is in the therapeutic relationship. The purposes of mature health care professionals are to listen carefully with the third ear; to evaluate; to assist; to support; to help problem solve alternatives that lead to healing; to apply therapeutic measures, aimed at alleviating pain and dysfunction; to teach; to help others discover how to maneuver successfully in the world; and to solve their own problems that interfere with the highest and deepest functioning possible.

Carl Rogers[4] suggested 7 key questions that lead to a form of self-examination that will help us evaluate the quality of one's helping:

1. **Can I behave in some way that will be perceived by the other person as trustworthy, dependable, or consistent in some deep sense?** Here, congruence is the key factor. Whatever feeling or attitude is being experienced must be matched by an awareness of that attitude, and actions must match feelings.

2. **Can I be expressive enough as a person that what I am will be communicated unambiguously?** The difficulty here is to be fully aware of who one truly is. Rogers[4] said this: "… if I can form a helping relationship to myself—if I can be sensitively aware of and acceptant toward my own feelings—then the likelihood is great that I can form a helping relationship toward another."

3. **Can I let myself experience positive attitudes toward this other person—attitudes of warmth, caring, liking, interest, respect?** This often engenders the fear that if we allow ourselves to openly express these feelings, the helpee might misinterpret our intentions, and the therapeutic distance might be blurred. The key here is to remain in our professional identities and still relate in a caring way to the other person.

4. **Can I be strong enough as a person to be separate from the other?** This question speaks to avoiding identification. I must be ever aware of my own feelings and express them as mine, totally separate from the feelings I may perceive that the helpee is experiencing. Likewise, I must be strong in my otherness to avoid becoming depressed when my patient is depressed, fearful in the face of my patient's fear, or destroyed by his or her anger.

5. **Can I let myself enter fully into the world of my patient's feelings and personal meanings and see these as he or she does?** The key effort here is to avoid judging the patient's perspectives but instead allow empathy to occur. In this way, once the world of the other is more fully experienced, the help that is offered can be based on this holistic level of knowing made possible by empathy. Meanings can be confronted with acceptance and modified to work toward healing. Judgment and criticism of meanings place a barrier between the helper and the helpee.

6. **Can I act with sufficient sensitivity in the relationship that my behavior will not be perceived as a threat?** A patient who feels free of external fear or threat feels free to examine behavior and change it. Patient care can be threatening in and of itself. Whatever we can do to lower anxiety will assist the effectiveness of our helping.

7. **Can I meet this other individual as a person who is in the process of becoming, or will I be bound by his or her past and by my past?** Buber and Rogers used the phrase "confirming the other"; this means accepting the whole potentiality of the other, the person he or she was created to become.[9] People will act the way we relate to them. The Pygmalion effect was described following the famous Broadway play in which a poor working girl showed that she could behave like a princess when she was treated like one and was taught carefully.

The more fully one comprehends the importance of the nature of the helping interaction, the more one will become committed to the growth required for consistent therapeutic use of self. Yes, our professional knowledge and skill are critical to our effectiveness, but without the ability to interact in healing ways, we sabotage most efforts.

No one is able to achieve all these characteristics as a new graduate health care professional. Many of these behaviors and attitudes develop over time with years of experience and a history of working with all kinds of people in all situations. The queries and lists are offered to you as a way of giving you a benchmark of sorts to aspire to and a personal self-evaluation tool as you grow along your way to becoming an effective helper. Revisiting this experiential manual throughout your professional growth and development as a health care professional, striving for best practice in patient-practitioner interaction, shall serve you well as you continue your journey and are influenced by mentors and your patients and clients. As you gain your own first-hand experiences in your new and changed role as a health care professional, you shall have an opportunity for new and refreshed learning, revisiting the chapters and exercises with the new lens of experience. Chapter 9 will further guide your skills and abilities in self-assessment.

AWARENESS THROUGH ACTION

The exercises that follow are aimed at helping you discover your currently held ideas about the nature of helping and why you are interested in becoming a health care professional. Your beliefs about your self are explored, and you are given the opportunity to practice one of the major factors of effective helping: **active listening**. You will be surprised how difficult it is to really hear what someone else is saying.

REFERENCES

1. Sackett DL. Introduction to evidence-based medicine. In: Sackett DL, Strauss SE, Richardson WS, Rosenberg W, Haynes RB, eds. *Evidence-Based Medicine: How to Practice and Teach EBM.* 2nd ed. Edinburgh, Scotland: Churchill Livingstone; 2000:1-20.
2. Law ME, MacDermid J. *Evidence-Based Rehabilitation: A Guide to Practice.* 3rd ed. Thorofare, NJ: SLACK Incorporated; 2014.
3. Davis CM. *A Phenomenological Description of Empathy as It Occurs Within Physical Therapists for Their Patients* [dissertation]. Boston, MA: Boston University; 1982.
4. Rogers C. The characteristics of a helping relationship. In: Rogers C, ed. *On Becoming a Person.* Boston, MA: Houghton Mifflin; 1961:39-58.
5. Stein E. *On the Problem of Empathy.* 2nd ed. The Hague, The Netherlands: Martinus Nijhoff; 1970.
6. Powell J. *Why Am I Afraid to Tell You Who I Am?* Niles, IL: Argus Communications; 1969.
7. Combs AW, Gonzalez DM. *Helping Relationships: Basic Concepts for the Health Professions.* 4th ed. Boston, MA: Allyn & Bacon; 1993.
8. Corey MS, Corey G. *Becoming a Helper.* 7th ed. Independence, KY: Cengage Learning; 2015.
9. Anderson R, Cissna KN. *The Martin Buber–Carl Rogers Dialogue: A New Transcript With Commentary.* Albany, NY: SUNY Press; 1997.
10. Covey SR. *The 7 Habits of Highly Effective People: Powerful Lessons in Personal Change.* New York, NY: Simon & Schuster; 2013.

EXERCISES

EXERCISE 1: SELF-AWARENESS: WHY DO I WANT TO HELP?

Respond to the following questions. Discuss with 2 or 3 others and then with the entire class. Note the variety of reasons why people are drawn to the helping professions and note the responses most of you share in common.

1. Why do I want to be a health care professional?

2. Whom do I most want to help?

3. What specific rewards do I get from helping people?

4. How do I want to be perceived by those I intend to help?

5. Do I believe people are essentially lazy and will want to have me do all the work for them, or do I believe people most of the time want to help themselves? Is there a category of patients/clients who I believe are mostly lazy? How did I decide this?

6. I feel most anxious when I'm helping—when?

7. Those who require the most help from others are—who?

8. Answering these questions made me feel—what?

Journal Reflections

As I reflect on my response to the above questions, what did I learn about myself? Who am I becoming?

EXERCISE 2: BELIEFS ABOUT SELF

Complete the following self-awareness continuum. Place a mark on the line that reflects your current belief about yourself. Be as honest as possible, rather than responding as you think you should respond.

What I Believe About Myself Today

1. Personal Strengths and Weaknesses

●━━━━━━━━━━━━━━━━━━━━━━━━━━━━━━━━━━━━━━━●

I feel unsure about what I am good at. Often not aware of weakness until someone else points it out.

I know myself rather well. Am clear about strengths and weaknesses. Recognize that who I am as a person is the most important instrument that I possess.

2. Basic Curiosity and Openness to New Learning

●━━━━━━━━━━━━━━━━━━━━━━━━━━━━━━━━━━━━━━━●

Most of what I am learning is not that interesting. Seems like old stuff that is just rehashed.

My learning at this stage is new and I recognize it as important to my patient care skills. I am open to most of it.

3. Seeing Through the Eyes of the Helpee

●━━━━━━━━━━━━━━━━━━━━━━━━━━━━━━━━━━━━━━━●

I have difficulty taking the view of the other. I just cannot seem to understand the point of view of the other person most of the time.

I am willing and able to put myself in the place of the other person that I am helping, even if their opinion is very different from mine.

4. Able to Challenge Clients to Dream

●━━━━━━━━━━━━━━━━━━━━━━━━━━━━━━━━━━━━━━━●

It is important for me to have the right answer, and I want to encourage my patients to do as I ask them to, without adding their own ideas.

I want to inspire my patients to be able to do what they dream they can do in their lives, and I try to also live up to my dreams.

5. Areas of Need and Function

———————————————————————————————————————

I take pretty good care of myself physically and intellectually, but my feelings and my spiritual needs don't get much attention.

I deal with my personal problems right away. I take care of the needs in all areas—physical, mental, emotional, and spiritual.

6. Adaptability

———————————————————————————————————————

I have studied long and hard to be able to be an effective helper. I expect my patients to be willing to follow my instructions the way I have decided is best for them.

I recognize that each patient or client brings his or her unique situation to me for my help and I am willing to adapt my approach and techniques to the client's situation.

7. Personal Beliefs and Values

———————————————————————————————————————

My personal beliefs and values have been thought about and refined over time and are a composite of the best that my family and religious beliefs can offer.

My philosophy of life and beliefs and values have been personally developed and are my own, not imposed on me by anyone else, and I am willing to examine and challenge them.

8. Relationships With Others

———————————————————————————————————————

I look forward to being able to find friends and colleagues with whom I can establish healthy relationships. So far most of my friendships have been pretty superficial.

I am blessed with good friends, and I take pride in the fact that I have established some very meaningful relationships with a few colleagues, friends, and family.

9. Has a Healthy Sense of Self-Love and Pride, but Is Not Self-Absorbed

———————————————————————————————————————

I am very proud of my accomplishments, which I have to say I pretty much have done on my own. I know I am good, and I have to look out for myself. No one else can really be counted on.

I am very proud of my accomplishments. I try to live a life that I can be proud of and I like myself, but I recognize that I have achieved what I have with the help of others, and I am very grateful.

(Adapted from Corey MS, Corey G. *Becoming a Helper.* Belmont, CA: Thompson Brooks/Cole; 2007.)

EXERCISE 3: EFFECTIVE LISTENING

According to Rogers,[4] good listening involves the following:

- Not only hearing the words of the speaker but hearing the feelings behind the words as well.

- Putting oneself in the place of the other, or self-transposal; feeling the other's feelings and seeing the world through the speaker's eyes.

- Suspending one's own value judgments in order to understand the speaker's thoughts and feelings as he or she experiences them.

Really listening is difficult and takes practice, especially if you disagree with what is being said. Most normal conversations involve talking at one another, rather than with one another. Covey[10] also noted that "most people do no listen with the intent to understand; they listen with the intent to reply." Hence, we are working on really listening to what is being said and not focusing on our reply.

Divide into groups of 3. One person serves as monitor, the other 2 as discussants. The monitor helps the discussants find a topic of mutual interest, but one on which they fundamentally disagree. For example, one person believes that people should have the right to assisted suicide and the other believes that life is sacred and only God can determine when it begins and ends.

The first discussant states his or her position. In the typical discussion, we are so concerned with what we are going to say next, or so involved with planning our response, that we often tune out or miss the full meaning of what is being said.

In this exercise, before any discussant offers a point of view, he or she must **first summarize the essence of the previous speaker's statement so that the previous speaker honestly feels that his or her statement has been understood**. It is the monitor's role to see that this process takes place with each exchange.

Discussion takes place for 10 minutes, with the monitor assuming the responsibility of ensuring that the procedure described above is followed. At the end of 10 minutes, discussants give each other feedback about how well they felt they had been heard, understood, and responded to during the time frame allotted.

The process is repeated with the monitor assuming the role of discussant and one of the discussants becoming the monitor. One more note: The role of the monitor is critical to the success of this exercise. The monitor must insist that each person summarize the other's statement before speaking. This is difficult to do but essential to the success of the exercise. Be insistent, and be brave!

The exercises at the end of this chapter are also available online.
Please refer to the sticker in the front of the book and enter the access code provided.

7

EFFECTIVE COMMUNICATION

PROBLEM IDENTIFICATION AND HELPFUL RESPONSES

Carol M. Davis, DPT, EdD, MS, FAPTA and
Gina Maria Musolino, PT, MSEd, EdD

"Tell me and I'll forget. Show me and I may remember. Involve me and I may learn." –Benjamin Franklin

OBJECTIVES

- To teach communication strategies for interactions that are confused and/or emotion laden.
- To define congruence and give the opportunity to examine one's own congruence or lack of congruence.
- To emphasize the importance of thoughts and feelings in communication.
- To point out the risks and rewards of communicating clearly in the presence of intense feelings.

Very often, the bulk of our communication throughout the day is quite superficial. Rarely do we communicate with the express purpose of trying to understand in order to be helpful. Even when we make a greater-than-usual attempt to listen carefully because we care and are concerned, it is rare that our interaction might be said to be truly helpful. **Therapeutic communication requires learning a new skill, but more than that, it requires unlearning habitual, nonhelpful ways of interacting.**

This chapter initiates the skill development components of this text. It is devoted to teaching you a new way of communicating with the express purpose of developing your abilities to use communication as an integral aspect of your therapeutic presence with patients. The remaining chapters are problem oriented and will help you apply skills with particularly difficult situations. Let's begin with a case example.

Jonathan was enjoying the seventh month of his first position as a physical therapist in a rehabilitation center. Each day, he was experiencing more confidence in his skills in evaluation and treatment, especially using therapeutic exercise for patients with spinal cord and brain injury. One of his favorite patients was a 14-year-old high school cheerleader, who had been referred to him 2 months ago while still in a coma in the intensive care unit. Diane had gone through the front windshield of her mother's car, a consequence of not having her seatbelt fastened. Her mother escaped injury but was feeling tremendous guilt. She and Diane had been arguing at the time, and she mistakenly ran a stoplight that resulted in the accident.

(continued)

Davis CM, Musolino GM. *Patient Practitioner Interaction: An Experiential Manual for Developing the Art of Health Care, Sixth Edition* (pp 103-116).
© 2016 SLACK Incorporated.

Just last week, Diane began to respond to light and sound, and yesterday, she opened her eyes and looked at Jonathan for the first time after he had transferred her to a chair at the bedside. He was feeling elated and was very hopeful that soon she would be responding to verbal commands.

Diane's mother, Mrs. Graham, visited every day and often was present while Jonathan treated Diane. Today, Mrs. Graham seemed particularly discouraged. Although Diane was showing obvious signs of recovery from her coma, she was still unable to move. When Jonathan came to treat Diane, Mrs. Graham left the room but returned as he finished and told him she wanted to speak to him. As they walked out into the hallway, Mrs. Graham turned to Jonathan and shouted, "You're not helping her! No one is helping her recover. I asked around and found out you're a new therapist and you can't know what you're doing or my daughter would have been well long before this! I want you to stop seeing her. I want a therapist with experience to treat my daughter. I never want you to set foot in her room again!"

This is an example of an emotion-laden interaction, similar to many that take place daily in hospitals and health care facilities. If you were Jonathan, how would you have responded? What would you have felt? Would you have quickly defended yourself? Would you have argued that Diane was showing remarkable signs of improvement? Would you have shouted, "Nobody speaks to me like that!"?

When people are ill and injured, emotions run high on the part of the ill, their families, and those caring for them. Illness and injury stir up feelings of vulnerability and fear. People generally feel out of control and must give over control of their lives to strangers, often in institutions that seem like strange, impersonal, frightening cultures all their own.

At the root of every emotion-laden interaction is a problem. **What, exactly, is the problem in this situation, and whose problem is it?** Mrs. Graham would say that the problem is that her daughter is being treated by an inexperienced physical therapist and is not recovering because of this fact. Therefore, Jonathan and his inexperience are the problem. Jonathan might say that the problem is that Mrs. Graham is feeling helpless and responsible for her daughter's pain and injury and lashed out at him in her frustration. Another analysis might offer that the problem is that Diane did not have her seatbelt on and, if she had, she would not be in a coma. **Again, oftentimes the source of all conflict is a missed expectation. Effective communication provides the opportunity for clarity of expectations.**

THE IMPORTANCE OF IDENTIFYING THE PROBLEM UNDER THE EMOTION

Now we are going to focus on identifying problems and clarifying problem ownership in interchanges that are characterized by intense emotions. In the midst of an interchange like the one between Jonathan and Mrs. Graham, it is often difficult to sort out what is happening and what might be appropriate responses that would help resolve the situation. Our reflex response is to defend ourselves from attack, which tends to just heighten the emotion and further obscure the problem. As a health care professional (HCP), one of the new attitudes that will be helpful to learn is that it is often not the most important thing to be right in a situation. Solving the problem, separate from assigning blame or assigning who is right and wrong, becomes critically important. Different skills are required depending on the nature of the problem and who "owns" the problem.

Hence, the theme for helpful responses in effective communication is the following: **Communicating in ways that help to solve problems, while at the same time respecting and honoring human beings, will facilitate the healing process.** Because we work with people who are ill and disabled, it is not enough to make the correct diagnosis and give the most appropriate treatment. Something more is expected of us. That something more includes helping the patient understand his or her illness or disability to the extent that he or she can make choices with regard to treatment and modifying lifestyle, to prevent further problems, and to live successfully with the problems that are not going to be resolved.

LEARNING NEW COMMUNICATION SKILLS

Each of us enters the helping professions having communicated all of our lives. Little patient care experience is needed to quickly learn that the communication skills that served us quite adequately in our private lives often fall short of helping us to relate adequately to patients, families, caregivers, and colleagues in day-to-day patient care. As Dr. Eric Cassell[1] wrote in his book, *Talking With Patients*, without effective communication, we are unable to acquire objective and subjective information in order to make decisions that are in the best interests of the patient, and, more important, we are unable to use the relationship between practitioner and patient for therapeutic ends. This chapter focuses on sorting out emotion-laden communication to help patients identify and solve their own problems. Chapter 8 extends this theme in teaching you the skills of assertiveness, and Chapter 13 instructs you in carrying out a helping interview.

EMOTION-LADEN INTERCHANGES

Communication connects us to the world. Humans are essentially social and need to feel a connection to others. Getting our basic needs met more often than not requires some form of communication.

Barriers to the effectiveness of communication might include the use of a foreign language (or the use of jargon), carelessness in choosing the words that convey exact meaning, and/or an inability or unwillingness to listen to each other carefully (hearing deficit, distraction by environmental noise, unwillingness to concentrate, multitasking, defensiveness). Many of us are rather unaware of how effective we are in day-to-day communication. It is difficult to come outside of ourselves and watch ourselves interact with others, reflecting on our feelings and the way in which we react to others. Others of us have been given direct feedback about our communication. Statements such as, "I love the way you listen so intently to what I say and wait until I'm finished before you respond" vs "I wish you'd hear me out instead of mentally practicing a quick comeback!" give us clear information about how we are doing as we communicate in that moment.

DIFFICULTIES INTRODUCED WITH
TEXTING, SOCIAL MEDIA, AND DIGITAL TECHNOLOGIES

The fundamentals of communication consist of a sender, a message, a receiver, and an environment. In an emotion-laden interchange, the message is obscured by the fact that someone is upset and unable to identify clearly what the heart of the problem is and how to best go about solving the problem. Communication is difficult enough when the conversation is face-to-face or by phone. The introduction of email, texting, and other means of communication through social media platforms and digital technologies presents an entirely new set of considerations and problems.[2]

It was 8:00 AM. Justin was waiting for his patient to arrive and decided to check his emails on his phone in the staff room. At 8:05 AM, his patient arrived, and the receptionist announced this to him, but it was 8:15 AM before he came out to greet his patient, who was quite upset for having to wait for 10 minutes and told him so in front of his clinical instructor.

Jason bit his tongue and apologized. Later, when he opened his emails at home, he found a note from his clinical instructor telling him that he needed to be more prompt in greeting his patients. Jason was furious. He fired off a response to his clinical instructor indicating that he was waiting for his patient to arrive at 8:00 AM, and when he was not yet there by 8:05 AM, he went back to the staff room for just a minute or so to check his emails.

Furthermore, Jason wrote, he resented his clinical instructor calling him on this and not giving him the benefit of the doubt when she herself checked her emails several times each day. He took this opportunity to also write that he resented her picking on him and felt that because he was not a student from the school from which she had graduated, he could do nothing right.

Suffice it to say that had that exchange occurred in person, rather than by email, it would have been different. Up to 75% of communication is conveyed nonverbally, and when you take away all the nonverbals (see Chapter 11) and have only the written word, there is a lot of room for miscommunication. Likewise, "speaking" (ie, texting) on a device allows one to not have to pay attention to how one's words are being received, and meanings can be misunderstood, blown out of proportion, or taken out of context.

What is most important is that you realize that the luxury of simply spontaneously reacting to others, which you experienced as a private citizen before you made a commitment to becoming a health care professional, must now be replaced by a commitment to use emotion-laden communication (even when you feel personally attacked) as an opportunity to practice your therapeutic effectiveness. Furthermore, as you become a health care professional and think about your future career, you shall want to rethink your social media activities and digital presentation. We shall discuss this more in Chapter 11.

Less-Than-Helpful Responses

The most unhelpful response is indifference. To fail to listen is indicative of an inability, or unwillingness, to be therapeutically present to the one in need of help. Next would be anger or defensiveness, which can soon escalate emotion to rage, which further buries the original problem (see Figures 8-3 and 8-4). Other less-than-helpful techniques include the following[3]:

- **Offering reassurances.** Statements such as "Oh, it can't be all that bad" or "If you think you have it bad, you should just look around you" do little but signal an unwillingness to listen to patients' perceptions of their problems. At the heart of this reply is a practitioner who is not aware of his or her own feelings about the topic or who pretends to offer more time and attention than there is to give and is trying to get away as rapidly as possible.

- **Offering judgmental responses.** Judgmental responses include those that convey approval or disapproval, verbally or nonverbally, at an inappropriate moment; those that convey advice at a time when it is more important for the patient to make his or her own decision; and those that are stereotypical: "Adults should know better than to act like children."

- **Defensiveness.** When we feel threat to the ego, we respond defensively. Defensiveness indicates a personalization and a refusal to listen carefully to what the patient is saying. A response such as "You're always late. I've got better things to do than wait for you, you know" may be true but does little to solve the patient's tardiness problem.

Values That Underlie Therapeutic Responses

Nonhelpful responses are often impulsive and reactive and do not reflect value-based behavior. The values that underlie therapeutic responses were described in Chapter 3. Attitudes such as caring, warmth, respect, compassion, and empathy will help interrupt an immature, impulsive response to an emotion-laden communication.

Acceptance of the other person as doing the best that he or she can in the moment and acceptance of the responsibility to be therapeutic in the midst of a chaotic situation are signs of a mature health care professional. These responses emanate from the essential self, not the ego or persona. Remember, the goal of rehabilitation is to help the patient regain control over his or her life such that independent function at the highest and deepest levels is restored. The role of the practitioner in emotion-laden communication is to ascertain **what the problem is, as well as whose problem it is.**

Identifying Problem Ownership

Learning to send clear messages and receive accurate messages in intense situations requires identifying who owns the problem.[4] Different skills are required for each. For the sake of learning this skill, the rule that applies in every case is that **the person exhibiting the intense emotion is the owner of the problem, even if he or she is trying desperately to inform you that the problem is really yours.**

For example, if the patient is upset with you for being late and shouts at you as you enter the clinic, "You're late!" you don't have a problem. You just walked into the clinic. The patient who is upset has a problem, even though he or she might be trying to convince you that you are his or her problem.

In this new process that you are learning—identifying problem ownership—the person with the emotion owns the problem. The first step to resolving the issue is to realize the different skills required depending on who owns the problem. Figure 7-1 illustrates the 2 sets of skills required: active listening and "I" statements.

Emotion-laden exchanges are cluttered with intense feelings, derogatory remarks, apologies, illustrations, etc. To sort out the problem, special listening skills are needed to defuse the emotion and get at the problem. Critical to this method is resistance to the desire for the unhelpful response of wanting to fix it right away to get rid of the anger or conflict. The alternative is to listen by resisting the quick advice or the defensive reply.

Active Listening—When the Other Has the Problem

Active listening is a form of therapeutic listening that helps the agitated person with the problem clearly hear what he or she is trying to say. It involves **paraphrasing the speaker's words rather than reacting to them to clarify if you have caught the intended meaning.** You must suspend your thoughts and attend exclusively to the words of the other person.

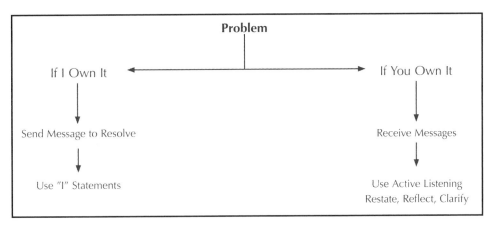

Figure 7-1. Identifying problem ownership.

Paraphrasing is not easy and requires development as a new skill. In a sense, it requires self-transposal, where you work to put yourself in the other person's shoes, to understand rather than judge or defend against. For some, it will require great effort to resist responding with a suggestion of what to do because the desire to fix it for others is so habitual.

Active listening is made up of 3 different processes[4]:

1. **Restatement**—Repeating the words of the speaker as you have heard them.

   Example: "I get so frustrated that I never have a day free from my back pain."

   Restatement: "You're frustrated because the back pain never leaves you?"

   Restatement can be annoying if not timed appropriately. When done well, it assures the patient that you have indeed heard the content of what he or she is saying. The main purpose of restatement is to help the person continue speaking and should only be used in the initial phases of active listening. Once you have reassured the patient that you are hearing his or her words, reflection and clarification become more useful responses.

2. **Reflection**—Verbalizing the content and the implied feelings of the sender.

   Example: "This pain has been going on for months. I just can't go on any longer."

   Reflection: "You're exhausted and feeling defeated from the constant pain?"

   The purpose of reflection is to express in words the feelings and attitudes sensed behind the words of the sender. This aspect of listening indicates you're hearing more than just the words; you're hearing the emotion behind them. Sometimes we guess incorrectly, but this gives the sender the chance to clarify for us and for him- or herself exactly what he or she is feeling. Awareness of feelings is critical to identifying the real problem. When the listener wants to help the sender to examine more extensively both thoughts and feelings, or to focus thoughts and feelings, clarification is used.

3. **Clarification**—Summarizing or simplifying the sender's thoughts and feelings and resolving confused verbalizations into clear, concise statements.

   Example: "When the doctor told me I needed physical therapy, I knew that you would be the person who would help me get rid of my pain. But it's been 2 weeks now and the pain just keeps coming back. I am afraid that I'll have this pain forever. I'm not sure what it is that I'm supposed to do. Do I just have to live with this or will somebody please help me?"

   Clarification: "When you first came to physical therapy, you thought the pain would be relieved immediately. Now you realize that ridding yourself of the pain is going to take longer than you expected and is more than a matter of somebody just fixing it?"

These skills take practice, as does resisting the answer that tends toward fixing it. The exercises at the end of the chapter will give you an opportunity to practice.

Clear Sending— Use of "I" Statements When I Own the Problem

When I feel the emotion and want to communicate to another person that I am upset, clear communication is facilitated when I am congruent. That is, my words clearly match my feelings. I express my feelings with "I" messages rather than the commonly used editorial "they," "you," or "everyone." First, let's look at congruence.

Congruence

Congruence is a term that indicates that the words and the music match. Congruence is present when **what I say matches what I do and what I feel**.[4] Incongruence appears ingenuine and dishonest and doesn't ring true. How often have we been caught in incongruence when someone asks for a compliment: "Well, do you like my new haircut or not?" "Yes, it's okay I guess." What was felt was less than okay, but no one likes to appear rude. When a person is congruent, he or she appears open, honest, genuine, and authentic. Nonverbal cues and tone of voice are consistent with the words spoken.

Congruence requires reflection. Before speaking, you must realize feelings and thoughts and reconcile such pulls as not wanting to be hurtful yet wanting to be honest. A congruent response to the requested compliment might be: "You know, I noticed you had a new haircut, but I believe I liked it better the old way." With this response, the person realizes that you value honesty and are willing to be honest and can avoid being rude. The message rings true, and you feel better. More important, the person knows you will resist responses aimed at trying to please others.

Congruence is best conveyed when it is communicated with sensitivity and thought. Congruent communication should never be used as a rationalization for insensitive and rude honesty.

"I" Messages

"I" messages are necessary when you feel emotion, you own the problem, and you want to get the problem solved. Our tendency is to blame when we feel uncomfortable. An example might be, "You always leave the dirty dishes in the sink! I'm getting sick and tired of cleaning up after you."

What is the problem, and whose problem is it?

Well, I'm upset, so the problem is mine and requires a clearer message than that if I want to get it solved in a helpful way. Using an "I" message is the way I would proceed: "I'm feeling very frustrated. This is the third night in a row that I've found dirty dishes in the sink, and I'm tired of doing them for you. Let's talk about this."

With "I" messages, I clearly own my frustration. Then, it's up to the other person to respond, hopefully with concern, perhaps even with active listening. Please note, however, that **use of an "I" statement does not guarantee that the other person will respond in a helpful way. What it does guarantee is that my feelings will be expressed and I will take responsibility for my upset, rather than blaming someone else.** Another person might never get upset over dirty dishes in the sink!

Using "I" statements involves taking a risk: I speak in the first person and I own my feelings rather than ignore, disclaim, or minimize them. It takes reflective thought to decide what it is that I'm feeling and how it is I can express that. Sending "I" messages tells the other person that you are owning your upset and that you and he or she are worthy and capable of solving this problem with appropriate, clear, respectful discussion. The exercises at the end of the chapter will help you practice this important skill.

Remember Jason in the earlier example. Emails are never a good way to communicate any sort of emotion, so I would recommend that Jason respond to his clinical instructor with a neutral message: "I understand that you are disappointed in my behavior. I would like to make an appointment to discuss this with you before we start tomorrow morning, say about 7:45 AM? Will that work for you?"

Face to face, Jason needs to own his frustration, and hopefully his clinical instructor will use active listening skills to respond. In the interim, he may come to the conclusion that his clinical instructor had every right to mention his lateness to him: "I feel frustrated that I was late with my patient because I got distracted with my emails when the patient did not arrive on time at 8:00 AM. I apologize and will work to not let it happen again. But I must also comment that my frustration is in part due to my perception that I feel singled out by you. Is that the case?"

CONCLUSION

Communication that is helpful resists the need to impulsively respond, become defensive, or offer quick advice or a quick solution to a problem. Instead, therapeutic communication strives to clarify the problem and assist the person with the problem to solve it for him- or herself. When we were children, we needed adults to fix it for us, to put a bandage on our bruised knees or our bruised egos. As mature health practitioners, we must unlearn the natural tendency to help by giving advice. We must respect and value the communication process as one more tool in our repertoire of therapeutic responses, where we help the other person help him- or herself.

Let's return to the case example at the beginning of the chapter. Jonathan and Mrs. Graham are standing in the hallway outside Diane's room, and Mrs. Graham has just let Jonathan have it. What is the problem and whose problem is it?

Clearly, it is Mrs. Graham's problem. Jonathan has practiced his therapeutic communication skills, and, instead of defending himself, he responds with, "You're obviously upset and frustrated at the apparent lack of progress on Diane's part, and you believe that is due to my inexperience."

Mrs. Graham says yes and goes on for another few minutes while Jonathan keeps up with her with active listening responses. Soon she calms down and, feeling really listened to, she looks at Jonathan and admits that the real problem is that she feels that this is all her fault and she feels so helpless. Jonathan explores with her what he believes her choices are in dealing with the guilt she feels and then promises to include her in his therapy sessions to a greater extent tomorrow so that she can provide minor aspects of treatment in the evenings. Mrs. Graham shakes his hand, thanks him, and agrees to see a counselor to work on her feelings of guilt.

Not all communications will end this amicably, but the majority will end far less amicably if the practitioner responds impulsively or simply reacts. Therapeutic communication is the most useful way to ensure a helping response to emotion-laden communication.

References

1. Cassell EJ. *Talking With Patients: Vol 1. The Theory of Doctor-Patient Communication*. Cambridge, MA: MIT Press; 1985.
2. Goleman D. Email is easy to write (and to misread). *New York Times*. October 7, 2007.
3. Kozler B, Erb GL. *Fundamentals of Nursing. Concepts and Procedures*. 6th ed. Reading, MA: Addison-Wesley Publishers; 1987.
4. Munson PJ, Johnson RB. *Humanizing Instruction, Or Helping Your Students Up the Up Staircase*. Chapel Hill, NC: Johnson Self-Instructional Package; 1972.

EXERCISES

EXERCISE 1: CURRENT PATTERNS

1. Think of a recent situation in which you felt emotionally upset or frustrated. Describe the situation briefly.

2. Whose problem was it? If you were upset, it was your problem. How did you communicate? Did you communicate at all, or did you swallow it and hope it would go away or at least change so that it was no longer a problem?

3. What did you communicate, exactly?

4. How would you change that now, using "I" statements or active listening? Do you think the outcome would have changed if you had used "I" messages or active listening?

5. Write an "I" statement designed to communicate you're upset.

EXERCISE 2: ACTIVE LISTENING AND "I" MESSAGES

Active listening involves restatement (of the words of the sender), reflection (of the words and underlying feelings of the sender), and clarification (summarizes and focuses the sender's message). Practice writing all 3 types of responses.

Restatement

SENDER	RESPONSE FROM YOU
I'm very worried about my shortness of breath.	You're worried about your shortness of breath?
I used to be able to jog for a whole hour, but now my joints start to ache.	
I wish I could swim for 100 laps without getting so tired.	

Reflection

SENDER	RESPONSE FROM YOU
This pain has been going on for months now. I just wish someone would fix it for me or someone would help.	Your pain just drags on and you wish to relieve it. Perhaps you're concerned that it will never go away?
Yesterday was a good day, but today I feel the same old way.	
It's hard remembering to do my exercises.	
I want to get better, but it's hard.	

Clarification

SENDER	RESPONSE FROM YOU
I wish someone would tell me what's going on with my knees. When I get up in the morning they're fine, but by noon they're swollen and feel tired. I'm too young to be suffering with joint problems. Is this arthritis or what? Do I have to live with this forever?	You're worried that your knee problem might be arthritis, and that you'll never be rid of it?
So when the chiropractor told me I had a curved spine and I had to keep coming back for more adjustments every day, I felt that surely there must be something I could do for myself. I got a little frustrated by having so little to do to help myself.	
I almost didn't make it here. I got a horrible headache as I was driving here. The traffic is so stressful in this city. Will it ever end? New cars every day on the road. I don't know if I can keep up driving with these headaches. Is there anything you can do for me?	

Read each situation and the "you" message (blaming response) and then write an "I" message in the third column.

SITUATION	"YOU" MESSAGE	"I" MESSAGE
The aide has neglected to clean the whirlpool for 3 days in a row.	What's the matter with you? Are you getting lazy or what?	I'm confused and frustrated. For 3 days the whirlpool hasn't been cleaned. What's the problem?
Your patient has arrived late and set your schedule back by a half-hour all day.	You're late again! Now I'm going to be a half-hour behind for the last 3 treatment sessions.	
The patient seems depressed and has been reluctant to speak up for several days.	You're so quiet lately. Did I do something to make you mad?	

EXERCISE 3: PATIENT-PRACTITIONER INTERACTIONS

A series of vignettes follows. Divide into groups of 3, where one person is the health care professional, one is the patient, and one is the observer.

Role-play the first vignette for 5 minutes or so or until an appropriate place to stop occurs. The observer should have in hand a copy of the Patient-Practitioner Interaction Checklist (located at the end of the exercise vignettes). At the conclusion of the vignette, the observer asks the patient how he or she is feeling and then asks the practitioner the same question. The observer then gives the practitioner feedback, as recorded on the checklist. At the end of the first round (approximately 15 minutes), remain in the same group of 3 but exchange roles and repeat the same vignette. After all 3 of you have role-played the practitioner, discuss the experience among yourselves. Take a risk and give each other helpful feedback, negative and positive, about your communication skills. Journal about the experience, focusing on what it felt like to be the therapist, the patient, and the observer giving negative feedback to a classmate or colleague.

Vignettes

Each person playing a role should see the description for that role only. Read the brief description and then act out the part as you would if it were happening to you. These vignettes are written for the role of physical therapist, but feel free to alter the descriptions to make them more applicable to the role that you are preparing for in your education if it is not physical therapy.

VIGNETTE 1

Physical Therapist

You've been working with this patient, who uses a wheelchair, for 4 months. The past 3 weeks, the 2 of you have focused on the patient's discharge home. The patient seems pleased to be returning home but also anxious. You notice lately that the patient is short tempered and cuts people off who try to help. You hate conflict and want to avoid it at all costs.

Patient

You must use a wheelchair to get about and have been working in physical therapy for 4 months with the same therapist. The past 3 weeks, the 2 of you have focused on your discharge home. You've begun to be very anxious about separating from the rehabilitation center and are experiencing intermittent episodes of chest pain. You're afraid to tell anyone about this because you fear that they will discount your symptoms and label you as overly dependent, and you're actually afraid that they might be right. You're exhausted because you haven't slept more than 1 or 2 hours for the past 3 nights. You decide to confide your fears in your physical therapist, but you're feeling exhausted and defensive. You decide to just blurt it all out and hope that your therapist will understand.

VIGNETTE 2

Physical Therapist

You are the therapist for a program for children with cerebral palsy. One mother brings her child 3 times a week to your center and stays and watches you treat her daughter along with the other children. This child is Black, and children of several races and ethnicities are represented at the center. You are White. This center is the only place where children with cerebral palsy can get treatment in this small town.

Patient's Mother

You are the mother of a child with cerebral palsy. You bring your child to physical therapy at the rehabilitation center in your small town 3 times each week and wait while she receives treatment. You notice that the physical therapist seems to spend less time with your daughter than she spends with 2 other children. You are Black and the others are White, as is the physical therapist. You've decided to confront the therapist with your suspicions. You're angry and hurt, but you fear that if you say the wrong thing, your daughter will be treated even less than before. This is the only center in town that offers treatment for your child. This is not the first time you've felt that you and your family were being discriminated against because of your race.

VIGNETTE 3

Physical Therapist

Your 20-year-old patient who had minor knee surgery 2 days ago is still complaining of pain. He keeps his knee elevated with ice, hates to do exercises, screams with pain, and uses his crutches only with assistance and only to go to the bathroom. The surgeon is anxious to discharge the patient home, but you're convinced that he is not ready and will surely fall. He has 10 stairs to climb just to get from the sidewalk to the front door of his house. You're subconsciously afraid that your lack of experience in caring for patients with knee surgery has contributed to his poor postoperative adjustment, so you're feeling guilty.

Patient

You just had knee surgery 2 days ago and are experiencing a lot of postoperative pain. You're protecting your knee, keeping it very still so it will heal faster and hurt less. Your physical therapist seems to think you should be discharged home today and is frustrated with your oversensitivity to the pain. You've never had surgery before, and no one really prepared you for this experience. You're afraid you'll be discharged suddenly, and you feel very shaky with your crutches. You have no idea how you'll climb up the 10 steps to your front porch, let alone the 15 to your bedroom. You're upset with yourself for being afraid, you hurt, and you're fearful of being thrown out in the cold with no help. You decide to talk to your therapist before physical therapy today. You feel angry at her for putting you in this position.

VIGNETTE 4

Physical Therapist

You are with a private practice assigned to cover the patient care needs at a nursing home and, although you love the patients and enjoy the interaction with them, you realize that much of their functional activity has to be supervised by the nursing staff when you are not there. The nurses love the patients also, but they are understaffed. They are constantly asking you to help them with nursing functions while you are doing therapy, and you cooperate but are becoming increasingly frustrated. You decide to talk to the head nurse about this after you discuss one of your patients who needs to be ambulated 3 times a shift to build endurance. You approach the nurse as she is making out her daily census report.

Nurse

You are in charge of a unit of elderly patients, and you are understaffed. The administrator has been criticizing you for inefficiency, and you feel that she is being unrealistic in her demands on you. Secretly, you fear that if one more thing goes wrong, you are likely to lose your job. The physical therapist has asked to see you, and you are angry at her because she seems to make more work for your nurses so that their nursing tasks do not get completed. The physical therapist is always asking the nurses to dangle patients to help ambulate them; you think they should hire another therapist and let your nurses do nursing care.

VIGNETTE 5

Physical Therapist

You are working with a young football player who is the star quarterback of his college team. He has had a tear of his adductor tendon in his right leg and is receiving physical therapy so that he can heal quickly and return to playing. You have a lot of pressure on you to help him return to the game as soon as possible, and so he has been assigned to rehab 2 hours in the morning and 2 hours each afternoon after his classes. He is a very popular person on Twitter, and each time you try to work with him, he delays his treatment several times so that he can text his fans.

Patient—Star Football Player

You are recovering from a groin injury sustained during a football game and are assigned to come to rehab 4 hours a day—2 hours in the morning and 2 hours after classes in the afternoon. You are so bummed about not to be able to play, and you are afraid that your fans will abandon you and forget about you, so your one hope is to hold onto them by Tweeting a moment-by-moment description of what rehab for a groin injury is like. It is very important for you to be able to maintain their attention so that you can count on their support when you return to playing.

Patient-Practitioner Interaction Checklist

The observer in the triad responds to these questions during each role-play situation and then uses this information to give feedback to the practitioner about his or her therapeutic communication.

How well did the practitioner:

1. Attend to the patient's (or nurse's) emotional state and feelings?

2. Identify what the problem was and who had the problem?

3. Use reflection and clarifying responses during active listening and use "I" statements when he or she owned the problem?

4. Use open-ended questions and statements to encourage the patient to talk more?

5. Remain silent when appropriate?

6. Respond to the patient with signs of sympathy and self-transposal?

7. Avoid judging, defensive, or blaming statements?

8. How could the therapist improve communication next time?

Journaling

At the conclusion of the exercises, journal your feelings about this new form of communicating. How do you feel about its usefulness? Do you believe that you will be able to develop skill in using "I" statements? Are you willing to practice at home? How about active listening skills? Make a commitment to practice using these skills at least once each day until you believe that you've developed some skill, and remember that this form of communication is now a choice for you in any situation.

The exercises at the end of this chapter are also available online.
Please refer to the sticker in the front of the book and enter the access code provided.

ASSERTIVENESS SKILLS AND CONFLICT RESOLUTION

Carol M. Davis, DPT, EdD, MS, FAPTA and
Gina Maria Musolino, PT, MSEd, EdD

"Of the many cues that influence behavior, at any one point in time, none is more common than the actions of others." –Albert Bandura

OBJECTIVES

- To identify the importance of using assertive communication in healing interactions.
- To distinguish between nonassertive, assertive, and aggressive communication.
- To describe situations in which each person tends to give up personal power.
- To describe how to defuse a hostile, angry reaction.
- To define bullying and identify bullying behaviors in the workplace.
- To identify the rights we all share as human beings.
- To offer the opportunity to contract for changing negative, reactive behavior to positive, assertive behavior.

ASSERTIVENESS TRAINING

In the previous chapter, we learned a new way of communicating in intense or emotional moments. This chapter expands on the skills previously learned and teaches a way of communicating that will improve one's sense of personal power and self-esteem in situations where stress would have us give up that power. Let's begin with a case example:

Davis CM, Musolino GM. *Patient Practitioner Interaction: An Experiential Manual for Developing the Art of Health Care, Sixth Edition* (pp 117-137).
© 2016 SLACK Incorporated.

Sheila Lester, registered nurse, was standing at the nurses' station reading her patient's chart before going into the patient's room to give her treatment. The patient's physician came to the station and was searching for the chart. When he saw that Sheila was reading it, he turned to her and said, "Give me the chart, Honey. That's my patient and I have to see her now." Sheila felt as if she were being treated in a nonprofessional way, to say the least. She felt her heart begin to race, she knew she was blushing, and she realized that she felt degraded and humiliated. Before she could stop herself, she turned to the physician and shouted, "My name is not Honey, and this is my patient as well!" The physician looked up with amusement and returned, "Well, well. What is your name then, Honey?" Sheila felt as if the battle were lost and put the chart down and walked away in anger.

Assertiveness training has become well known in the past decade, and many people claim its benefits as a communication skill, but it also carries a negative connotation in some circles. Images of the "uppity" woman or the aggressive man come to mind. These images result from our socialization, from the messages we heard from our parents as we grew up. As rambunctious children, many of us were taught that we should "know our place" and practice humility. As we grew older, we heard other messages: "Children should be seen and not heard!" "Go to your room until you can come out with a smile on your face!" "If you can't say something nice, don't say anything at all!" Certainly Traditionalists and Baby Boomers and families from strong ethnic cultural backgrounds heard, "Women belong in the supportive role to their husbands." More recently, we hear phrases such as, "Don't worry, be happy!" and "Don't sweat the small stuff!"

The accumulative effect, especially on all those who suffer from low self-esteem and those who feel disempowered in the community, can result in communication that is not healthy or healing in nature. Following rules that do not encourage genuine and appropriate expression of feelings results in multiple unhealthy behaviors, including the bottling up of genuine emotion and the repression of feelings over time that often results in stress-related illness, passive-aggressive silence or manipulation, and inappropriate outbursts of anger, rage, defensiveness, and frustration. At the extreme, we see the rampage killings at high schools in the United States committed by adolescents who were enraged by bullies and felt powerless to communicate their feelings to others. Today bullying has become a greater issue in the workplace.

BULLYING DEFINED IN THE WORKPLACE

The Workplace Bullying Institute[1] defines workplace bullying as "repeated, health-harming mistreatment of one or more persons (the targets) by one or more perpetrators. It is **abusive conduct** that is:

- Threatening, humiliating, or intimidating; or

- Work interference—sabotage—that prevents work from getting done; or

- Verbal abuse."

The bully's behavior is deliberate and targeted to a specific victim, occurring frequently and with a level of intensity over a period of time. Bullying behaviors are overt and covert, which often make it difficult for the victim to recognize, identify, respond to, and report bullying. Being bullied at work has also been attributed to resemble the first-hand experience of a battered spouse. The Workplace Bullying Institute states that "not calling bullying 'bullying,' to avoid offending the sensibilities of those who made the bullying possible, is a disservice to bullied individuals whose jobs, careers, and health have been threatened as the result."[1] Raynor and Hoel[2] identified 5 categories of bullying behaviors (Figure 8-1).

The American Nurses Association House of Delegates adopted a resolution regarding Hostility, Abuse, and Bullying in the Workplace in 2010,[3] which was a reaffirmation of its existing principles from the 2006 resolution, related to workplace abuse and harassment of nurses. The 2010 resolution included additional recommendations for action to proactively reduce the growing problem of workplace abuse, harassment, and bullying of nurses and to explore collaborative solutions with other disciplines and organizations to leverage resources for research and education. Although your professions code of ethics may address the topic in a general manner, bullying today is very specific in that it is directed toward control and clear destabilization of another person within the workplace, and the need to create safer workplaces has become increasingly evident.

The Joint Commission, in *Sentinel Event Alert*,[4] proclaimed its intolerance of intimidating and disruptive behaviors in the document "Behaviors That Undermine a Culture of Safety." The Joint Commission implemented a Leadership Standard (LD.03.01.01) that addresses disruptive and inappropriate behaviors in 2 of its elements of performance[4]:

> *"Element of Performance 4: The hospital/organization has a code of conduct that defines acceptable and disruptive and inappropriate behaviors; and*

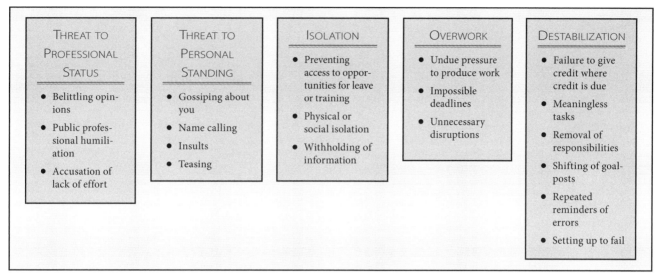

Figure 8-1. Raynor and Hoel's 5 categories of bullying behaviors. (Adapted from Raynor C, Hoel H. A summary review of literature relating to workplace bullying. *J Community Appl Soc Psych.* 1997;7:181-191.)

Element of Performance 5: Leaders create and implement a process for managing disruptive and inappropriate behaviors. This document also includes 11 suggested actions to ensure compliance."

The Healthy Workplace Bill,[5] which provides protection from bullying to employees and employers, was initiated in 2001. As of mid-2015, 28 states and 2 territories have introduced the bill, but no laws have yet been enacted. Five states currently have a bill active, recently Virginia in January 2015. In 2010, the New York and Illinois state senates passed the bill. Discussions about a federal law were begun in 2010 with members of the US House of Representatives and the US Senate. Bullying is an issue that is often ignored or swept under the rug because it is underreported and difficult to address. As President Maltby of the National Workrights Institute stated, "Bullying is the sexual harassment of 20 years ago; everybody knows about it, but nobody wants to admit it."[6] (Title VI of the Civil Rights Act currently covers sexual harassment and discrimination.)

THE CHALLENGE OF COMMUNICATING WISELY IN HEALTH CARE

As health care professionals (HCPs) move away from more traditional assistive roles and into more prominent primary care responsibilities, such as in the clinical doctoral degree programs for physical therapists (DPT), occupational therapists (OTD), and nurse practitioners (DNP), more assertive communication styles are required to be effective as a health care leader. These skills do not come automatically with the conferring of the degree.[7] In addition, health care calls for a great deal of practice when dealing with fellow practitioners who are often working under stress and when dealing with patients and their families who are feeling intensely vulnerable. Emotional communication, including anger, is very prevalent in the practice of health care. Many situations occur daily in which a person is stimulated to react, either in anger or in giving up personal power and feeling helpless.

GENDER DIFFERENCES

Women predominate in all of the health professions except medicine and surgery, and medical school admissions data indicate that they are quickly catching up to balance male applicants. However, we live in an evolving society that has been, and continues to be, essentially male dominated and patriarchal. The culture of the West has been slow to accept the balancing of the opposites, although the reality of the need for both is well established in all cultures. Despite the fact that health care consists of much more than physician care, medicine was created by men to be practiced by men. Nurses, who are predominantly women, feel especially affected by this disparate power structure. In a study conducted by Friedman[8] on nurse-physician relationships, nurses reported that they had to deal with the following:

- Condescending attitudes
- Lack of respect as either a person or a professional

- Public humiliation as physicians rant and rave in front of patients, families, or anyone who will listen
- Temper tantrums
- Scapegoating (nurses are blamed for everything that goes wrong)
- Failure to read nurses' notes or listen to nurses' suggestions
- Refusal to share information about the patient
- Frequent public disparaging remarks

The continuum of insensitive behavior, issuing from people in power to those in less powerful positions, can run from poor taste and bad manners to outright sexist abuse, bullying, and harassment. The sources of verbal abuse to nurses described in Friedman's[8] article were primarily physicians, then patients' families, and lastly the nurse supervisor. Although it is true that part of the power struggle in health care has to do with the difficulties in our culture of men and women relating equally with each other, it is not as simple as that.

As much as all children are alike, developmentalists have shown us that boys and girls are different in the way they are treated by adults, their goals and ideals, the way they see their place in the world, and the way they make decisions about right and wrong. But, all people have a genderless essential self, a core identity that is good, that underlies the public self or persona and the ego. All people have the natural desire to become more, to grow, to learn, to increase self-esteem, to have influence, and to feel capable and able to facilitate change for the better. For the most part, people in health care, men and women, want to help others, to change conditions of illness and pain or the inability to function fully as a human being in the world. To help in healing ways, one must exercise personal and professional power for the good. The goal must be to mature beyond the need for the ego to defend itself and to reach down to the essential self, where we are confident of our personal rights and assured of our equality and from where we can communicate with empathy and understanding.

CULTURAL DIFFERENCES

As our country becomes more and more diverse in population, health care professionals' classrooms reflect this broad diversity. As you will learn in Chapter 12, some cultures emphasize the inappropriateness of asserting oneself in a leadership role, deeming assertive behavior as rude or selfish, and emphasize more passive ways of achieving goals that would not be effective in the health care system in our country. These behaviors, such as not making eye contact or speaking in a very low tone of voice, would seem out of place and weak to colleagues and patients and would be ineffective as healing behaviors in the United States and other Western countries.[9]

EXERCISING OUR PERSONAL POWER

In previous chapters, we learned that how we feel about ourselves has everything to do with how we view the world and how we view other people. How we feel about our own self-worth is directly connected to how much personal power we feel we have and how we use that power. Webster's Dictionary defines power as a possession of control, authority, or influence over another; the ability to act or produce an effect; legal or official authority, capacity, or right; physical might; or political control or influence.[10] Notice that power is a neutral term, having neither positive nor negative value connotations. If we want to facilitate change to make the world better, we have to learn how to exercise power.

Women in our society have been taught to play a role secondary to or supportive of men. Men have been taught to seek out and expect the support of women. But we are all born equal. **We learn to give up our power.** Some beliefs that we develop that result in a giving up of personal power include the following:

- I am not as important as the other person (often the physician or supervisor).
- I am lucky to be treated with respect by others (those in authority).
- I have years of training and experience, but they still do not compare to medical school.
- I must act in ways that indicate I know my place so that I can keep my job, keep referrals coming, and keep peace for others' sake.
- When criticized by a superior, I must not respond but agree to save face and avoid further criticism.
- My needs are not as important as others'.

Some situations seem inherently more apt to stimulate stress than others; thus, we can predict that we might be tempted to give up power, or respond defensively with anger, when we find ourselves required to respond. Ten such situations that may cause stress for some or all of us include the following:

1. Command—Someone orders us to do something
2. Anger—Includes name calling, using obscenities, shouting
3. Negative criticism—Someone judges us as being less than adequate, without suggestions for improvement
4. Unresponsiveness—Indifference to us or to our request
5. Depression—A feeling of gloom in another, extreme sadness
6. Impulsivity—Someone flies off the handle, acts crazy
7. Affection—Someone expresses love and affection or asks us for it
8. Making mistakes—Fear that you cannot make a mistake; feeling as if you must always have the right answer
9. Sexual content—Someone makes an overt or covert sexual comment or sexual advance
10. Pain—Feelings of wanting to flee in the face of pain

PERSONAL RIGHTS

When we hear terrifying stories of people's inhumanity to each other, we are often moved to righteous indignation. For example, none of us can hear recounting from Holocaust victims without cringing with horror. Likewise, prisoner of war stories recently revealed from the Iraq War and Guantanamo, and Islamic State of Iraq and Syria human rights abuses, terrorists actions, and war crimes move us to anger and outrage. Human beings deserve to be treated in certain ways, simply because we are human. What rights do all people have as human beings? What does each human being deserve, simply by virtue of the fact that he or she is a person alive on this Earth? Make a list of the basic rights of all human beings. Do you act in ways that are consistent with your beliefs about your rights? Are there certain rights that you fail to claim for yourself? If so, why is that? How does this list change when a human being becomes ill or disabled?

Thoughts or beliefs we developed even before we could talk lead to feelings (rational or not), which then lead to behaviors or reactions. It is a universal right that every person is entitled to act assertively and to express honest thoughts, feelings, and beliefs. Assertiveness training teaches us that we have a choice of communicating in a way that allows us to convey our thoughts and feelings with tact and respect for others and honor for ourselves. As human beings, each one of us has the right to the following[11]:

- Being treated with respect
- Having needs and having those needs be as important as other people's needs. We have the right to ask (not demand) that other people respond to our needs and to decide whether we want to respond to others' needs.
- Having feelings and expressing those feelings in ways that do not violate the dignity of others
- Changing our minds
- Determining our own priorities
- Asking for what we want
- Refusing without making excuses
- Forming our own opinions and expressing them or having no opinion at all on a certain topic
- Giving and receiving information as fellow health care professionals
- Acting in the best interests of the patient

When we allow our rights to be overlooked, we assume a dependent role, which lowers self-esteem and fosters nonassertive behavior. Recognizing that we have rights is the first step in the cognitive retraining that is essential to assertiveness.

ASSERTIVENESS

What exactly is assertiveness? The concept of assertive behavior can best be described in comparison with what it is not—nonassertive (passive) and aggressive behavior.

Nonassertive Behavior

- Failing to get your point across by remaining quiet or passive. Perceived by others to be weak, easily taken advantage of, or manipulated.
- Key message conveyed: I don't count. My feelings are not as important as yours.

Aggressive Behavior

- Getting your point across but perceived by others as hostile, angry, offensive, sarcastic, or humiliating.
- Key message conveyed: This is what is true. Any reasonable person would agree. You are stupid to disagree. What I want is most important; what you want, feel, or think does not matter.

Assertive Behavior

- Getting your point across without offending others. Direct, congruent expression of thoughts, feelings, beliefs, and opinions in a nonoffensive way.
- Key message conveyed: This is how I view the situation. This is what I think and feel at this moment.

Alberti and Emmons[12] noted 10 key elements to assertive behavior:

1. Self-expressive
2. Respectful of the rights of others
3. Honest
4. Direct and firm
5. Equalizing, benefiting self and relationship
6. Verbally appropriate, including the content of the message (feelings, rights, facts, opinions, requests, limits)
7. Nonverbally appropriate, including the style of the message (eye contact, voice posture, facial expression, gestures, distance, timing, fluency, listening)
8. Appropriate for the person and the situation, not universal
9. Socially responsible
10. Learned, not inborn

EXAMPLES OF ASSERTIVE RESPONSES

Many of us have found ourselves in the situation when, dining out, we order our meal and something happens to make it less acceptable than we had expected. We find ourselves in a situation where we feel that it is necessary to speak up to enjoy the meal that we've requested. Let's say that the dinner is completely cold. What are our choices in this situation?

- Passive—Say nothing at all. When the waitress asks, "How's your dinner?" you respond, "Fine." (The person you're dining with, however, receives the brunt of your hostility all evening.)
- Aggressive—Stand up, shout for the waitress or waiter, and say in a loud and angry voice, "This meal is ice cold. I'm willing to pay good money for a good dinner, but you have the nerve to bring me a meal that has been sitting around for half an hour, and I resent it. Take this meal back immediately and bring me some hot food."
- Assertive—Motion for the waiter, state calmly that your food has become cold, and request that it be heated and brought back to you as quickly as possible.

Upon comparison, it is easy to value assertive communication as superior to nonassertive and aggressive modes. Difficulty in acting assertively in appropriate situations with any consistency stems from the real or perceived threat of rejection, anger, or disapproval. Often, this reluctance to be assertive is based more on habit and subconscious fears that we learned long ago and that now guide our responses in an automatic way. Assertiveness helps us realize that we have a real choice to stand up for ourselves and to hold onto our power in difficult situations. Why in the world would anyone sit and eat a cold dinner while not enjoying it and be willing to pay for it? What is the fear behind speaking up to ask for your rights? For many of us it is simply a matter of overlearning the dictate, "Don't make waves, don't cause a fuss, and don't do anything that will bring attention to yourself." Behind this admonition is the basic feeling that others' rights are more important than mine—that I don't count.

Likewise, why would someone stand up and shout at a waiter in anger for something that is easily remedied? Usually this kind of behavior is acting out anger or frustration with something not related to the meal at all. Or the customer carries a sense of entitlement and feels that it is his or her responsibility to teach others the right behavior.

TYPES OF ASSERTIVE RESPONSES

There are 8 types of assertive responses that can benefit us in the practice of health care and in our day-to-day interactions[12]:

1. Being confrontational
2. Saying no
3. Making requests
4. Expressing opinions
5. Initiating conversation
6. Disclosing self
7. Expressing affection
8. Entering a room of strangers willing to get to know others and allowing ourselves to be known

The first 2 areas can be described as assertive responses that express what commonly appear to be negative emotions, the next 3 responses are emotionally neutral responses that are task specific, and the last 3 responses call for expressing positive emotions. In the exercises at the end of the chapter, you will be given the opportunity to draft assertive, passive, and aggressive responses to each situation.

ATTRIBUTION AND THE DESIRE TO ACT ASSERTIVELY

A person can be quite knowledgeable about assertiveness but will not think to use these skills for any number of reasons. For example, if one believes that no matter what is done the attempt will end in failure, assertiveness does not seem important. This problematic way of thinking illustrates one aspect of behavior, which can partially be explained by attribution theory.[13] The exercise in Figure 8-2 will help you discover the nature of your attributions, or how your lenses are set today. Chart your numbers in the grid at the bottom of the figure.

Note the differences in your perceptions of the causes of success and failure. If you are like most people, you tend to attribute success to causes that are different in nature from those to which we attribute failure.

Attribution theory provides a framework to understand the ways that a person's lenses are set. An attribution is what we feel or think caused an outcome we have experienced.[14] How we view outcomes, as successful or failing, is critical in determining our expectations and our future actions. The 3 dimensions of the causes to which we attribute success or failure are the *locus* (due to something inside or outside of me), *stability* (lasting or temporary), and *controllability* (to what extent I can control this) dimensions.

Attributions that we assign to outcomes have a great deal to do with how we think about ourselves or relate directly to how our lenses are set with regard to self-esteem. If we have good self-esteem, we are likely to attribute the cause of our successes to something inside of ourselves, something that is stable or controllable. If we have low self-esteem, we are likely to see our successes as due to forces outside of ourselves that are unstable and uncontrollable, such as luck or the difficulty of the task. In contrast with failure, a person who indicates a cause that is internal, unstable (changeable), and controllable, such as the amount of effort we expended or the strategy we chose, will be more likely to expect success in the future by increasing effort or changing the ineffective strategy.[13]

In other words, with high self-esteem, we choose to believe that we are going to succeed directly because of our actions, and if we fail, it is not because of a fixed internal trait (we have low ability or a poor personality) but because of circumstances that can change if we apply a different, more successful strategy to the task.

In summary, when failure is attributed to stable, external, and uncontrollable events, there is little we can do to effect change and we are unlikely to use assertiveness or any other strategy to get the job done. This is a loser's or victim's "script."

It is important to describe the nature of success and failure in ways that allows success to be judged realistically and over the long term.[14] The most adaptive attributions occur when success is defined in other than all-or-nothing terms, are realistic in the circumstances, and are attributed to one's personal ability, effort, or good judgment.[15] In health care, many frustrating situations are unlikely to change, but we can change how we think about them and how we deal with them to experience success over the long term. If success is seen as having all patients be discharged from our carefully cured or having Medicare pay for 100% of treatment in 100% of eligible cases, few practitioners would ever feel as if they succeeded. Compromise, realistic expectations, and acceptance of long-term strategies are necessary, along with avoiding dualistic right-wrong judgments.

Put yourself in a time when you've done a project that was highly praised. What did you do? Who praised you? How did you feel? How did this influence future activity? Write down one major cause of your success.

1. Is the cause due to something about you or due to something outside of you?
Internal   1   2   3   4   5   6   7   External
(Inside you)   (Other resources)

2. Is the cause something that will remain stable or be only temporary?
Lasting   1   2   3   4   5   6   7   Temporary
(Stable)   (Unstable)
(Constant [IQ])   (Changing [weather])

3. Do you see this cause as something you can control or is this beyond your control?
Controllable   1   2   3   4   5   6   7   Uncontrollable
(Whether I study or not)   (Other person's mood)

4. How likely are you to experience the same outcome in the future?
Highly likely   1   2   3   4   5   6   7   Unlikely

Now, think of a time when you have experienced a failure, for example, given an important talk and the audience reacts negatively or cooked a meal that no one liked. Write down one major cause.

5. Is the cause due to something about you or something outside of you?
Internal   1   2   3   4   5   6   7   External

6. Is the cause something that will remain stable or be only temporary or changing?
Lasting   1   2   3   4   5   6   7   Temporary
(Stable)   (Unstable)

7. Do you see this cause as something you can control or is this beyond your control?
Controllable   1   2   3   4   5   6   7   Uncontrollable

8. How likely are you to experience the same outcome in the future?
Highly likely   1   2   3   4   5   6   7   Unlikely

Now chart your numbers on this grid:

	Success	*Failure*
Internal/External		
Stable/Unstable		
Controllable/Uncontrollable		

Figure 8-2. Attribution exercise. (K. Curtis, personal communication.)

In sum, we must change the way we define failure and think about the causes of failure for assertiveness to be useful and successful. If we believe that failure is attributed to external events that are uncontrollable and stable, we will be unlikely to use assertiveness. But, if we reframe our thoughts, decide that our goal might have been a little too unrealistic, and decide to use another strategy to work for success, assertiveness can be a useful tool to solve problems.

LEARNING TO ACT ASSERTIVELY

The skill of assertive behavior is not inborn; to develop it requires learning 5 new behaviors[12]:

1. **Recognize situations in which you are tempted to become passive or aggressive in your communication.** Develop the skill of observing yourself. Be conscious of situations where you automatically give up your power, have irrational thoughts that do not relate to the present moment, or feel the necessity to put the other person down.

2. **Recognize when you are tempted to attribute failure to forces that are uncontrollable and stable, such as a powerful person's unpleasant personality traits or a medical system that fails to acknowledge patient needs.** Challenge yourself to think of a strategy to replace feelings of hopelessness or negativity.

3. **Replace these old thought patterns with different, more positive and powerful thoughts.** Cognitively interrupt the old thought patterns of "You're right, I'm no good" or "How dare you attack me, you arrogant fool?" or "It's no use!" Alone or with another trusted person, do the following:

   - Discuss the nature of the situation that aroused the emotion
   - Confront the tendency to react passively or aggressively
   - Identify the belief that lies behind your reaction
   - Replace the erroneous belief with a counteracting right
   - Identify a more positive thought that will bring more confident feelings

4. **Practice thinking new thoughts as a first step in changing the feelings that go with the old thoughts, thus deflating the energy behind the old reaction.** You will know that you are on the right track when the new thoughts make you feel positive and hopeful.

5. **Practice the new behavior that goes along with the ownership of the right.** Be assertive. Count your blessings and feel good about your ability to make a positive difference in the world.

How might Sheila, the nurse in the example at the beginning of the chapter, communicate assertively? Chapter 7 taught one aspect of assertive communication, the use of "I" statements. This mode of communicating transforms an aggressive, blaming, or accusatory response to an assertive, responsible, and clear expression of feeling, essentially telling the other person what effect his or her behavior has on you. In many cases, an "I" statement alone initially is sufficient to get your assertive message across. The situation Sheila found herself in calls for a confrontational assertion. Sheila feels diminished, less than a colleague and more like a slave being asked to do the master's bidding. Her feeling response is anger at being treated so poorly, and her initial reaction is to be angry. When her anger does not get her what she wants, the messages in her head revert to "See. You're just not as good as the physician. Your rights are not important here." She gives up and walks away in frustration. What she hoped for was a collegial relationship with the physician because both of them carry out their clinical responsibilities with the patient. This calls for a confrontational response aimed at helping her avoid becoming aggressive in anger and avoid passively giving up her power to silently comply with the physician's rude request.

First, Sheila must be aware of her feelings in the situation and her tendency to react in anger and give up her power. She must be aware of what causes she attributes the outcomes in this situation to. Next, she must pay attention to the messages she gives herself and challenge the negative thoughts with more affirming, positive thoughts that confirm her rights as a human being. Then she is ready to respond with an assertive reply aimed at exercising her right to express her honest thoughts, feelings, and beliefs around this situation. One format for an effective response is through the *describe, express, specify, and consequences (DESC) approach* of framing your response.

DESC Response as a Format for Assertive Communication

The DESC format described by Bower and Bower[16] incorporates "I" statements but expands them and is useful when a more detailed interaction is required to get the other person's attention to your point of view. DESC is an acronym for:

       D—**Describe** the situation.

       E—**Express** your feelings about the situation: "I feel _____ ."

       S—**Specify** the change you want: "I'd like for you to _____ ."

       C—**Consequences.** Identify the results that will occur: "In that way _____ ."

Let's compose a DESC response for Sheila in the situation outlined at the beginning of the chapter:

       D—"Yes, Dr. Dutton, I realize that this is your patient. She's my patient as well; I'm her nurse."

       E—"My name is Sheila Lester. When you call me 'Honey,' it demeans me, and I do not appreciate it."

       S—"I'd like you to call me Sheila or Ms. Lester because I'd like to discuss this patient with you as a colleague would, and I would like you to treat me as a colleague."

       C—"In that way, I feel the patient will receive better care because we are working together with her in a more respectful and collegial way."

Sheila took a big risk with this physician by speaking up to tell him how his behavior made her feel. She must have trusted that this was a risk worth taking. We would hope that the physician would respond in a mature way and treat her request with respect. Assertive communication does not guarantee this, however, as we'll discuss in a moment.

Sometimes you know that the risk is not well placed. An alternative to the DESC confrontation is the *describe, indicate, specify, and consequences (DISC) confrontation*, which is used when you are confronting a person who will not care what you feel, so you eliminate the expression of feeling and substitute I for "indicate," indicating the problem the behavior is causing. DESC and DISC are just amplifications of the effective "I" statement, but using them in a practiced, disciplined way provides an opportunity to erase an old, ineffective way of responding by replacing it with an assertive response.

An illustration of the DISC response for a physical therapist would be a powerful physician who refers a patient with low back pain to you, a physical therapist, and specifically orders the following: evaluate and treat with heat and massage and no exercise, no mobilization. Upon evaluation, you realize that this back pain is the result of an acute muscle spasm that occurred recently and was facilitated by poor body mechanics and weak flexor and extensor muscles. Your professional knowledge requires that you treat with ice and teach exercises to relax the current problem and prevent recurrence.

Your DISC confrontation might go something like this:

       D—"I'd like to talk with you about Mr. Doughty's back problem."

       I—"Your physical therapy referral for heat and massage is a logical place to start for a chronic problem, but my examination reveals this to be an acute spasm, which the literature indicates responds faster and more effectively to ice. Likewise, his back extensor and abdominal muscles are quite weak, and he needs gentle relaxation exercise to reduce the spasm and eventual instruction in proper body mechanics."

       S—"I'd like for you to approve my plan to treat with ice and massage, then follow with gentle pelvic tilt and bridging exercises to tolerance to release the spasm, and eventually teach him stretching and strengthening exercises and proper body mechanics and posture to prevent recurrence."

       C—"That way, perhaps we can help him recover and get him strong enough and wise enough to keep him from reinjuring himself."

Organizing your thoughts will be more difficult at first, so the exercises for this chapter will provide practice following this 4-step method by writing out your response to a past situation that was particularly difficult for you. The key to your success will be paying attention to the way you feel. When you feel negative feelings, reach for a more positive thought. Thoughts are very creative, and we have a built-in indicator of how well we are doing with moving in a positive and growing direction. Good thoughts feel good. It's as simple as that.

You're probably wondering how you'll learn to respond quickly and on the spot with such a detailed DISC or DESC format when an assertive response is indicated. At first, you will not be so organized. The most you can hope for is to recognize your feelings, avoid giving up your power angrily or passively, and buy time before responding at all. Eventually, however, it will become second nature to speak up with an "I" statement or a DESC response.

Assertively Dealing With Anger

Once in a while, you will have to deal with an angry, defensive person. Feeling trapped in another's lashing out usually stimulates a fight-or-flight response or passive or aggressive behavior. The ego is stimulated into defending itself, or the

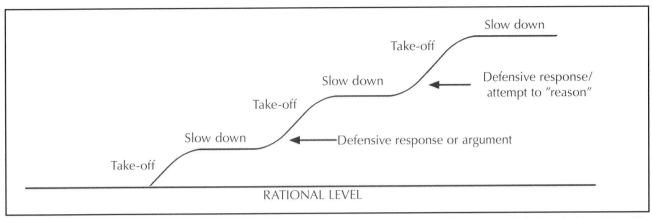

Figure 8-3. Hostility/rage pattern of escalation. (Adapted from Allaire B, McNeil R. *Teaching Patient Relations in Hospitals—The Hows and Whys.* Chicago, IL: American Hospital Association; 1983.)

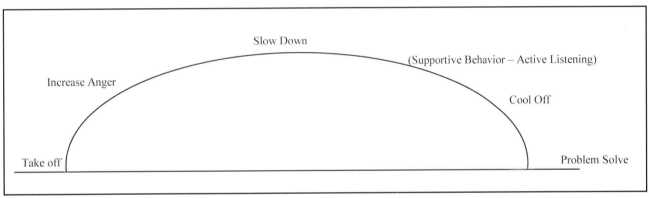

Figure 8-4. Hostility curve handled skillfully. (Adapted from Allaire B, McNeil R. *Teaching Patient Relations in Hospitals—The Hows and Whys.* Chicago, IL: American Hospital Association; 1983.)

ego caves into fear and wants to run away. In the previous chapter, we learned to use active listening when the other person has the emotional outburst; this continues to be the most effective response in an assertive mode. Using active listening skills to help the person defuse the energy behind the outburst, which is most often secondary to fear, allows you then to use "I" statements to offer your assertive response. In other words, be a Teflon sponge; absorb the emotion by using restatement, reflection, and clarification and let it slide off of you.[17]

HOSTILITY CURVE

A hostile, angry person will use a predictable pattern when raging that looks somewhat like what is shown in Figure 8-3.[18] When you argue or respond defensively with someone who is raging, this will only fuel his or her fire and produce another take-off, escalating the argument to higher levels. Likewise, if you interrupt the hostile person and appeal to him or her to "be reasonable," a similar response will result. One person just keeps setting off the other, and no problem is identified, let alone solved.

Skillful handling of a person who is raging (Figure 8-4) involves the active listening skills we practiced in Chapter 7. During the raging person's irrational phase, it is best to simply wait and listen carefully but not say anything. Wait for the moment when the angry person seems to run out of steam and then demonstrate that you have been listening and say something supportive, such as "If the same thing had happened to me, no doubt I would be angry too" or "I know this has been a very difficult experience for you."

Being supportive does not require your agreeing with the person but simply hearing him or her. This eventually will serve to defuse the increasing emotion, and he or she will begin to cool off. Very often he or she will apologize for losing composure. At this point, it is important to help the angry person save face and lead him or her to a private area, where you can sit down and use your neurolinguistic psychology match, pace, and lead skills that you will learn in Chapter 11.

What people are asking for most is recognition and understanding. Active listening gives you the chance to stand still and offer a therapeutic response, which will increase the chances for a positive outcome to the interchange. Once emotions have dissipated, offer your assertive point of view and offer to work together to solve the problem.[16] It is important that you vent your own feelings with a trusted friend after the incident is over, and keep in mind these important words from Mother Teresa:

> *People are often unreasonable, irrational, and self-centered. Forgive them anyway. If you are kind, people may accuse you of selfish, ulterior motives. Be kind anyway. … The good you do today will often be forgotten. Give your best anyway. In the final analysis, it is between you and God. It was never between you and them anyway.*

BENEFITS OF ASSERTIVENESS

In a study with nursing and medical students, students' assertiveness and self-esteem at posttest and 1-month follow-up measurements of the experimental group after training were significantly increased compared with the pretest measurement.[19] There are several benefits to using assertive behavior:

- It is our ethical and healing responsibility.
- It increases our self-respect.
- It increases our self-control.
- It improves self-confidence.
- It helps us develop more emotionally satisfying relationships with others.
- It increases the likelihood that everyone's needs will be met.
- It allows us to exercise our personal rights without denying the rights of others.

To exercise our personal rights relates to competency as a citizen, a consumer, a member of an organization or school or work group, and a participant in public events to express opinions, work for change, or respond to violations of one's own rights or those of others.[12] In the health professions, we must work side-by-side with colleagues, helping our patients regain their feelings of confidence and ability to function independently in the world. To make sure this happens, everyone's rights become important, and the exercise of those rights is critical to the healing process.

COMMON MYTHS ABOUT ASSERTIVENESS

As valuable as assertive communication is, there are some common myths that accompany this process:

- **If I speak up with assertiveness, others will like what I say and do what I ask.** Using assertive communication is no guarantee for anything, except that you have expressed yourself with dignity, honesty, and regard for others. How others respond to you is always a question and has much to do with the other person. Most important, you never have the right to violate another person's rights, even when you use assertiveness.

- **All I have to do is say the assertive words and I will be perceived as being assertive.** Assertive words are critical to an assertive message. But assertive words spoken passively or aggressively destroy the basic message of assertiveness. The posture of assertiveness is an appropriate tone of voice, a steady voice, open posture, and good eye contact.

- **Once I learn assertiveness skills, I must use them all the time in every situation that tends to make me feel powerless.** There are times when the best assertive response is to simply walk away and say nothing. One good example is deciding not to retaliate to an aggressive person. Then it is best to say nothing. Always remember, you are free to choose not to assert yourself in a situation. Ask yourself:
  - How important is this situation to me?
  - How am I likely to feel afterward if I don't assert myself?
  - What do I gain by being assertive? What do I lose?
  - What do I gain by not being assertive? What do I lose?

- **One assertive reply is all that is needed.** The first assertive response is the easiest. It is the comeback response that is more difficult. People will argue with your assertive response and try to get you to give up your power despite your effectiveness. For example, saying no when you mean no often takes several repeats of the no, and you may decide to end the conversation with "Don't try to make me feel guilty. I told you I care about you, but I will not say yes this time. I said no. I mean no. End of discussion."

PRACTICE LEADS TO ACTION

As discussed in the beginning of the chapter, bullying has been defined[1,2] and specifically linked with resultant medical errors in patient care within a variety of health care enviornments.[3-5] Bullying in health care settings has been identified as an international problem,[20-29] with guidelines to address bullying now being provided by professional societies to address and assist in mitigating the problem.[3-5,30] In a qualitative study of 8 final-year physiotherapy students in the United Kingdom, only 1 of the 8 subjects reported experiencing a specific incident of abusive bullying on clinical internship.[29] In the United Kingdom study, 4 main themes were identified by the researchers[29]:

(1) external and situational influences of bullying; (2) students' reactions to the experience of bullying; (3) inability to reveal the experience; and (4) overcoming problems. Bullying had a range of adverse effects on the students, with many expressing self-doubt in their competence and viewing their supervisor as unapproachable and unsupportive. Five students were not initially able to recognize the experience as bullying. In addition, students did not feel able to report the experience and use the support mechanisms in place. This may have been a result of having concerns that the problem would escalate if they reported the experience and, as a consequence, have a negative effect on their grade. Students were keen to offer a range of strategies for clinical practice in order to prevent bullying for future generations of students.

The authors concluded that "students' health, security, and confidence in their ability as a physiotherapist can be at great risk from bullying. Steps are needed to ensure that students are better protected from bullying and feel more able to address bullying behavior during clinical internships."[29]

Through this chapter on appropriate assertive behavior, you now have the tools to confront bullying and stop it before it becomes an insurmountable concern. Utilize your newly acquired DISC and DESC assertive behavior skills to confront potentially abusive behaviors in an appropriately assertive manner. A student recently contacted me regarding some "mild" concerns that her clinical instructor might be being a bit inappropriate. She was not sure and was reaching out for support. In her description, she relayed that her instructor had made her uncomfortable with some of his statements on several occasions. I asked her to describe the statements. She revealed that the instructor said, "Your hair looks better brown than blonde" when he was examining her identification badge with respect to her current hair color. Then, a few days later, after walking through an area of construction within the hospital grounds, he said, "You look hot in that construction hat." Finally, while walking to the parking garage together, he said, "Let's have dinner together sometime and we can discuss your cases."

After debriefing, the student felt that overall the clinical experience was going well and she was learning a lot from the instructor with the patient encounters, but she was beginning to become quite concerned and rather uncomfortable at times regarding the instructor's comments. He was a married man with children, and she felt the comments were completely inappropriate. She was correct and was instructed to implement her DESC response of assertive communication. She practiced the response with me and successfully relayed her concerns to the clinical instructor. The clinical instructor responded appropriately and received the constructive critique in the manner intended. The clinical instructor immediately adjusted his behavior and communication and apologized to the student, without further interventions required. In follow-up, the student no longer felt uncomfortable and had no further issues or matters of concern. She did have lunch in the hospital cafeteria with her clinical instructor to debrief following her midterm review, in an area that was not within earshot of others but was within eyesight of others. She successfully completed her internship, met all learning goals, and accomplished additional abilities in her forthright and appropriate assertive communication with her supervising instructor. Imagine if the student had not elected to report and take appropriate action.

Bullying has been described as the sexual harassment of this generation.[1] Do not be one who allows any type of bullying to thrive. Trust yourself that you have the ability to address bullying behavior, whether it is your being subject to inappropriate language (cussing, foul language) by someone ranting and raving or your being purposefully embarrassed in front of others by those charged to provide constructive feedback. You should no longer just ignore bullying behavior, yet appropriately confront the abuse or potentially abusive behavior so that it does not escalate and the workplace is healthier for you, the rehab team, and the patients/clients we serve. Remember that, as a student, you are in a partnership with the clinical affiliate and the university or school, and you should seek support in the process for the important conversations that need to occur in a professional manner. Seek additional counseling and support services and security measures to be taken, if needed.

The following exercises begin with self-awareness about your own tendencies to respond passively or aggressively in certain situations. The exercises proceed into opportunities for you to practice assertive communication with your classmates in role-playing situations. Don't forget to journal about the impact that the readings and exercises have on you. How does all of this make you feel? For some of you, at first your new behavior will feel awkward and disingenuous. For many of us, we've overlearned the feelings that accompany low self-esteem and need to dramatically break up harmful, reactive behaviors to false beliefs, so assertive communication may be very challenging for you. Practice. Ideally, we could all experience the necessary inner transformations quickly and congruently. Life is a bit more complex, so start the process from outside-in rather than from inside-out. The goal is the same. The outer behavior, as inauthentic as it feels—for example, to be equal to a physician or experienced colleague—is still in everyone's best interest. Act as if you have every one of those rights, and eventually you will accept it as the truth. Act as you believe someone you admire would act in this situation. Soon you will feel the inner confidence needed to ensure authentic assertive and kind behavior under the greatest of stress. Believe in yourself; imagine your success and it will come quickly.

REFERENCES

1. The Workplace Bullying Institute. The WBI definition of workplace bullying. www.workplacebullying.org/individuals/problem/definition/. Accessed June 15, 2015.
2. Raynor C, Hoel H. A summary review of literature relating to workplace bullying. *J Community Appl Soc Psych*. 1997;7:181-191.
3. American Nurses Association 2010 House of Delegates Resolution: Hostility, Abuse and Bullying in the Workplace. Summary of Proceedings. https://nursing2015.files.wordpress.com/2012/04/hostilty.pdf. Accessed December 22, 2015.
4. The Joint Commission. Behaviors that undermine a culture of safety. Sentinel Event Alert. July 9, 2008. www.jointcommission.org/assets/1/18/SEA_40.PDF. Accessed May 5, 2015.
5. Healthy Work Place Bill. www.healthyworkplacebill.org/bill.php. Accessed May 5, 2015.
6. Daniel TA. Bullies in the workplace: a focus on the "abusive disrespect" of employees. http://thepeoplegroup.com/wp-content/uploads/2008/04/article-bullies-in-the-workplace1.pdf. Accessed March 15, 2015.
7. Timmins F, McCabe C. Nurses' and midwives' assertive behaviour in the workplace. *J Adv Nurs*. 2005;51(1):38-45.
8. Friedman FB. A nurse's guide to the care and handling of MDs. *RN*. 1982;45(3):39-43,118-120.
9. Bosher S, Smalkoski K. From needs analysis to curriculum development: designing a course in health care communication for immigrant students in the USA. *English for Specific Purposes*. 2002;21:59-79.
10. Merriam-Webster Online Dictionary, 2015. www.merriam-webster.com/. Accessed May 1, 2015.
11. Chenevert M. *STAT: Special Techniques in Assertiveness Training for Women in Health Professions*. 4th ed. St. Louis, MO: CV Mosby; 1993.
12. Alberti RE, Emmons ML. *Your Perfect Right*. 9th ed. San Luis Obispo, CA: Impact Publishers; 2008.
13. Anderson C, Jennings DL. When experiences of failure promote expectations of success: the impact of attributing failure to ineffective strategies. *J Pers*. 1980;48(3):393-407.
14. Weiner B. Attribution theory and attributional therapy: some theoretical observations and suggestions. *Br J Clin Psychol*. 1988;27(pt 1):93-104.
15. Curtis K. Altering beliefs about the importance of strategy: an attributional intervention. *J Appl Soc Psychol*. 1992;22(12):953-972.
16. Bower SA, Bower GH. *Asserting Yourself: A Practical Guide for Positive Change*. Boston, MA: DeCapo Press; 2004.
17. Silber M. Managing confrontations: once more into the breach. *Nurs Manage*. 1984;15(4):54-58.
18. Allaire B, McNeil R. *Teaching Patient Relations in Hospitals: The Hows and Whys*. Chicago, IL: American Hospital Association; 1983.
19. Lin YR, Shiah IS, Chang YC, Lai TJ, Want KY, Chou KR. Evaluation of an assertiveness training program on nursing and medical students' assertiveness, self-esteem and interpersonal communication. *Nurse Educ Today*. 2004;24(8):656-665.
20. Stubbs B, Soundy A. Physiotherapy students' experiences of bullying on clinical internships: an exploratory study. *Physiotherapy*. 2013;99(2):1781-180.
21. Askew DA, Schluter PJ, Dick ML, Régo PM, Turner C, Wilkinson D. Bullying in the Australian medical workforce: cross-sectional data from an Australian e-Cohort study. *Aust Health Rev*. 2012;36:197-204.
22. Crutcher RA, Szafran O, Woloschuk W, Chatur F, Hansen C. Family medicine graduates' perceptions of intimidation, harassment, and discrimination during residency training. *BMC Med Educ*. 2011;11:88.
23. Bairy KL, Thirumalaikolundusubramanian P, Sivagnanam G, Saraswathi S, Sachidananda A, Shalini A. Bullying among trainee doctors in Southern India: a questionnaire study. *J Postgrad Med*. 2007;53:87-90.
24. Frank E, Carrera JS, Stratton T, Bickel J, Nora LM. Experiences of belittlement and harassment and their correlates among medical students in the United States: longitudinal survey. *BMJ*. 2006;333:682.
25. Ahmer SYA, Bhutto N, Alam S, Sarangzai AK, Iqbal A. Bullying medical students in Pakistan: a cross-sectional questionnaire survey. *PLoS One*. 2008;3:e3889.
26. Mukhtar F, Daud S, Manzoor I, et al. Bullying of medical students. *J Coll Physicians Surg*. 2010;20:814-818.
27. Department of Health. Bullying of staff within the National Health Services Trust. London, UK: Department of Health; 2008.
28. Cheema S, Ahmad K, Giri SK, Kaliaperumal VK, Naqvi SA. Bullying of junior doctors prevails in Irish health system: a bitter reality. *Irish Med J*. 2005;98:274-275.
29. Whiteside D, Stubbs B, Soundy A. Physiotherapy students' experiences of bullying on clinical internships: a qualitative study. *Physiotherapy*. 2014;100(1):41-46.
30. Chartered Society of Physiotherapy. Dealing with bullying: a guide for physiotherapy students on clinical placement. London, UK: Chartered Society of Physiotherapy; 2010.

EXERCISES

EXERCISE 1: SELF-AWARENESS: ASSERTIVENESS INVENTORY

Complete the Assertiveness Inventory from Alberti and Emmons's *Your Perfect Right*.[12] As directed at the bottom of the survey, circle the 3 statements that most often result in your giving up your power and becoming passive or so angry that you become aggressive.

1.   Look at your responses to questions 1, 2, 4, 5, 6, 7, 9, 10, 11, 12, 14, 15, 16, 17, 18, 19, 21, 22, 24, 25, 27, 28, 30, and 35. These questions are oriented toward nonassertive behavior. Are you rarely speaking up for yourself? Or is there one situation that gives you more trouble than the others? If so, journal about it starting with the earliest memories you have about that incident.

2.   Look at your responses to questions 3, 8, 13, 20, 23, 26, 29, 31, 32, 33, and 34. These questions are oriented toward aggressive behavior. Are you pushing others around more than you realized? Does one question give you more trouble than the others? Again, journal about it.

3.   Few people are assertive, aggressive, or passive all the time. The situation often dictates the response. On rereading your total responses, do you see a pattern? Do you favor one way of responding over the others? Draw some conclusions about yourself from the inventory and journal about them. Which situations cause you the most trouble? Which situations do you handle with no trouble at all? Why is that?

4.   Can you identify obstacles that stand in the way of asserting yourself confidently? What beliefs do you hold about yourself and the world that make it difficult or easy to assert yourself? What is the worst thing that could happen? Journal about your learning.

5.   Ask family members and trusted friends to give you honest and specific feedback about their observations of your behavior under stress. Do you show patterns of passivity or aggressiveness? Ask them to illustrate their points with examples. Resist the natural desire to defend yourself as they respond. Just listen and take notes, then journal about what you learned and about your feelings.

ASSERTIVENESS INVENTORY

The following questions will be helpful in assessing your assertiveness. Be honest in your responses. All you have to do is draw a circle around the number that describes you best. For some questions, the assertive end of the scale is at 0, for others at 4. Key: 0=no or never, 1=somewhat or sometimes, 2=average, 3=usually or a good deal, 4=practically always or entirely.

1.   When a person is highly unfair, do you call it to his or her attention? 0 1 2 3 4
2.   Do you find it difficult to make decisions? 0 1 2 3 4
3.   Are you openly critical of others' ideas, opinions, behavior? 0 1 2 3 4
4.   Do you speak out in protest when someone takes your place in line? 0 1 2 3 4
5.   Do you often avoid people or situations for fear of embarrassment? 0 1 2 3 4
6.   Do you usually have confidence in your own judgment?..0 1 2 3 4
7.   Do you insist that your spouse or roommate take on a fair share of household chores?.........0 1 2 3 4
8.   Are you prone to "fly off the handle"? 0 1 2 3 4
9.   When a salesperson makes an effort, do you find it hard to say "no" even though the merchandise is not really what you want? 0 1 2 3 4
10. When a latecomer is waited on before you are, do you call attention to the situation?...........0 1 2 3 4
11. Are you reluctant to speak up in a discussion or debate? 0 1 2 3 4
12. If a person has borrowed money or a book/garment/thing of value and is overdue in returning it, do you mention it?..0 1 2 3 4
13. Do you continue to pursue an argument after the other person has had enough? 0 1 2 3 4
14. Do you generally express what you feel? 0 1 2 3 4
15. Are you disturbed if someone watches you at work? 0 1 2 3 4
16. If someone seems to be kicking or bumping your chair in a movie or a lecture, do you ask the person to stop?..0 1 2 3 4
17. Do you find it difficult to keep eye contact when talking to another person?.........................0 1 2 3 4
18. In a good restaurant, when your meal is improperly prepared or served, do you ask the waiter/waitress to correct the situation?..0 1 2 3 4
19. When you discover merchandise is faulty, do you return it for an adjustment?.......................0 1 2 3 4
20. Do you show your anger by name-calling or obscenities? 0 1 2 3 4
21. Do you try to be a wallflower or a piece of the furniture in social situations?........................0 1 2 3 4
22. Do you insist that your landlord/mechanic/repairperson make repairs, adjustments, or replacements that are his or her responsibility? 0 1 2 3 4
23. Do you often step in and make decisions for others? 0 1 2 3 4
24. Are you able to openly express love and affection? 0 1 2 3 4
25. Are you able to ask your friends for small favors or help? 0 1 2 3 4
26. Do you think you always have the right answer? 0 1 2 3 4
27. When you differ with a person you respect, are you able to speak up for your own viewpoint?...0 1 2 3 4
28. Are you able to refuse unreasonable requests made by friends? 0 1 2 3 4
29. Do you have difficulty complimenting or praising others? 0 1 2 3 4
30. If you are disturbed by someone smoking near you, can you say so? 0 1 2 3 4
31. Do you shout or use bullying tactics to get others to do as you wish?....................................0 1 2 3 4
32. Do you finish other people's sentences for them?..0 1 2 3 4
33. Do you get into physical fights with others, especially with strangers? 0 1 2 3 4
34. At family meals, do you control the conversation? 0 1 2 3 4
35. When you meet a stranger, are you the first to introduce yourself and begin a conversation?...0 1 2 3 4

Now go back and circle the 3 statements that most often result in you giving up your powers and becoming passive or that anger you so much you become aggressive.

(Reprinted with permission from Alberti RE, Emmons ML. *Your Perfect Right.* 2nd ed. San Luis Obispo, CA: Impact Publishers; 1974.)

EXERCISE 2: ASSERTIVE, AGGRESSIVE, AND PASSIVE RESPONSES

Practice making responses to the following situations. The first situation is done for you as an example.

Saying No

The head nurse stops you on the floor as you are just about to evaluate a new patient. "Mr. Johnson needs to be supervised in the use of his walker as he goes to the bathroom, and none of us have time. I wonder if you'd mind walking with him right now."

1. Passive: "Well, I'm very busy, but if he has to go right now, I suppose I can help."

2. Aggressive: "Look, I taught him how to use that walker. It's your job to supervise him in bathroom activity. I've got a patient to evaluate, and I don't appreciate your inconsiderate views of the value of my time."

3. Assertive: "No, I can't do that right now. Mrs. Adams is able to help him, as can his family members. I have a new evaluation that can't wait."

Making Requests

It's the end of the day and you have 3 more patients to evaluate before leaving. You're going to need some help or you'll be working very late. How do you ask for it?

1. Passive:

2. Aggressive:

3. Assertive:

Expressing Opinions

An edict comes down from above that all staff must treat at least 4 "units" of patient care per hour. You feel that this is unreasonable and interferes with establishing a therapeutic presence with your patients. How do you respond?

1. Passive:

2. Aggressive:

3. Assertive:

Initiating Conversation

You're attending a workshop and you've always wanted to talk with the speaker about a topic of great interest to you. You feel shy and somewhat intimidated by the speaker and his reputation.

1. Passive:

2. Aggressive:

3. Assertive:

Self-Disclosing

Your parents are in the midst of a year-long divorce battle that has brought great grief to your younger brother. Last night, he called you and spoke of thoughts of suicide. They live far away, and you feel frightened and helpless. At work, you seem distracted and upset. A friend asks, "Is there anything wrong? You seem preoccupied today."

1. Passive:

2. Aggressive:

3. Assertive:

Expressing Affection

A patient who you have been working with is being discharged. You go to the room, and his family is there packing to help him move back home. He asks to speak to you privately and takes your hand and thanks you for everything you've done for him and gives you a warm hug.

1. Passive:

2. Aggressive:

3. Assertive:

Entering a Room of Strangers

You've just moved to a new city to begin your first position after graduating. A new colleague invites you over for a party. You walk into the apartment and you realize you do not know one person in the room except the host. Everyone else seems to have known each other for years. No one is dressed the way you are.

1. Passive:

2. Aggressive:

3. Assertive:

Reflect in your journal which of these situations was easiest for you to envision handling assertively and which was most difficult. Which responses were easiest to come up with? Do you find that how you might respond has very much to do with your perception of the stress inherent in the situation?

EXERCISE 3: ASSERTIVE COMMUNICATION

In this chapter, you learned about DISC and DESC communication. Now you have a chance to role-play various assertive responses to the following vignettes. Before role-playing, however, you are asked to write the DISC or DESC response. The practitioner or student is in the assertive response position; the other person should use this opportunity to practice the active listening skills learned in Chapter 7. A third person serves as the observer, giving feedback at the end of the dialogue on the effectiveness of the communication. Use the Observer Response Guidance that follows to jot down your observations as they occur. Each person should choose an appropriate vignette and write a DISC or DESC statement before breaking up into groups of 3. For each vignette, write a DESC response and then role-play practicing the DESC/DISC communication.

Vignette 1

You are a student on your first of 2 final clinical assignments. The clinical facility is very high-powered, with a superior reputation. You feel that no matter what you do, you could never achieve the level that is expected of the staff. You truly feel that you're doing your best, but you are under constant stress to prove yourself. You are to be checked out on a knee evaluation, but you've forgotten some of the basic steps, and you've asked for help from the orthopedic star of the staff, who always says, "Yes, but I'm too busy. Catch me tomorrow." Your clinical instructor stops you as you are ready to go home and relax at the end of the day and says, "I've let you off the hook long enough. You should have that knee evaluation down by now. Come with me and let me check you out."

Vignette 2

You are a clinical instructor. You've observed your student for 3 weeks and feel that she may be weak in evaluation skills, and you feel that she is not taking the assignment seriously. When you suggest a check-off session, your student always asks for more time. Yet all you hear is talk about lots of parties and after-hours fun, and you notice a real reluctance to read or show initiative in looking things up or asking for help. You think she might be trying to squeeze through without the appropriate amount of responsibility. You've decided to confront your student and ask for check-off on a knee evaluation.

Vignette 3

You've just accepted a position at a health care facility that also has an active student program. The staff seems to ignore the dress regulations and everyone wears what he or she wishes, so you decide you will wear what you wish as well and come to work in comfortable clothes: hip-huggers and a tunic top. Your supervisor tells you to go home and change your clothes and come back in the "regulation uniform." You decide to confront him or her.

Vignette 4

In the middle of a treatment, your patient, a young and rather seductive member of the opposite sex, grabs your arm and tells you that he or she has very strong sexual feelings for you and wonders if you might meet privately at the end of the day.

Vignette 5

You are a professional on the staff for more than a year. You still lack skill in one treatment technique that an aide knows how to do flawlessly. In front of the patient, the aide comes up to you and chastises you for not knowing how to do even the simplest procedures. You are embarrassed and decide to confront the aide.

Vignette 6

Your colleague, who always takes advantage of others, comes up to you in front of a patient and asks you to cover for her because she has to make an important phone call. She disappears and does not return for 2 hours. When she returns, you decide to confront her.

Vignette 7

You are instructing a 35-year-old woman in pelvic stabilization exercises, and the patient is having difficulty recruiting her lower abdominals and pelvic floor. Suddenly, the patient begins to cry, saying that her back hurts so much that she and her husband have not been able to be intimate for 6 months and she feels as if he no longer desires her. How do you respond? (Hint: Resist the common desire to fix patients' problems, and remember active listening skills.)

Vignette 8

Your supervisor notices that you are taking longer than is common for a patient treatment with one of your patients who has suffered a stroke. She suggests you delegate the care of this patient to an assistant. You believe the patient requires the attention of a professional. What do you say?

Vignette 9

KYLE

Chuck has been your clinical instructor/fieldwork supervisor for the past 4 weeks on your final clinical education internship and has already identified you as a potential for some opportunities at the hospital in the future. Chuck is easy to work with and has given you a great deal of autonomy. You feel comfortable making your own decisions and are quite satisfied with your style of patient care management. You are happy to be entering practice in a few more months.

CHUCK

You are Kyle's instructor and you are pleased with Kyle's overall progress and patient care. However, lately you have noticed that Kyle has been letting his long hair and facial hair become excessive, and even though he pulls his hair back in a ponytail for patient care, you noticed it getting caught up in the patient's underarm when he was instructing the patient with crutch training and again when he was doing shoulder mobilizations. Kyle's beard has grown out excessively, and some of your coworkers say he is looking "criminal." How can you, as his clinical instructor, confront Kyle using the DESC/DISC method to assure that he understands not only the safety and hygiene factors but also the consequences in terms of his professionalism ratings?

Vignette 10

Your student, LaTonya, has just decided to poke the patient in intermediate care with her long fingernails to check for pain sensation. You recommend to your student that she use monofilaments for testing sensory status. The recommendation was not accepted. Later after lunch, you overhear LaTonya gossiping about another staff member in a negative light to other students in a disrespectful manner. Use the DESC/DISC to confront the student and affect a change.

Vignette 11

Review your responses from the Assertiveness Inventory in Exercise 1. Create a vignette that typifies a situation that is predictably problematic for you. Teach your partner how to act in a way that is sure to elicit passive or aggressive behavior from you. Then write a DISC or DESC response and role-play.

Observer Response Guidance

As an observer, your role is to facilitate a dialogue that has an adequate assertive response. The dialogue may begin with the aggressor making the statement that requires the assertive response, or it may begin with time having elapsed since the incident and the assertive response is occurring now. Keep track of time, and keep the interchange to 2 or 3 minutes. At the conclusion, **ask the assertive responder how he or she feels and then ask the other partner the same**. Proceed to give feedback to both on these various aspects of their communication.

1. How well did the assertive communicator:

    a. Communicate using "I" statements and DISC or DESC responses?

    b. Stay nonaggressive, nonjudgmental, and nonaccusatory?

    c. Listen and respond in an assertive way to the other's response?

2. How well did the aggressor use active listening skills and still stay in character?

3. How would you suggest each could improve his or her communication?

The exercises at the end of this chapter are also available online.
Please refer to the sticker in the front of the book and enter the access code provided.

READINESS FOR REFLECTIVE PRACTICE

PEER AND SELF-ASSESSMENT

Gina Maria Musolino, PT, MSEd, EdD

"An unexamined life is not worth living." –Socrates

OBJECTIVES

- To understand the concept of self-assessment (SA) and reflective practice (RP) theories.
- To apply and practice self-assessment and peer assessment (PA) to facilitate reflective practice.
- To point out the barriers, challenges, and support for peer and self-assessment.
- To explore students' awareness and perceptions of reflective practice, self-assessment, and peer assessment capabilities as determinants for development as a health care professional (HCP).
- To appreciate the professional responsibilities and gifts of peer and self-assessment, along with potential impacts for patient care and development toward expertise in practice.
- To consider career development and lifelong learning opportunities, in relation to peer and self-assessment, including the role of clinical education instruction.

YOUR THOUGHTS AND ASSUMPTIONS

Let's start by thinking about peer and self-assessment. Jot down or share your thoughts and assumptions for the following queries:

- What is self-assessment? Peer assessment?
- Why should you consider doing self-assessment? Peer assessment?
- What might be some of the challenges and barriers to doing self-assessment? Peer assessment?
- What might be some of the support and rewards for doing self-assessment? Peer assessment?
- What is reflective practice?

What does a health care professional need to know about reflective practice to develop one? Is any health care professional able to be a reflective practitioner? How can merely reflecting on one's work improve practice? How does the theory of reflective practice relate to the profession's values and professional codes of ethics, which you learned about in Chapter 3?

Davis CM, Musolino GM. *Patient Practitioner Interaction: An Experiential Manual for Developing the Art of Health Care, Sixth Edition* (pp 139-157).
© 2016 SLACK Incorporated.

REFLECTIVE PRACTICE: CONCEPTS

When the concept of reflective practice is first encountered, many wonder why it is of value or worth taking the time and energy to complete. Initially, you may find this novel, foreign, esoteric, or just plain peculiar or strange. The concepts of self-assessment and tenets of reflective practice theories do not necessarily match with how you think you should be taught or learn. Many think that being a clinician is all about knowing skills and applying techniques.

Certainly, appropriate skill levels and proper techniques are needed and required elements for professional practice; however, how we arrive at the best choices for our evidence-based practice skills and become more proficient with our techniques are what distinguishes us from nonprofessionals. To become the best health care professional, this is a matter of reflective practice. Try to be open-minded because becoming less reliant on traditional, passive teaching as an emerging health care professional and enhancing your self-assessment abilities as a developing reflective health care professional will lead to expertise in practice sooner rather than later for the willing health care professional. Reflective practice leads to improved academic performance and enhanced metacognitive skills for a novice health care professional, which benefits your patients' clinical outcomes.[1-7]

Remember to be journaling along the way as you develop your reflective practice abilities as a new health care professional. In relation to reflective practice, cogitate on the key words of Sir William Osler (1849-1919), Canadian medical physician and founder of Johns Hopkins Hospital, who stated that when education is done right, the learner "begins with the patient, continues with the patient, and ends with the patient."

Let's look more closely at the concepts and tenets of self-assessment and examine the theories of reflective practice. Osterman and Kottkamp[8] defined the purpose of reflection as two-fold: "(1) to initiate a behavioral change, and (2) to realize an improvement in professional practice." Kirby and Teddlie[9] defined a reflective practitioner as one who has "the ability to integrate research with practice in response to uncertainty and complexity that, citing, according to Russell and Spafford,[10] qualifies the practitioner for professional status. This theory is vital to occupations where theory is incomplete or where multiple, even conflicting theories confront the practitioner."

Does the definition of a reflective practitioner match up with your profession? The theory and tenets of reflective practice have been examined and continue to be studied in the professions of architecture, art, teaching, law, medicine, nursing, physical and occupational therapy, pharmacy, dentistry, etc. According to Brookfield,[11] the concept of reflective practice is defined as:

> *Rooted in the Enlightenment idea that we can stand outside of ourselves and come to a clearer understanding of what we do and who we are by freeing ourselves of distorted ways of reasoning and acting. There are also elements of constructivist phenomenology in the understanding that identity and experience are culturally and personally sculpted, rather than existing in some kind of objectively discoverable limbo.*

Hence, reflective practice is not a passive process but an active one that challenges us to see ourselves as others see us. As reflective practitioners, we are challenged to think about what we do and how we act, to consider alternatives and reason through the possibilities, and to consider options while simultaneously noting the environmental and cultural influences.

Dewey,[12] an American philosopher, psychologist, and educational and social reformist, purported reflection as a cognitive activity that begins in perplexity and "forked-road" situations but is an active, persistent, and careful consideration of any belief or knowledge. Dewey[12] first identified reflection as a cognitive activity with 5 stages of reflective thought:

1. Perplexity, confusion, doubt;
2. Attentive interpretation of the given elements;
3. Examination, exploration, and analysis to define and clarify the problem;
4. Elaboration of the tentative hypothesis; and
5. Testing the hypothesis by doing something overtly to bring about anticipated results.

The cognitive activity of reflection includes a responsibility for future consequences and is retrospective and progressive. Osterman and Kottkamp[8] shared 6 key assumptions for reflective practice:

1. Everyone, regardless of age, stage, or attitude, needs professional growth opportunities.
2. All professionals have a natural desire to want to improve.
3. All professionals want to learn.
4. All professionals are capable of assuming responsibility for their own professional growth and development.
5. All people need and want information about their performance.
6. Collaboration with other professionals enriches one's professional development.

Kolb[13] advanced reflection a step further and noted that reflection should be to take action to a new and changed behavior. He detailed this concept in the experiential learning cycle, where a learner flows through concrete experiences, reflective observation, abstract conceptualization, and active experimentation. Kolb's[13] learning style approach provides the opportunity for input and processing of information. He described how learners reflect on experiences, learn from these experiences, then try out what they have learned and cycle through again on subsequent practice attempts, leading to enhanced metacognition through reflection activities. Oftentimes, we may get hung up in one aspect of the cycle, and that is where it is of benefit to consult with colleagues or those who think differently from our preferred style or approach to learning.

REFLECTIVE PRACTICE: METHODS AND MODELS

Why is this critical reflection so important? Brookfield[11] asserted that it helps professionals to make informed decisions and take informed actions and to develop a rationale for practice. Brookfield[11] believed that it "helps professionals avoid self-laceration, serves for emotional grounds, enlivens professional practices, and increases democratic trust." The importance was elaborated on by Donald Schön,[14,15] an influential thinker who developed the theory of reflective practice for professional learning in the 20th century. He asserted that managing the complexity is the challenge for the reflective practitioner.[14,15] He also maintained that a reflective practitioner has an unprecedented requirement for adaptability and is cognizant of the tension between theory and practice.[15] He alluded to the balance of the art and science in the health professions.[14,15] Schön[14,15] believed in the reflective practice concepts of *reflection-in-action*, *knowing-in-action*, *reflection-on-action*, and *recognizing surprise* in terms of professional work interactions. These frameworks serve us well to foster reflective practice abilities. We can reflect within these frameworks and ask ourselves guiding questions to facilitate our abilities in reflective practice using the tenets of theory as a guide (eg, "How do you think that went while you were performing the technique?").

- **Reflection-in-action:** As you performed the grade I to grade II mobilizations, you realized, based on prior experience with mobilization and on the patient's response and joint movement perceived, that you could proceed with the next level of mobilization and moved readily to grade III without hesitation.

How did you know that you would get the expected result from the technique?

- **Knowing-in-action:** As you performed rhythmic stabilization with the patient, how did you know that the technique would illicit the outcome you expected?

How do you think you did? Did you get the outcomes you were hoping for with the techniques? What could you have done differently? Is there another approach?

- **Reflection-on-action:** Over the weekend, while taking your morning swim, you are thinking back about the patient you worked with last Thursday. You realized that you could likely have reached her better by using a visual approach to her learning when instructing her in the home exercise program and that you may have overloaded her with too much written information. You forgot to ask her about her preferred learning style in her history, but you recalled how well she responded when you first demonstrated proper lifting techniques, first showing her and then allowing her to repeat-demonstrate to you the proper technique.

How could you have done better? What is going well? How can you progress from here?

Schön[15] stated that "good practice generates new knowledge." He looked critically at how a professional readjusts in day-to-day practice as key for development.[14,15] Hatcher and Bringle[16] echoed Schön's[14,15] sentiments, with clear linkages to self-assessment. They noted that reflection activities develop self-assessment skills, as a life-long learner, and explore and clarify values that can lead to civic responsibility. They believed reflection activities serve to "...engage students in the intentional consideration of their experiences in light of particular learning objectives and provide an opportunity for students to do the following:

- Gain further understanding of the course content and discipline;
- Gain further understanding of the service experience;
- Develop self-assessment skills, as a life-long learner; and
- Explore and clarify values that can lead to civic responsibility."

The reflection activities incorporate learning from experiences in society, such as through clinical and fieldwork education, in the health professions, and service learning activities that meet objectives for those served and the learners. Eyler et al[17] considered the "4 Cs of reflection" as viable activities for the development of reflective practice, including the following:

1. Continuous reflection
2. Connected reflection

3. Challenging reflection

4. Conceptualized reflection

Likewise, Williams and Driscoll[18] proposed the following guidelines for facilitating reflection: "Structured as ongoing aspects of a course (or clinical), offered in multiple forms, included in assessment, modeled by the instructor, connected to the course content, and supported by class context." Hatcher and Bringle[16] offered the following examples of reflection activities: personal journals, directed readings and writings, case studies with guiding questions, portfolios with self-assessments, rubrics with self-assessment techniques, experiential research, service-learning with opportunities for reflection, and personal narratives.

Osterman and Kottkamp[8] defined reflective practice as a "professional development strategy designed to enable professionals to change their behavior, thereby improving the quality of their performance." They contended that reflective practice is neither a solitary nor a relaxed meditative process; rather, it is a demanding practice that is most often successful in a **collaborative mode**.[8] Reflective practice exposes the discrepancy between theory and practice and creates a self-awareness of the unacceptable outcomes and drives toward a new behavioral change for development. Hence, reflective practice is not only an active and collaborative process, it is one of maturation as a health care professional and peer colleague. Provided in appropriate contexts, as a peer colleague, peer assessment provides an invaluable gift for professional growth.

May et al[19] identified that students in physical therapy, according to clinical instructors and clinical coordinators of clinical education, need to be able to demonstrate the ability to **self-assess**, **self-correct**, **and self-direct** in their commitment to learning as shared in the developed professional behaviors abilities instrument. The Professional Behaviors Assessment Tool will be further examined in Chapter 11 (see Table 11-1). The American Physical Therapy Association (APTA) Clinical Performance Instrument[20] (APTA CPI) and American Occupational Therapy Association (AOTA) Fieldwork Performance Evaluation Form[21] require that students in clinical education or fieldwork experiences self-assess their abilities in terms of performance criteria for professional development and professional practice management, along with the clinical instructor's or fieldwork instructor's assessment. Students who do not develop requisite professional behaviors are more likely to be deficient in terms of the critical behaviors and skills that are foundational elements for practice and essential to professional competence within the professions.[19] The evaluative tools require quantitative ratings and narrative statements with respect to SAs.

The APTA and AOTA national professional member associations provide the opportunity for licensed practitioners to use tools for self-assessment of their clinical/fieldwork instructor abilities. To assist new and experienced clinical instructors, both national associations offer basic and advanced training for the instructors through the AOTA Fieldwork Educators Certificate Workshop[22] and the APTA Credentialed Clinical Instructor Programs (CCIP)–Basic and Advanced[23] to address identified needs from the self-assessment for continuing competency to enhance clinical educators' skills and abilities. Many of the skills are translatable to administration, management, and supervision of support staff, as well as enhanced patient/client management, especially in terms of education and conflict negotiation. The AOTA and APTA trainings, to credential clinical and field work instructors, incorporate peer and self-assessment. Although the time may seem far away when you are deeply immersed in your new health care professional education, as an early career health care professional, you should consider the credentialing training in your career pathway to further develop your reflective practice skills and abilities and to continue the opportunity to pay it forward as a future clinical or fieldwork instructor.

Once you are a licensed health care professional, assessments for continuing competence entail various formats of self-assessment and often incorporate peer assessment for maintaining contemporary knowledge and licensure; hence, fostering reflective practice capabilities remains relevant throughout your career and for pursuing advanced specializations.

Today, more than 50,000 physical therapists and physical therapist assistants are APTA Credentialed Clinical Instructors. Musolino et al[24] examined why more than 300 licensed health care professionals in the state of Florida sought the APTA CCIP credential and determined their learning goals and outcomes postcourse. They discovered that the participants overwhelmingly would recommend the continuing competency course to a colleague.[24] Musolino et al[24] reported that CCIP participants readily achieved learning outcomes that facilitated the subject's reflective practice skills as a clinical instructor, especially in the areas of communication, feedback and assessment methods, teaching and learning styles, goal setting, and goal-writing skills, along with formative feedback methods for the student's learning and progression as a reflective practitioner.

Let's now consider reflective practice statements, modified from Kirby and Teddlie's[9] reflective teaching instrument. As you reflect on each statement, please consider your level of agreement in your own practice or in your observations of other health care professionals:

- I feel that it is important for me to integrate theory and research into my health care professional practice.

- It is incumbent upon me as a good health care professional to be familiar with current research in my profession.

- I often revise my practice methods after trying them with a patient.
- I want my patients to question my way of looking at things.
- I often think about the hidden agenda (ie, does my practice help my patients adopt the values and attitudes I want them to acquire for their health?).
- I sometimes find myself changing practice strategies in the middle of a treatment session.
- If I can't get through to a particular patient, I experiment with different approaches.
- If my patients are having trouble in the health care setting, it is up to me to find a solution.
- I have a great deal of influence on the personality and attitudes of my patients.
- I can make the least motivated patient like therapy.
- If my patients do poorly in therapy, I blame myself.
- I'm responsible for the behavior of the patients under my care.
- In my practice setting, I should have the final decision in determining what is to be done and how.

While considering each of these statements, you likely had varying levels of agreement based on your experiences or that of observing others or the amount of accountability and responsibility you may consider to be in or out of your control as a health care professional. You also likely acknowledged the need for problem-solving capacities and clinical decision-making skills as hallmarks for reflective professional practice.[25-27] You probably also noted aspects of personal causation within the reflective practice statements relative to the health care professional's ability to influence the patient and practice settings. As a health care professional, one cannot be totally personally responsible for all aspects of care, yet one can work to influence and change the multifactorial impacts of care. True reflection and experience are parallel to achieving action and a new and changed behavior with reflective practice,[13-15,19] and as you will soon learn, the environment also has a large impact on our abilities to peer and self-assess.

Schön's[15] work describes reflective practice as the "ability to critically and deliberately think about the things that happen in daily practice in order to learn from them, in action, as well as after the events happen." Peters[27] built upon Schön's works and offered the following:

> *Reflective practice involves more than simply thinking about what one is doing and what one should do next. It involves identifying one's assumptions and feelings associated with practice, theorizing about how these assumptions and feelings are functionally or dysfunctionally associated with practice, and acting on the basis of the resulting theory of practice.*

Smith et al[28] devised a method to assist in simplifying one's abilities to introduce reflective practice through the *Describe, Analyze, Theorize, and Act (DATA) model*. Although this framework is simple, it helps promote the novice's ability to begin the concept of reflective practice through self-assessment. Each step in the model is interrelated to the others. The DATA model makes the reflective practice steps straightforward and overlaps with some of the thought processes while practically bridging theory into real-world practice. An adapted summary of the DATA model is shown in Table 9-1[28]; we shall revisit it with the chapter exercises. You will likely find it helpful when applied to problem-solving with patient/client cases and when your self-assessment may be incongruent with others' assessment of you and/or in conflicting situations in relations with others.

REFLECTIVE PRACTICE: PEER AND SELF-ASSESSMENT

So what is self-assessment exactly? At the beginning of the chapter, you were asked to consider how you defined self-assessment, what you believed were barriers or challenges to self-assessment, and why you might want to do this thing called self-assessment.

Practice in peer and self-assessment shall assist you in developing as a mature health care professional. Musolino[29] stated that self-assessment skills are not only essential for health care professionals but are crucial to becoming a reflective practitioner[14,29,30] and highly relevant for moving along the professional development continuum from novice to expert practice.[2-8,11,24,25,27,29,31] Musolino[29] reported, in her qualitative research study of self-assessment abilities, that to foster self-assessment for reflective practice, physical therapy students and new graduates required professionalism, reflection, time management, support, and change management. Musolino[29] discovered self-assessment was improved and promoted through a variety of self-starting, self-steering, self-directed, and self-pacing activities with subjects' motivation for professional competence and self-improvement. Related to practice effects, the greatest barriers to self-assessment, noted by the research subjects, were time, complacency, negativity, self-esteem, and lack of objectivity. However, the

TABLE 9-1
DATA Model
Describe: Identify and specify the situation at hand in detail, reflecting on the whole context and the setting; describe what has occurred and answer the following queries: *What is going on in this situation? Who is involved? What is the context? What happened?*
Analyze: Examine the "why" as a central focus; examine one's and other's beliefs, assumptions, biases, and preconceived notions. Consider practical questions: *How can I solve this dilemma? What is the best way to deal with the situation? Why are things going the way they are going? What are my assumptions and beliefs in this situation? What are/were your feelings and emotional responses? What was good? Bad?*
Theorize: Practical theory or practice-based reasoning addressing questions such as: *What do I believe is needed? Why is this solution better than other potential solutions? What has worked before and how well? Is there relevant literature to indicate this option is better than others? What sense can you make of the situation, and what resources might you need?*
Act: Determine the theoretically best solution to address the situation. Answer the following queries: *What are you going to do about it specifically? What is the developed plan of action? What steps are needed? What will you do differently in the future? What is your plan of action now?*
Adapted from Smith FL, Barlow PB, Peters JM, Skolits GJ. Demystifying reflective practice: using the DATA model to enhance evaluators' professional activities. *Eval Program Planning.* 2015;52:142-147.

greatest support for self-assessment included taking the time, seeking feedback, being honest and objective, creating a safe environment for feedback, setting goals, having supportive peers and faculty, and using the guides for written and oral assessments. Musolino's[29] study findings paralleled not only Schön's[14,30] concept of reflective practice but also supported Bandura's[32-35] social learning theory in the resulting developed, conceptual model of self-assessment (Figure 9-1).

Albert Bandura,[32] an innovative scholar who did pioneering work in social cognitive theory, related that people's level of motivation, affective states, and actions are based more on what they believe, rather than on objectivity, and that human behavior can only be understood in terms of a reciprocal interaction between external stimuli and internal cognition. Bandura[32-35] proposed that a fundamental way humans acquire skills and behaviors is by observing the behavior of others. The learner must be able to reproduce the behavior that has been observed. Sometimes the reproducible behavior stems from a lack of requisite cognitive or motor skills but often reflects the learner's lack of feedback about what the learner is actually trying to accomplish. Bandura[35] called this "reciprocal determinism": the world and a person's behavior cause each other, or one's environment causes behavior and behavior causes the environment. Converting reflective practice didactic skills into actual clinical abilities likely requires a transformative process for novice clinicians.

In my role as Director of Clinical Education, I see the transformation from novice to more experienced reflective practitioner when students take self-assessment and reflective practice seriously. Students work from initial unconscious incompetence toward more conscious competence in their professional development and practice management skills and abilities through self-assessment. Initially you will not know exactly what you don't know because you have never before been asked to be the professional you are becoming, and your clinical or fieldwork instructor is your guide on the side, facilitating your abilities and providing you with benchmarks and guidance. Your Director of Clinical Education and others may ask you to complete reflective practice activities in formative and summative ways to assist you in becoming more consciously competent. As you progress in your abilities with reflective practice, you shall become more enlightened, progress in your conscious competence, and ultimately realize how much more there is yet to know, even once you know what you do and do not know in practice!

An often-cited barrier to self-assessment abilities is time. Frankly, self-assessment does not take a lot of time. Certainly there are recesses when contemplating your navel and letting your mind wander are welcome reprieves from the hectic world we live in today. Self-assessment does not demand hours, but frequent moments and the opportunity to stop and reflect, and thus eventually makes it more of a habit or natural occurrence. Notably, people learn through experience and training, with unlearning occurring simultaneously. Deliberate efforts to learn involve action, reflection, and self-monitoring. Learning to learn becomes more of an awareness of self and active examination of what happens as learning

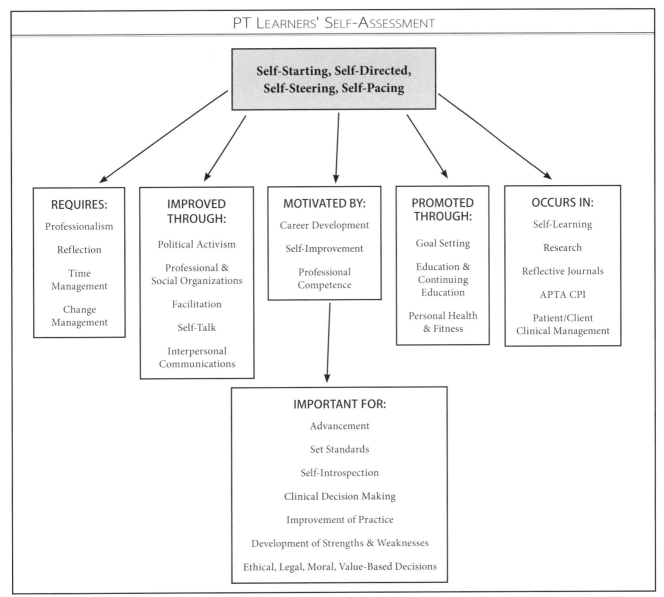

Figure 9-1. Conceptual model of physical therapy learners' perceptions of SA activities. APTA CPI = American Physical Therapy Association Clinical Performance Institute; PT = physical therapy. (Reprinted with permission from Musolino GM. Fostering reflective practice: self-assessment abilities of physical therapy students and entry-level graduates. *J Allied Health*. 2006;35[1]:37.)

occurs. Self-assessment, therefore, is not a laissez-faire approach to awarding the self, but the ability to critically self-evaluate in a systematic fashion. The heart of the learning process is developing the awareness and capacities for effective self-monitoring and active reflection.

Self-assessment is the ability to assess one's own skills, identify one's own educational needs, evaluate one's own progress, and determine one's performance.[36] Self-assessment is "not merely one who minimally qualifies, but one who seeks an ever more perfect understanding and performance of one's work."[37]

Peer assessment is essentially self-assessment, except it involves being constructively critical of your peer's performance and abilities, helping them to see themselves as you do, usually in relation to a set of standards or criteria. Peer assessment also improves your own metacognitive skills and abilities to provide constructive feedback, which you also need to do for your patients. The peer assessment process correspondingly provides the opportunity to further reflect on your work in a comparative manner as well. Peer and self-assessment may be initiated by simply asking thought-provoking questions verbally or in a guided journal reflection: *What went well? It would be even better if? The next step would be? How could you approach differently? What else could be the problem or going on? How did you incorporate your findings with your decision making along the way? Thinking back now, how might you approach differently? Thinking back, what additional information,*

TABLE 9-2		
SUMMARY OF BARRIERS AND SUPPORT FOR SELF-ASSESSMENT		
SUPPORT	**BARRIERS**	**BARRIER AND/OR SUPPORT**
Honesty	Awareness/complacency	Time
Observation/comparing	Dishonesty	Feedback/networking
Self-focus/self-talk	Unsafe environments	Peers and teamwork
Goal setting	Lack of goals	Faculty feedback or not
Objectivity	Pressure	
Written and oral SA	Negativity	
Cases/patients/projects	Payer demands	
Clinical faculty queries and debriefing	Lack of cultural competence	
Clinical performance instruments	Incongruent philosophy	
Portfolios and reflective journals	Low self-esteem	
Family	Ambiguity	
Positive self-esteem		
Ambiguity in practice		
Safe/supportive environment		
Reprinted with permission from Musolino GM. Fostering reflective practice: self-assessment abilities of physical therapy students and entry-level graduates. *J Allied Health.* 2006;35(1):30-42.		

if any, would you like to have gathered that you may have missed? Where in the learning do you think you might have been challenged? Explain your thought process in your approach before, during, and after the encounters.

Your peer and self-assessment should be substantive and not just simple, easy comments, but deeper assessment providing a true, meaningful gift of feedback for improvement and reinforcement. Do not just gloss over the feedback and introspection opportunities. Be hard on the problems or areas for improvement, not the person. Guide yourself and your peers.

Frequently, I ask my students and their instructors in clinical/fieldwork education to complete the **2-Minute Clinical Instructor activity**. I ask them to share with each other, **in 2 minutes' time, 2 things they are doing well and 2 things they need to work on** and then reverse roles the next time. The 2-Minute Clinical Instructor: Student learner exchange provides a platform for self-assessment and becoming more consciously competent of where you are, or are not, on the learning curve for your clinical/fieldwork education and, voila, it only takes 2 minutes! Rapid reflection also leads to enhanced abilities with deeper reflection.

Try it out! Have the 2-minute conversation with a peer. The brief time-out for fostering self-assessment is reassuring for you as the learner, to receive feedback and insights, and for your instructor to see that you are proactive in your learning processes. The 2-Minute Clinical Instructor is a formative feedback opportunity and is likely positive because it is meant to be informal, constructive, and transformative. Through the 2-Minute Clinical Instructor activity, you are provided with the gift of constructive feedback about your self-assessment and abilities to progress toward reflective practice and of achieving your clinical learning goals for patient care.

Once you have graduated, unless you have a strong mentor or colleague, which I hope you will, you will need to be more self-reliant on your abilities for self-assessment, and ultimately reflective practice, for the benefit of your patients and clients. The formative work of self-assessment, as you continue your professional development, shall guide you to achieving more understanding and insight into the performance of your work as a health care professional as you progress in your capabilities as an autonomous practitioner for your patients and society. Peer and faculty assessment can also be followed up by showing a peer what you were to improve, explaining or demonstrating how you have improved, and then asking for their additional feedback.

Time was mentioned previously as a perceived barrier for self-assessment, and additional barriers to self-assessment were discovered by Musolino,[29] which were also sometimes perceived as potentials for self-assessment support (Table 9-2). Being aware of the potential barriers and/or supports for self-assessment shall assist you in overcoming barriers and assuring you have the needed support for progressive self-assessment. Let's consider some reflective quotes from those who have gone before you in their professional development. For example, self-talk reflections of a new graduate clearly demonstrate tenets of Schön's[14,15] theory of reflective practice, noted in parentheses[29]:

> *I look at what I'm doing and what I've done and try to decide if it's the right thing, the wrong thing, how I can change, how I can make it better...am I prepared to treat this person, was I prepared to handle this situation or that situation (recognizing surprise), this new person that came in, this returning person that...what do I need to know...what did I do good (knowing-in-action)...what should I have done differently, what would have helped for the future...I think about this during the situation (reflection-in-action), at the end of the day, driving home in the car (reflection-on-action), it spans everything from treatment sessions to time management or administration of care...reviewing step-by-step how to improve to be ready for the next morning.*

> *I think as far as ethics, values, and morals, it is important too because if you don't reflect on those things you can make bad decisions or sometimes not necessarily bad, but not as good as they could be for the patient, or the best for your company or coworkers.*

Reflecting on these thoughts and potential barriers and/or support aspects of self-assessment will assist you on your journey to becoming a reflective practitioner and being present and capable of best serving your patients/clients and supporting your peers and colleagues in the process of self-assessment for best practice. Now, let's consider the reflective thoughts of a few professional students immersed in training regarding their support and/or barriers to doing self-assessment in the classroom or laboratory[29]:

> *Sometimes people are afraid to give constructive criticism and this might hurt another when actually it is helpful when done correctly, but there has to be time and people can't say "that's a bunch of BS" or it is immediately stifled or they might say, "Just hurry up and get it over with"...the time crunch factor.*

> *In labs it can be kind of embarrassing, I don't like to admit that I'm really weak in this area, I compare myself to others and this can be a barrier because you may gain strengths and weaknesses and it's really hard to catch my own weaknesses...but if I have a video of myself that helps a lot to see a vision of yourself as a whole person and be able to break things down...especially with low self-esteem or someone who is joking around or making culturally derogatory statements that might be supposed to be in fun, but it is a big barrier.*

> *Sometimes you are lazy and just don't want to do it, it is a matter of putting forth the effort and taking the fifteen minutes during the day or night before I go to sleep, on the long drives on the commute home to just think and not letting others discourage you from doing self-assessment because it is important and can make a difference. ... I ask what have I learned, what do I need to learn, where do I need to go now to learn.*

In addition, let's also contemplate the importance of educators in the role of facilitating self-assessment from the learner's perspective[29]:

> *When I am "forced" to write down my peer and self-assessment or if others ask me that is helpful to self-assessment, when faculty pushes it and group interactions help too.*

> *It is the obligation of educators to make sure that they are not sending out people who are only going to be good for the next 6 months, but for the duration of their careers. And that's much like patient education, I can train someone how to walk with crutches down the busy hall, but if I don't educate them how to fall and other safety related issues, then I have not done them much justice either. Just like our patient, we need to think about what we are doing, how we are doing it, and what might need to change physically and behaviorally...constantly considering the changing environment.*

Some authors[2,11,29,31,38,39] have noted the influence of critical thought and reflective action through the process of self-assessment and the need for guided feedback to affect a change toward what Epstein[38] refers to as mindful practice. The novice learners and new graduates echoed the sentiments that professional education will be overshadowed by "unreflective doing"[38] if self-assessment does not remain at the forefront of day-to-day educational processes through the "teachable moments"[38,39] in clinics and classrooms. Students do not begin to learn until asking questions of themselves.[1] Much of what future clinicians may need to know for practice is not even known today and, consequently, cannot necessarily be taught. Hence, the importance in education lies in being able to teach learners how to acquire knowledge and to critically assess. Learners must master how to do self-assessment in relation to contemporary expectations and meeting the needs and responsibilities of patients and clients.[36-42]

As a novice practitioner, you may be more stressed by the fast-paced clinical environment; therefore, practice may, unfortunately, be more routine than reflective.[31] Similar to Orest's[43] findings with practicing physical therapist clinicians,

Musolino[29] discovered that learners in physical therapy and recent graduates were motivated to perform self-assessment through the desire for self-improvement, through career development, and through efforts for clinical and professional competence. These processes included advancement efforts; setting or achievement of practice standards; self-introspection efforts; clinical decision making; development of strengths and weaknesses; and ethical-, legal-, moral-, and value-based decision making. Learners believed that self-assessment is improved through self-talk, interpersonal communications, and mentoring in professional and social networks, and, in some cases, that it may lead to or be fostered through political activism.[29]

In Figure 9-1, the developed conceptual model for self-assessment is summarized.[29] **Consider how the conceptual model agrees or disagrees with your thoughts and assumptions regarding self-assessment from the beginning of the chapter.** The conceptual model of physical therapy learners' self-assessment may assist you in becoming increasingly sophisticated in your abilities to actively assess your own performance and that of your peers and enhance your lifelong learning through conscious and genuine efforts along your learning continuum for reflective practice.[29] To enhance your self-assessment abilities, several recommendations should be considered, including the following: videotaping, with reviews[39]; experiential guides and workbooks, such as the *Patient Practitioner Interaction* one you are using; learning style (eg, Kolb's Learning Style Inventory)[44] and personality inventories (eg, Myers-Briggs Type Indicator)[45]; self-assessment with clinical education evaluative instruments; facilitation of active training for teaching and learning; provision of time to complete self-assessment; guided reflective journals; guided debriefing inquiries; and practice sessions with immediate feedback, such as from standardized patients, the 2-Minute Clinical Instructor activity, and peer and self-assessment, along with instructor feedback.[46] Effective peer and self-assessment capabilities provide the foundation for progression to sound clinical reasoning abilities, which are expected of the doctoring professions.[46-50]

CONCLUSION

We have now considered the concept of self-assessment and theories of reflective practice. Shortly, we will provide the opportunity for you to practice peer and self-assessment and to facilitate your abilities specifically. However, as you have noted from considering the pithy quotes of professional learners who have gone before you and the related research, it is important to not only be positive in the effort to enhance self-assessment, but to be mindful of your own impact on the learning and teaching environment to support peer and self-assessment. The influence of the learning environment is key for peer and self-assessment success as evidenced through Bandura's social learning theory.[34]

You have had the opportunity to explore, change, and/or adapt your perspectives and considerations for self-assessment and are now cognizant of the gifts of peer and self-assessment for best reflective practice for those we serve in health care. My hope for you is that you are able to continue to translate your newly acquired knowledge for your progression of learning in the affective, cognitive, psychomotor, and spiritual domains (see Chapter 14) as you continue your professional development journey toward reflective practitioner because your patients and clients are counting on you! The work of self-assessment is challenging, yet the rewards are worth the time and effort. Self-assessment is a viable process, and you shall ultimately have greater learning gains in this mode of active learning with serious thought and considerations than with more passive learning methods; the process of self-assessment shall promote your continuous learning.

It is time now for you to try thinking on your feet (reflection-in-action), working to make sense of your experiences after they occur (reflection-on-action) to learn more deeply, and scaffolding your learning (knowing-in-action) for reflective practice.[14,15,29,30,46] We want you to now challenge your assumptions as learners; ask new questions; make sense of your experiences; not be afraid to admit errors and make course corrections (recognize surprise) through self-assessment and feedback; put what you are learning into deeper memory as active, engaged learners; and assist your peers and colleagues in the process.[14,15,29,30,46] Make it a point to thrive on constructive feedback and gently provide the gift of peer assessment for others to succeed. Perhaps Bandura[32-35] said it best: "Of the many cues that influence behavior, at any one point in time, none is more common than the actions of others."

As you transition from classroom to clinics and hospitals, you may find it helpful to complete guided self-assessment in relation to specific aspects of your patient-practitioner interactions. Gremigni et al,[51] Italian researchers, investigated how health care professionals self-evaluate their ability to relate to patients in day-to-day practice from a patient-centered perspective. Gremigni et al[51] tested the psychometric properties of a developed instrument called the Provider-Patient Relationship Questionnaire (PPRQ). They studied 50 nurses from a sample of 600 in 8 hospitals (6 in northern Italy and 2 in southern Italy) and determined good reliability and validity of the 16-item PPRQ instrument, rating each statement using a scale from 1 to 5, where 1 = not at all and 5 = very much. Although the study is novel, it has merit in examining communication, interest in your patients, empathy, and care involvement from a self-assessment standpoint. The PPRQ reports on 16 common considerations when working with patients in a hospital setting. Consider the PPRQ's 16 items, provided here, as you transition to patient-centered care and use the framework to facilitate your self-assessment of your patient-provider interactions in these specific areas:

1. I provided clear information.

2. I was interested in what the patient feels about his/her current health status.

3. I turned to the patient in a calm and quiet tone.

4. I understood the emotions that the patient may have.

5. I was interested in what the patient knows about the disease/prognosis.

6. I respected the patient as a person.

7. I was interested in what the patient wants from care.

8. I was able to listen.

9. I was paying attention to what the patient said.

10. I was able to put myself in his or her shoes.

11. I gave the patient time to ask and to talk about the disease.

12. I inspired confidence and security when touching the patient and being nearby.

13. I asked questions that allowed the patient to express his or her view.

14. I was interested in what the patient expects from care.

15. I gave the patient encouragement and transmitted optimism.

16. I offered the patient the opportunity to discuss and decide together the things to do.

REFERENCES

1. West KM. The case against teaching. *J Med Educ*. 1966;41(8):776-771.
2. Jensen GM, Gwyer J, Shepard KF. Expert practice in physical therapy. *Phys Ther*. 2000;80:(1):28-43.
3. Jensen GM, Shepard KF, Hack LM. The novice versus the experienced clinician: insights into the work of the physical therapist. *Phys Ther*. 1990;70(5):314-323.
4. Shepard KF, Hack LM, Gwyer J, Jensen GM. Grounded theory approach to describing the phenomenon of expert practice in physical therapy. *Qual Health Res*. 1999;9(6):746-758.
5. Jensen GM, Shepard KF, Gwyer J, Hack LM. Attribute dimensions that distinguish master and novice physical therapy clinicians in orthopedic settings. *Phys Ther*. 1992;72(10):711-722.
6. Yusfuff KB. Does self-reflection and peer-assessment improve Saudi pharmacy students' academic performance and metacognitive skills? *Saudi Pharm J*. 2015;23(3):266-275.
7. May BJ, Dennis JK. Expert decision making in physical therapy—a survey of practitioners. *Phys Ther*. 1991;71(3):190-202.
8. Osterman KF, Kottkamp RB. *Reflective Practice for Educators: Professional Development to Improve Student Learning*. 2nd ed. Thousand Oaks, CA: Corwin Press; 2004.
9. Kirby PC, Teddlie C. Development of the reflective teaching instrument. *J Rsch Dev Educ*. 1989;22(4):45-51.
10. Russell TL, Spafford C. Teachers as reflective practitioners in peer clinical supervision. Paper presented at AERA; April 1986; San Francisco, CA.
11. Brookfield S. *Becoming a Critically Reflective Teacher*. San Francisco, CA: Jossey-Bass; 1995.
12. Dewey J. *How We Think*. Boston, MA: Heath; 1933.
13. Kolb DA. *Experiential Learning: Experience as the Sources of Learning and Development*. Englewood Cliffs, NJ: Prentice Hall; 1984.
14. Schön DA. The theory of inquiry: Dewey's legacy to education. *Curriculum Inquiry*. 1992;22(2):119-139.
15. Schön DA. *The Reflective Practitioner: How Professionals Think in Action*. New York, NY: Basic Books; 1983.
16. Hatcher JA, Bringle RG. Reflection: Bridging the gap between service and learning. *College Teaching*. 1996;45(4):153-158.
17. Eyler J, Giles DW, Schmeide L. The impact of a college community service lab on students' personal, social and cognitive outcomes. *J Adolescence*. 1994;17:327-329.
18. Williams D, Driscoll A. Connecting curriculum content with community service: guidelines for student reflection. *J Public Service Outreach*. 1997;2(1):33-42.
19. May WW, Morgan BJ, Lemke JC, Karst GM, Stone HL. Model for ability-based assessment in physical therapy education. *J Phys Ther Educ*. 1995;9(1):3-6.
20. American Physical Therapy Association. Clinical Performance Instrument, 1997, 2006. Alexandria, VA: American Physical Therapy Association. http://www.apta.org/PTCPI/TrainingAssessment/. Accessed December 22, 2015.
21. American Occupational Therapy Association. Understanding the OT/OTA fieldwork performance evaluations. http://www.aota.org/Education-Careers/Fieldwork/Supervisor/Inservice.aspx. Accessed July 1, 2015.

22. The American Occupational Therapy Association. Fieldwork Educators Certificate Workshop. www.aota.org/Education-Careers/Fieldwork/Workshop.aspx. Accessed May 1, 2015.

23. American Physical Therapy Association. Credentialed Clinical Instructor Program (CCIP). http://www.apta.org/CCIP/. Accessed July 1, 2015.

24. Musolino GM, van Duijn J, Noonan AC, Eargl LK, Gray DL. Reasons identified for seeking the American Physical Therapy Association-Credentialed Clinical Instructor Program (CCIP) in Florida. *J Allied Health*. 2013;42(3):e51-e60.

25. Alspach JG. *The Educational Process in Nursing Staff Development*. St. Louis, MO: Mosby; 1995.

26. Bridges EM, Hallinger P. Using problem-based learning to prepare educational leaders. *Peabody J Educ*. 2002;72(2):131-146.

27. Peters JM. Strategies for reflective practice. *New Directions for Adult and Continuing Educ*. 1991;51:89-96.

28. Smith FL, Barlow PB, Peters JM, Skolits GJ. Demystifying reflective practice: using the DATA model to enhance evaluators' professional activities. *Eval Program Planning*. 2015;52:142-147.

29. Musolino GM. Fostering reflective practice: self-assessment abilities of physical therapy students and entry-level graduates. *J Allied Health*. 2006;35(1):30-42.

30. Schön DA. *Educating the Reflective Practitioner: Toward a New Design for Teaching and Learning in the Professions*. San Francisco, CA: Jossey-Bass; 1987.

31. Jensen G, Denton B. Teaching physical therapy students to reflect: a suggestion for clinical education. *J Phys Ther Educ*. 1991;5:33-38.

32. Bandura A. *Self-Efficacy: The Exercise of Control*. New York, NY: W.H. Freeman; 1997.

33. Bandura A. Self-efficacy: toward a unifying theory of behavioral change. *Psychol Rev*. 1997;84(2):191-215.

34. Bandura A. *Social Learning Theory*. Englewood Cliffs, NJ: Prentice-Hall; 1977.

35. Bandura A. The self-system in reciprocal determinism. *Am Psychologist*. 1978;33(4):344-358.

36. Watts NT. *Handbook of Clinical Teaching: Exercises and Guidelines for Health Professionals Who Teach Patients, Train Staff or Supervise Students*. New York, NY: Churchill Livingston; 1990.

37. Jonsen A. *The New Medicine and the Old Ethics*. Cambridge, MA: Harvard University Press; 1990.

38. Epstein RM. Mindful practice. *JAMA*. 1999;282(9):833-839.

39. Seif GA, Brown D. Video-recorded simulated patient interactions: can they help develop clinical and communication skills in today's learning environment. *J Allied Health*. 2013;42(2):e37-e44.

40. Barrows HS. *Practice-Based Learning: Problem-Based Learning Applied to Medical Education*. Springfield, IL: Southern Illinois University School of Medicine; 1994.

41. Barrows HS. *What Your Tutor May Never Tell You: A Medical Student's Guide to Problem-Based Learning*. Springfield, IL: Southern Illinois University School of Medicine; 1996.

42. Jensen GM, Shepherd KF, Gwyer J, Hack LM. Attribute dimensions that distinguish master and novice physical therapy clinicians in orthopedic settings. *Phys Ther*. 1994;72(10):711-722.

43. Orest M. Clinicians' perceptions of self-assessment in clinical practice. *Phys Ther*. 1995;75(9):824-829.

44. Kolb DA. Kolb Learning Style Inventory. Version 4. Philadelphia, PA: Hay Group; 2007. www.haygroup.com/leadershipandtalentondemand/enhancing/kolb.aspx. Accessed December 22, 2015.

45. Briggs KC, Myers IB. Myers-Briggs Type Indicator (MBTI). The Myers & Briggs Foundation. www.mbtionline.com/. Accessed February 3, 2015.

46. Musolino GM, Mostrom E. Reflection and the scholarship of teaching, learning, and assessment. *J Phys Ther Educ*. 2005;19(3):52-66.

47. Dreyfus HL, Dreyfus SL. The relationship of theory and practice in the acquisition of skill. In: Benner P, Tanner CA, Chalsa CA, eds. *Expertise in Nursing Practice*. New York, NY: Springer; 1986:29-48.

48. Dreyfus SE, Dreyfus HL. A five-stage model of the mental activities involved in directed skill acquisition. Berkeley Operations Research Center, University of California, Berkeley; 1980. http://www.dtic.mil/dtic/index.html. Accessed July 13, 2015.

49. Furze J, Black L, Hoffman J, Barr JB, Cochran TM, Jensen GM. Exploration of students' clinical reasoning development in professional physical therapy education. *J Phys Ther Educ*. 2015;29(3):22-33.

50. Furze J, Gale JR, Black L, Cochran TM, Jensen GM. Clinical reasoning: development of a grading rubric for student assessment. *J Phys Ther Educ*. 2015;29(3):34-45.

51. Gremigni P, Casu G, Sommaruga M. Dealing with patients in healthcare: a self-assessment tool [published online ahead of print January 25, 2016]. *Patient Educ Couns*.

SUGGESTED RESOURCES

Examples of Self-Assessment on the American Physical Therapy Association Clinical Performance Instrument

Professional Practice–Safety: *I consistently attempt to establish a safe working environment prior to each patient session. I put down mats in cases where patients will be swinging and will need to land on cushioned ground. I remain vigilant of changes in patient conditions by asking them about their pain using pain scales, in addition to observation of physiological changes, such as skin color or respiratory rate. In cases where a patient may have a shunt, I ensure that I do not perform* *activities where a patient would be placed in an upside-down position. When I feel uncomfortable performing an intervention due to lack of experience, I ask for assistance from my clinical instructor to ensure the patient remains safe. I consistently utilize proper body mechanics in order to protect myself and my patients. I am well versed in the facility's safety procedures as well. I am continuously learning about how to keep pediatric patients safe and that it requires constant vigilance on my part. Over the next few weeks, I will continue to expand my safety skills by efficiently learning where to keep my hands so they can be ready in case a patient has an outburst or movement alteration that could make him or her a fall risk.*

Professional Practice–Communication: *When working with a complex patient, I seek communication from my clinical instructor during that patient's session to ensure I am being safe and my reasoning with treatment is logical. When I feel uncomfortable or unsure of the quality of my service, I am able to communicate this to my clinical instructor immediately and efficiently with verbal cues. I consistently actively listen to my patients and their parents and commonly review what they have stated to me to ensure all parties are on the same page. My verbal and nonverbal messages are consistent, and I strive to have the tone in my voice match what I am asking a patient to perform. When a patient performs a task correctly, I utilize a positive, encouraging tone. My clinical instructor has educated me on what tones and level of wordiness are appropriate for different diagnoses, and I have since applied this on a more consistent basis. I still require further practice using a more authoritative voice with a patient whose behavior is inappropriate. When communicating with a patient and parent about what his or her home exercise program consists of, I commonly perform the exercises with him or her in the clinic. I also offer pictures and take-home worksheets to help the patient visualize the exercises and give him or her a way to remember and replicate the exercises I am asking him or her to perform at home. In cases where a patient may not be able to verbalize his or her needs, I utilize nonverbal signs, such as crying or parental cuddles to determine what the patient needs. In some cases, I also utilize sign language, as demonstrated by speech therapists on staff.*

Patient Management–Clinical Reasoning: *I offer a logical rationale for my clinical decisions. If a patient has sensory deficits, I will be sure to include some aspect of sensory input into that day's session. If a patient exhibits trunk and lower extremity weakness, I will include fun muscle-building activities in the session. I select my interventions based on results from pediatric examination tools and patient preferences. For a patient who has a fear of therapy balls, I avoid interventions that utilize transitioning or stretching on the ball. I consistently integrate patient needs, such as being able to ride a bike or jump to play with friends, into their plan of care. When an intervention is ineffective for a child, I am able to recognize this and implement a new variation of the intervention instead. I consistently and efficiently utilize peer-reviewed articles, textbooks, parents, medical records, and other members of the therapy staff to formulate plans of care and make clinical decisions for patients.*

After reviewing these examples, remember to journal about your thoughts on reflective practice.

EXERCISES

EXERCISE 1: WARMING UP WITH PEER AND SELF-ASSESSMENT— CHECK YOURSELF BEFORE YOU WRECK YOURSELF

All health care professionals work to maintain good body mechanics throughout all our work activities and in daily living. We also educate our patients in proper postural alignment for good musculoskeletal health and their work, recreational, and daily activities. The environment does not allow us to maintain proper body mechanics at all times, yet maintaining strength and flexibility provides the ability to adjust to the demands of gravity and challenges with body mechanics on a daily basis. Many students initially struggle with maintaining their own safety when first entering a practice setting due to the competing demands and being novices. So let's check your posture and your peer and self-assessment abilities for the psychomotor skills of good posture and body mechanics as a warm-up self-assessment activity.

Part A

Find a partner and ask your partner to lift a readily available item (chair, books, backpack, trash can, or similar) from the floor to the table and back down again. While the lifting trial is being completed, review the checklist, answer yes or no, and make notations. When your partner is finished with the lifting trial, have him or her complete a self-assessment using the ratings, and then you should compare your responses and discuss. Then reverse roles and complete it again.

BODY MECHANICS LIFTING TRIAL—PEER AND SELF-ASSESSMENT

1.	Overall good postural body alignment throughout the activity:	Yes	No	Note:
	a. Maintains slight cervical lordosis	Yes	No	Note:
	b. Maintains slight thoracic kyphosis	Yes	No	Note:
	c. Maintains slight lumbar lordosis	Yes	No	Note:
2.	Appropriate base of support:	Yes	No	Note:
	a. Too wide	Yes	No	Note:
	b. Too narrow	Yes	No	Note:
3.	Carries the load close to the body within the base of support	Yes	No	Note:
4.	Avoids twisting of the trunk	Yes	No	Note:
5.	Avoids bending from the waist	Yes	No	Note:

Now, consider if mobile devices are wreaking havoc on your body? Heads up—are you developing text neck?

Part B

The person evaluating first in Part A should now be the one to initiate the activity while the partner evaluates. As you are likely aware, poor posture while texting places pounds of pressure on your neck. Just as we teach our patients regarding proper body mechanics with the use of computer terminals, we wish to avoid having degenerative cervical spine problems and the corresponding associated neurological issues. Although overuse injuries are also causative factors, associated with prolonged texting or computer use with poor posture repeatedly over time, we can work to prevent musculoskeletal imbalances by checking ourselves before we wreck ourselves. Poor posture causes tension headaches, neck and shoulder pain, and breathing difficulties.

Ask your partner to send a few text messages and/or complete some work at his or her laptop, notebook, iPad, or other mobile electronic device. After he or she has been engaged for a while, describe what is good or not so good regarding his or her posture (you need not limit yourself to just the cervical spine). Complete your visual assessment, asking your partner to complete his or her self-assessment, and then debrief and later reverse roles (when he or she doesn't think you are watching) and provide your recommendations.

Posture while using an electronic mobile device:

Good:

Not So Good:

Recommendations:

EXERCISE 2: PONDERING FOR PRACTICE: GUIDED REFLECTION ALONG THE WAY

Consider a recent concrete experience in your learning, classroom or clinical. Reflect on your experience and respond to the following queries:

1. What was the muddiest point in your learning experience?

2. What percentage of mud was due to the following:

   a. Unclear presentation?

   b. Lack of the opportunity to ask questions?

   c. Your lack of preparation?

   d. Your lack of participation?

   e. Your lack of setting a specific goal?

3. What theories or concepts did you draw upon or discover from the experience?

4. How could you have been more present and available to the learning experience?

5. Who are you becoming as a professional?

(Adapted from Musolino GM, Mostrom E. Reflection and the scholarship of teaching, learning, and assessment. *J Phys Ther Educ.* 2005;19[3]:52-66.)

Exercise 3: DATA-Driven Model—Reflection

Recall the DATA model.[28] Refer to the DATA steps. Recall a specific interaction—classroom, practical, or clinical—and apply the model.

- Describe—the situation:

- Analyze—examine the why:

- Theorize—practice-based reasoning:

- Act—the best solution:

EXERCISE 4: REFLECTIVE JOURNALS— APPLYING SCHÖN'S REFLECTIVE PRACTITIONER THEORY

The following are sample reflective journal entries in response to Schön's queries of recognizing surprise and reflecting-on-action, which also contains an element of surprise. As you continue your learning journal, the next time you are surprised, take a moment to respond to the queries.

Part 1

RECOGNIZING SURPRISE

Reflect on a recent patient interaction or learning encounter and share your biggest surprise and how you adapted.

Example A: *"I also believe that I have adapted and changed in the way I approach every patient interaction. When I first began this program, I approached each clinical mentoring, exam, standardized patient encounter, and practical as a pressure situation and a memorization exercise. As I have progressed in this program, I have learned that this is not the case and that building trust and having compassion is just as important as stating facts. It is more important to go with the flow of each evaluation and interaction."*

Example B: *"Recently, I have had the opportunity to work with a stroke survivor in his early 60s with significant left-side neglect and weakness. I interact with not only this patient daily, but also his son. During my session with him, my biggest surprise was to see how much my patient and his son trusted me and my knowledge base while working with him. I know that I have studied, prepared, and worked hard to get to this point, but I don't think I had actually put into perspective how much my patients appreciate my help. It was an eye opener for me and very rewarding to be able to work with this patient daily and see how he progresses and how I can challenge myself to be a better clinician for him and his functional progress."*

Example C: *"We recently had a patient who did not want to be evaluated or observed by a student. I respectfully understood her opinion and left the evaluation room while my clinical instructor performed the evaluation. This was a big surprise to me because I have never encountered this with any patient in all of my clinicals. I asked the other physical therapists if they wanted any help with their patients and worked with 2 other patients that hour."*

Example D: *"Yesterday, I had a new outpatient evaluation with a patient status post stroke. The patient had global aphasia, which made the entire evaluation difficult to complete because the patient was unable to provide the information I needed to successfully complete it. I surprised myself by my ability to adapt to this situation. I used simple steps, first by remembering to take his baseline vitals and repeating them during the exam, and then by using one-step commands and tactile cues to complete the majority of the evaluation. After 20 minutes, while he was in a rest mode, I noticed that he was becoming more unresponsive, was flushed, and began sweating. I quickly went to the patient and assisted him to hook-lying with the assistance of my clinical instructor. We rechecked his vitals, the paramedics were called, and the patient was transferred to the hospital for further workup. I surprised myself again by my ability to remain calm, help calm the patient's spouse, and act quickly to ensure the patient had the care he required."*

Example E: *"In the past few weeks, I saw a patient whom my clinical instructor had evaluated and deemed as difficult due to his prescription drug–seeking behaviors and multiple inappropriate comments during his evaluation. When I treated him, I was very nervous as to how he would act toward me as a student. Surprisingly, he acted appropriately, with only some signs of symptom magnification that we were able to work through. This instance helped me to learn that it is always important to go into treating each patient with an open mind and to be nonjudgmental, despite anything I may have heard about the patient. By being friendly and treating the patient as I would have despite my clinical instructor's warnings, I was able to have a productive and appropriate treatment session with him."*

Now it's your turn. Reflect on a recent patient interaction or learning encounter and share your biggest surprise and how you adapted.

Part 2

REFLECTION-ON-ACTION

Consider a recent patient or personal encounter that did not go the way you had anticipated. Reflecting on the encounter, describe the following:

- What happened?
- What were you thinking/feeling?
- What sense did you make of the situation?

- What else could you have done?
- What was good and bad about the experience?
- If the same would arise again, what would you do?

Example

What happened? *"A patient was admitted for continued management of respiratory failure with multiple comorbidities, had an extensive past medical history, and was being evaluated for physical and occupational therapies. Upon chart review, I imagined the patient as being in need of total assist with very poor functional mobility. When I got in the room, the patient was able to roll in bed with minimal assistance and could even perform a stand pivot transfer with moderate assist of 2 people. This was contradictory to what I had imagined the patient interaction would be during the initial encounter."*

What were you thinking/feeling? *"I felt as though I had overlooked something in the chart. I knew the patient's prior level of function was pretty good, but the recent change in medical status led my mind to imagine a patient who would present in far worse condition from a functional perspective. I felt a bit embarrassed, thinking back now."*

What sense did you make of the situation? *"I just went with it and acted as if I had expected the patient to perform this well all along. After the encounter, it made me realize that, in the long-term/acute care setting, the patient's status can change drastically in 24 hours or less and that I should only rely on the documentation for clarification. Also, this situation taught me to never get so focused on a mental image; it's good to have going in, but it's never the same image you imagined once you leave the room. Whether it's better or worse than you originally imagined, it's always impacted by the patient encounter."*

What else could you have done? *"I could have allowed the patient to do more at the beginning of the encounter, rather than acting as if the patient was dependent with everything. After the evaluation, I felt as though I was too cautious and that the patient might have been capable of more than I allowed him to do on his own; the session could have been maximized more in terms of progression."*

What was good and bad about the experience? *"The patient felt comfortable and performed better than I expected. I wish I would have acted as if the patient was completely independent or much more capable, rather than initially acting as if he were dependent with everything."*

If the same would arise again, what would you do? *"I would not allow my chart review prior to the patient interaction to cloud my judgment of how I perceive the patient's functional capabilities. Also, going into the room, I would first see what the patient could perform on his or her own rather than being quick to assist with everything."*

Now it's your turn. Consider a recent patient or personal encounter that did not go the way you had anticipated. Reflecting on the encounter, describe the following:

- What happened?

- What were you thinking/feeling?

- What sense did you make of the situation?

- What else could you have done?

- What was good and bad about the experience?

- If the same would arise again, what would you do?

**The exercises at the end of this chapter are also available online.
Please refer to the sticker in the front of the book and enter the access code provided.**

LEADERSHIP AND ADVOCACY FOR HEALTH CARE

Gina Maria Musolino, PT, MSEd, EdD

"Education is the kindling of a flame, not the filling of a vessel." –Socrates

OBJECTIVES

- To comprehend the importance of incorporating concepts of leadership for patient/client health care.
- To value Covey's *The 7 Habits of Highly Effective People: Powerful Lessons in Personal Change.*[1]
- To proactively investigate one's own leadership queries for personal and professional leadership development.
- To appreciate the benefits of every person's abilities to lead and follow.
- To examine and reflect upon leadership principles and leaders.
- To discover leadership resources to explore and develop as leaders
- To realize the need to advocate for the health care needs of society and the health care professions through legislative and political processes.
- To participate in mechanisms to take action for advocacy for those we serve.

Most people want to make a difference in this world, whether it is through teaching others, scrubbing floors, changing bandages or diapers, or herding cattle—most people want to do a good job and make a difference. Everyone has the opportunity to be a leader in life to create an even grander difference.

IGNITING YOUR THOUGHTS ON LEADERSHIP

- Describe the kind of leader you want to be.
- As a leader, what do you want to be able to achieve?

I recently visited the Smithsonian National Museum of American History in Washington, DC, and I was pleasantly surprised to see an entire display dedicated to the First Ladies of the United States (FLOTUSs), exploring the unofficial, yet ever-important and often influential, position of the FLOTUS. The displays included many of their first inaugural

Davis CM, Musolino GM. *Patient Practitioner Interaction: An Experiential Manual for Developing the Art of Health Care, Sixth Edition* (pp 159-180).
© 2016 SLACK Incorporated.

ballgowns (the oldest displayed is Martha Washington's), lovely portraits, and how each FLOTUS contributed to the work of the nation during the presidential administrations of her husband. The role of the FLOTUS is not specifically defined, is an unofficial title, and carries no specific official duties; however, each FLOTUS has contributed in meaningful ways. FLOTUSs are much more than dresses or adornments; they served the nation with specific agendas, often not completely uncovered until they were in the history ("herstory") books.

Leadership is not necessarily a formal position or role; one does not need an official position of leadership to be a leader. Leadership is action to guide and direct. Every day, we provide guidance for our patients, families, and caregivers to direct their abilities for movement and function. Leadership remains an important aspect of every health care team and is a foundational skill for the development of health care professionals (HCPs) who lead their patients and families/caregivers. Incorporating the concepts of leadership throughout didactic and clinical education is important for fostering leadership skills in novice health care professionals. Every health care professional, at one time or another, shall be called upon to lead in everyday patient care encounters for the management of patient care. Our profession's futures shall be positive or dismayingly inadequate depending on our abilities to serve as everyday leaders in health care. In a moment, we are going to begin with a pre-exercise that allows adult learners in the Millennial generation to explore leadership concepts and skills through a proactive leadership[2] reading, reflection, and writing. The activity is a catalyst for personal and professional change for health care professionals, and as Covey[1] stated, you will "begin with the end in mind."

Initially in this chapter, we are going to reverse our approach and thinking now that we are diving into the second half of *Patient Practitioner Interaction*. We are going to apply the leadership constructs of *Leading With Soul: An Uncommon Journey of Spirit*[3] and, through social influence, begin to proactively work toward supporting future patient health care needs, examine our abilities to collaborate in health care teams, and thrive through application of evidence-based practice[4] leadership concepts and frameworks.[5,6] We are going to explore some of the theories of leadership, including Bolman and Deal's[5] frameworks, Kouzes and Posner's[7] challenges, and Covey's[1] *The 7 Habits of Highly Effective People: Powerful Lessons in Personal Change* as you begin to examine your foundational capacities for everyday leadership.

Bolman and Deal,[3] in *Leading With Soul: An Uncommon Journey of Spirit*, ask the reader to consider Jesus's words when thinking about the direction of a true leader, paraphrasing: "What do we profit if we gain the whole world, but lose our own soul in the process?" (Matthew 16:26). Bolman and Deal[3] reminded us not to lose our heart and soul in the process of our work as leaders. We consider these concepts at the outset of the chapter to benefit from the leadership insights from their lifetime of work as educational leaders and researchers. In the often challenging yet highly rewarding works as health care professionals, it remains relevant for you to not lose sight of the emotional side of leadership nor compromise professional values (as discussed in Chapter 4). Staying in touch with your affective domain and the emotional aspects of care allows for a strong leader to be sensitive to the rhythms of the people we lead and influence, be it patients, clients, and/or peers. We shall further address aspects of spirituality related to patient care in Chapter 14; however, we will touch upon it briefly here with respect to leadership.

Mitroff and Denton[8] conducted a landmark study examining spirituality in the workplace. The researchers defined spirituality as "the basic feeling of being connected with one's complete self, others, and the entire universe." Mitroff and Denton[8] discovered that "people do not want to compartmentalize or fragment their lives. The search, meaning, purposes, wholeness and integration is a constant, never-ending task. To confine this search to one day a week or after hours violates people's basic sense of integrity, of being whole persons. In short, soul is not something one leaves at home." An example shared from a research participant's interview was when a chemical worker awoke one morning and decided his work was wounding his soul because he could not reconcile the fact that the chemicals he was using to manufacture and treat furniture were highly toxic and very lethal to the environment.[8] The worker's spirit could no longer cope with the mismatch of his occupation with his own self-concept.

More than likely, you elected to pursue your dream to become a health care professional because the professional career allows you to marry your soul with a higher calling to provide for others in the service of health care delivery. Thus, you can give of yourself more fully as a health care leader, sharing your genuine spirit while helping to transform others' lives through helping others. Consider these selected quotes from Bolman and Deal's[3] *Leading With Soul: An Uncommon Journey of Spirit*:

> *Perhaps we lost our way when we forgot that the heart of leadership lies in the hearts of leaders. We fooled ourselves, thinking that sheer bravado or sophisticated analytic techniques could respond to our deepest concerns. We lost touch with a most precious human gift-our souls. If you show people you don't care, they'll return the favor. Show them you care about them, they'll reciprocate. When people know that **someone really cares, you can see it**. It's there in their faces. And in their actions. Love really is the gift that keeps on giving. The essence of leadership is not giving things or even providing visions. It is **offering oneself and one's spirit**.*

How do these perspectives relate to your school, health care institution(s), and home environment?

Do you think the concepts could apply to any situation? Why or why not?

Do you think the concept of spirituality belongs in health care? Why or why not?

Now that you have warmed up to the idea of leadership, let's consider the habits of those who are highly effective through Pre-Exercise 1.

PRE-EXERCISE 1: PROACTIVE READING, REFLECTION, AND WRITING: *THE 7 HABITS OF HIGHLY EFFECTIVE PEOPLE: POWERFUL LESSONS IN PERSONAL CHANGE*

As Covey[1] stated, we are going to "begin with the end in mind" and start with a proactive pre-exercise related to leadership and engaging your developing self-assessment and peer-assessment skills, which you gained from Chapter 9. You will need to obtain a copy of the internationally popular text, *The 7 Habits of Highly Effective People: Powerful Lessons in Personal Change*, a seminal work on the universal and timeless habits for the foundations of leadership, written by Stephen R. Covey (1957-2012). If you have had the pleasure of previously reading it, it is worth revisiting. However, if you have read it within the last year or so, you may wish to select another contemporary leadership text for the reading and reflection (resourced at the end of the chapter); however, you should revisit Covey's book as a refresher because we shall be discussing the impact of the habits related to you as a developing health care professional. Most learners find *The 7 Habits of Highly Effective People: Powerful Lessons in Personal Change* a timeless text that provides for new learning at any point along life's journey.

Once you have obtained a copy of *The 7 Habits of Highly Effective People: Powerful Lessons in Personal Change*, you are going to complete what is called a proactive reading, reflection, and writing. Reading proactively is a skill I learned while working on my doctor of education degree in my leadership coursework and subsequently used successfully over the past decade with my DPT students' leadership learning.[2] Proactively reading—reading actively with questions in mind—is an important skill to develop now. It serves as a way to remain current in the contemporary literature, which may be helpful to your work as a health care professional. Yet, you may not always have the time to delve deeply into the popular readings and self-help contemporary texts; hence, you can read them proactively.

Similar to being an effective health care professional, an effective, proactive reader is able to look at the big picture of the text (as you do with the whole-to-part considerations with your patients) and then consider questions to search for answers in the reading (similar to how we conduct a focused history with our patients), subsequently scanning the front matter, back matter, prologue, table of contents, and index (as you would with screening a patient). Then, begin to actively search for answers, diving into the content (your more focused exam components with your patient, discovering answers and problem solving to affirm and support your clinical decisions), learning as you go how the findings apply to your leadership capabilities and abilities.

As a real-world health care professional, one cannot possibly keep current on all evolving concepts in leadership and management; the proactive reading and writing is one approach to facilitate your critical thinking while consuming contemporary media that may or may not be viable for practice. What do you want to get out of the resource text? What's most important for you to learn right now (ie, you won't be able to conduct every test in the book with your patients either)? The method involves first posing critical questions from your preview, then proactively reviewing the contemporary text, looking for crucial responses and supporting with pithy quotes and concepts from the text, fostering currency in contemporary leadership principles, all in an efficient manner. Health care professional students enjoy this exercise because it gives them the opportunity to learn about *The 7 Habits of Highly Effective People: Powerful Lessons in Personal Change*, learn how to proactively read, and incorporate the lessons learned for their current and preferred futures while experiencing the opportunity to critically perform peer and self-assessment and then develop and revise the writing until satisfied with the final product.[2]

Proactive Reading, Writing, and Reflection Steps to Follow

First, **preview** the information about the text and the author. Then, based on the preliminary information about the book and author, reflect on this information.

Second (**query**), write down 3 specific questions that you are interested in learning more about regarding the perspectives the author is presenting. One question should relate to you personally, one should be about your own professional development along the journey, and the third should be about your own preferred future; the final question may relate to your personal and professional future but must include consideration about your preferred professional future.

Third (**review and write**), review the text proactively, skimming for answers with your 3 questions in mind related to personal development, professional development, and preferred future (which may include personal perspectives and must include professional). Then, write out your well-considered responses based upon the author's guidance. Do not copy long quotes from the text; rather, incorporate key concepts from the author and synthesize with your thoughts to respond to your query. The responses should not read like a book report but should be a thoughtful and meaningful discussion incorporating what you have learned from the book in a proactive manner from posing a query first, then searching the text for how it is guiding you for your personal and professional growth and development, and your preferred future query. Your proactive, reflective writing should not exceed 5 to 7 pages in total. Be certain to cite any notable quotes or unique ideas attributable to the author and include a reference page (including any other text you may have referenced).

Finally (**assess**), prepare your self-assessment and plan for peer assessment and faculty assessment. Once you have completed your proactive reading, writing, and reflection, complete your own self-assessment using the proactive assessment form (Figure 10-1). Be prepared to exchange and peer review, and consider the learning shared by your peers. Be prepared to debrief regarding the book and leadership lessons in class discussions. Based upon peer feedback, you may wish to revise your proactive writing before seeking final instructor review of your last draft.

Once you have completed Pre-Exercise 1, with your first draft of the proactive reading, reflection, and writing and self-assessment completed, continue reading Chapter 10.

TIME AND COMPETENCY FOR LEADERSHIP HABITS

In a January 2015 report from the Educational Testing Service (ETS),[9] it was conveyed that Americans born after 1980 are lagging behind their peers within countries ranging from the continent and country of Australia to the northern European country of Estonia. The study looked at scores for literacy, technology problem solving, and numeracy from a test called the Program for the International Assessment of Adult Competencies, which tested the abilities of people in 22 countries, comparing the United States with 21 other member countries, in the Organization for Economic Cooperation and Development. Goodman et al[9] illustrated that although Americans between the ages of 20 and 34 years are achieving higher levels of education, they are falling behind their cohorts in other countries, such as high schoolers in Japan, Finland, and the Netherlands.

The authors urged policy makers and stakeholders to shift the conversation from educational attainment to one that acknowledges the growing importance of skills and examines these more critically.[9] American Millennials also scored poorly on problem solving in technology-rich environments and failed to meet basic proficiency, ranking them last among the 22 countries. The youngest segment in the ETS research study of US Millennials, from 16 to 24 years of age, ranked dead last in numeracy and near the bottom for countries in the problem solving in the technology-rich environment category. According to ETS researchers, they were surprised with the results because the hypothesis was that the Millennial generation would score better than older workers due to growing up digitally tech savvy. The researchers noted that not only did the US Millennials score worse, but their scores were abysmal.[9]

The Pew Research Center's Internet & American Life Project[10] also reported that young adults are the most avid texters. In 2011, cell phone owners between the ages of 18 and 24 years exchanged an average of 109.5 messages on a normal day—or about 3200 texts per month—with a typical cell owner in the age group sending or receiving up to 50 messages per day or about 1500 messages per month. Voice calling has changed little on a year-to-year basis. Cell phone owners make or receive an average of 12.3 voice calls per day, with a median average of 5 voice calls daily. The most active texters prefer text messages, whereas the majority of cell phone owners prefer a voice call when they want to be reached. Cell phones are virtual umbilical cords for many helicopter parents in today's society, making it more challenging for children to mature and make their own decisions, and also affecting their overall psychological well-being.[10] However, today's leaders should be responsive and embrace the unique diversity of thought that presents in the workplace and use it to innovatively solve problems and improve.

The study by ETS[9] and the project report from the Pew Center[10] demonstrated the current status of the rising generation of Millennials. It shall be incumbent upon each of you to not be in the averages on the aforementioned points. As a health care professional, you must demonstrate competency and proficiency with technical standards, ensure you have time to devote your full attention to your patients, and not be too distracted by technology and social media to focus on your studies and patient care. Technology may be used as an asset for health care, such as with telehealth; however, it can also be a barrier. I have had students incorporate decreased social media as a personal behavior change goal (which you will soon have the opportunity to formulate in Chapter 15) because they quickly realized with the demands of professional school and adjustments needed to dedicate themselves to becoming the type of professional they hoped to become, a personal change was needed. With a few setbacks along the way, the students were able to achieve their goals to decrease their social media use, be device-free in the clinic, and be more responsible in their time management.

As a developing leader in health care, you will need to be able to lead and model the way[7] when it comes to reducing the non-health care–oriented use of technology in your practice and learning environment while assuring that you are

1. **Name/Date** ☐ Included? Comments:

2. Includes **3 Questions** (underlined) with Responses ☐Included? Comments:

3. **Underline major headings:** Introduction *(1-2 paragraphs)*, Questions and Response, Conclusion, References *(1 page)* ☐ Included? Compliance? Comments:

4. **Length:** Excluding the reference page, the Proactive Reading & Writing should fall between 5-7 pages *(double spaced, 11-12 pt font)* ☐ Compliance?   Comments:

5. Paper includes all **inclusion items**, as indicated above Yes ☐ No ☐ Comments:

6. <u>**Substantive Content Review**</u>: *Each question (Q) response has sufficient* **breadth** *(wide range) and* **depth** *(complexity and reflective) of* **personal thought** *to answer the question &* **provides substantive support** *from the* **text** *within the response; consider each Q response individually:*

    a) Q 1 Yes ☐ No ☐ <u>**Provide your rationale /guidance-**</u> **Why or Why not?**

    b) Q 2 Yes ☐ No ☐ <u>**Provide your rationale/guidance**</u> **-Why or Why not?**

    c) Q 3 Yes ☐ No ☐ <u>**Provide your rationale/guidance**</u> **-Why or Why not?**

7. Appropriate reference citations are utilized where needed and direct quotes when required to provide appropriate citation format (AMA) include any additional references that you may cite or reference in addition to Covey; does not rely on long quotes, per directions; form and style also includes spelling, grammar, punctuation, capitalization, et al. **Form & Style Compliance:** Yes ☐ No ☐ Comments:

Signature of Peer Reviewer, Faculty Reviewer or Self-Assessment:_____

Figure 10-1. Proactive reading, reflection, and writing assessment feedback rating.

actively present and engaged so as not to miss firsthand learning application opportunities. I concur with the study findings due to the need to monitor personal devices for learners being on task and challenges when students transition from classroom to clinical education/fieldwork environments. For example, even though I advise students to begin a regular walking endurance program prior to initiating clinical/fieldwork, in addition to students being physically tired during their first week in clinical/fieldwork education (sitting in the classroom and periodic workouts do not prepare one for the

TABLE 10-1
COVEY'S *THE 7 HABITS OF HIGHLY EFFECTIVE PEOPLE:* *POWERFUL LESSONS IN PERSONAL CHANGE*
Habit 1: Be Proactive—The Habit of Choice
Habit 2: Begin With the End in Mind—The Habit of Vision
Habit 3: Put First Things First—The Habit of Integrity & Execution
Habit 4: Think Win-Win—The Habit of Mutual Benefit
Habit 5: Seek First to Understand, Then to Be Understood—The Habit of Mutual Understanding
Habit 6: Synergize—The Habit of Creative Cooperation
Habit 7: Sharpen the Saw—The Habit of Renewal
Adapted from Covey SR. *The 7 Habits of Highly Effective People: Powerful Lessons in Personal Change.* New York, NY: Simon & Schuster; 2013.

physical demands of health care practice), students have challenges acclimating to many of the environmental demands of the clinical setting requirements (time management, responsible or device-free use, physical endurance, safety awareness for self and others, multitask management, prioritization).

Covey[1] provided important lessons for change that lend to the required skill sets that translate for clinical practice success. We must shift to deeper learning and reduce distractions for learning. Remember how challenging it was to get into your program?

Your education, right now, is your investment in your future and that of society. Your future patients/clients and colleagues are counting on you, and the value for your monetary investment is only as good as the work you put in behind the effort. Make certain you have time for learning; do not allow others to hinder or sabotage your learning through negativity or distracting your time needed to learn and develop or by hovering too closely, and allow yourself the opportunity to develop competency to be a leader.[1,3,5-12] How do you intend to keep the *The 7 Habits of Highly Effective People: Powerful Lessons in Personal Change*[1] at the forefront, model the way,[7] and resist and stay out of the unproductive quadrants?

Leadership remains an important aspect of every health care team and is a foundational skill for development that you will need to demonstrate in your patient-practitioner interactions as a health care professional. As you incorporate *The 7 Habits of Highly Effective People*, as well as the 4 Quadrant time management lessons regarding where you spend your time, in your daily life and as a health care professional, they will become just that—helpful habits, providing a strong foundation for your success and leadership. As a reminder, habits 1 to 3 are related to **self-management**; habits 4 to 6 to **leading others** and **teaming**; and habit 7 to **unleashing your potentials** and **renewal of ourselves in body, heart, mind, and soul** (Table 10-1).[1]

LEADERSHIP QUALITIES AND CHALLENGES: MANAGERS, LEADERS, AND SERVANT LEADERSHIP

Real leaders genuinely care about the success of others and are open to new ideas, not just their own. True leaders appreciate others and do not steal credit; they genuinely and openly credit others in public ways. True leaders are humble, have appropriate self-insight, and recognize the importance of teamwork. Great leaders instill trust, connect with people, and are good listeners. Fearless leaders are not afraid to confront the tough problems and do so with grace. Real leaders are never too self-important to jump in and get their hands dirty. Most effective leaders often step in to determine function and capacities firsthand so as to not lose sight of all perspectives of those being led. Leaders know when to follow and let others lead and how to turn problems into solution-oriented opportunities. Leaders will never hesitate to improve themselves and role-model the same for their teams. Leaders are not afraid to ask for help. Kouzes and Posner[7,13] also believed that "leaders are most often ordinary folks demonstrating extraordinary courage, skill and spirit to make a significant difference." Bennis[14] provided clear distinctions between managers and leaders (Table 10-2). Being a good manager is not negative, but in order to be a strong leader, one must be transformational. Real leaders take risks and reach across generations, all while encouraging and modeling authenticity.

As a health care professional, you will be called upon to be a strong manager and an innovative leader within your organization, with your patients and their families, and with coworkers. Both skills sets and activities of managers and

TABLE 10-2	
BENNIS'S DISTINGUISHING QUALITIES	
MANAGERS	**LEADERS**
Administer	Innovate
Ask how and when	Ask what and why
Focus on systems	Focus on aligning people
Maintain	Develop and set direction
Rely on control	Inspire trust
Short-term perspectives	Long-term perspectives
Accept status quo	Challenge status quo
Have an eye on the bottom line	Have an eye on the horizon
Imitate	Originate
Emulate the classic good citizen	Are their own person
Copy and organize	Create strategy

Adapted from Bennis W. *On Becoming a Leader: The Leadership Classic.* 4th ed. New York, NY: Basic Books; 2009.

leaders are necessary for an organization to succeed; the challenge is continuing to find the best balance of management and leadership in order to respond to be able to handle the complexities and change needed in health care environments.

You will also be asked to serve as an advocate for your patients and clients through letters of necessity; appeals for non-payment of services; and with local, state, and federal government authorities that influence how we are able to practice and serve our patients through federal and state laws and rules. You may also take advantage of opportunities to serve in leadership roles with your membership organizations in your districts, regions, states, and nationally, and with other community-based and support groups that value your expertise and leadership capacities for health care.

Consider: What is best leadership practice for the patients and clients our profession serves? Why?

According to Ebener[15]:

Leadership is an interactive process where leaders and followers influence each other to bring about change. Leaders and followers move toward a common goal. Leadership is a voluntary and interactive relationship to bring about a change in thinking, action, attitude, policies, structures, culture and strategy.

Leadership is very distinct from management. Ebener[15] stated that "[m]anagement is positional, while leaders can emerge from anywhere. Management can and does use authority. Leadership is not coercive. Leaders inspire, invite, and influence. When we rely solely on positional authority, we are not leading." Leaders transform self, others, organizations, and society. Maxwell[16,17] concurred and said that the "true measure of leadership is influence—nothing more nothing less…it's about disposition not position." Kotter[18] agreed, stating that "Most organizations are over-managed and under-led." Ebener[15] further explained that "[l]eadership is a function, not a position."

Leadership is about being a transformative agent of change. Leadership also requires lifelong learning, which is why the concept of self-assessment and reflective practice, discussed in Chapter 9, is central for your development as a leader. Leaders stimulate change and serve as catalysts to effect change. Leadership is constantly influenced by external and internal factors and demands. The fast-paced, multigenerational society we live in today demands that we become increasingly more flexible as leaders. Ebener[15] shared the need for teaming with leadership and said that the essence of leadership is this:

Leaders bring about change. They feel passionate about something that needs to change and influence others to join them in creating and carrying out a strategy to change. They realize they cannot do it by themselves. They then develop their followers into leaders, because most big things need many leaders.

This should speak to you as a health care professional today. The "big thing" is the triple aim of health care[19]: improving the individual experience of care, improving the health of populations, and reducing the per capita cost of care. The triple aim will only happen through strong managers and leaders in health care working toward the triple aims.

	TABLE 10-3	
	KOUZES AND POSNER'S LEADERSHIP CHALLENGE	
5 LEADERSHIP PRACTICES	**10 COMMITMENTS**	
Model the way	• Clarify **values** • Set the **example**	
Inspire a shared vision	• Envision the **future** • Enlist others for a common **vision**	
Challenge the process	• Search for opportunities for **innovation** • Experiment and take **risks**	
Enable others to act	• Foster **collaboration** • Strengthen and develop **competence**	
Encourage the heart	• Recognize **contributions** • Celebrate the **value and victories**	

Adapted from Kouzes JM, Posner BZ. *The Leadership Challenge: How to Make Extraordinary Things Happen in Organizations*. 5th ed. San Francisco, CA: Jossey-Bass; 2012.

Stop now and reflect a moment. Can you think of ways right this moment how you, either from your own firsthand experiences or those of others you know, might effect a change in the triple aim? Considering Bennis's distinguishing qualities (see Table 10-2), what would your approach be as a manager vs a leader in order to do the following?:

- Improve health care experiences
- Reduce health care costs
- Improve the health of a population

Kouzes and Posner[7,13] shared that leadership is more about behavior and inspiring others to lead and follow. Leadership qualities that are most welcome and needed in health care systems today include appropriate interpersonal skills, the ability to work on a team, strong ethics and integrity, and solid analytical/problem-solving skills. In *The Truth About Leadership*, Kouzes and Posner[20] shared that it doesn't matter what generation you represent in order to produce positive work attitudes; good leadership is good leadership. They noted that the context of leading may change a lot, but the content of leading changes very little. The true fundamentals of leadership have not changed over the past 25 years. Kouzes and Posner[7,13] provided the fundamental challenges of leadership, which hold true today, to guide us in our own personal and organizational leadership development (Table 10-3).

In addition to using Kouzes and Posner's practices and commitments as guideposts along the leadership roadmap, I have found Maxwell's[16] 360 leadership principles particularly helpful in the process steps for effective leadership. Maxwell's[16] 360 method involves multipoint influences, checks along the way, and the need for formative and summative evaluative information, considering all stakeholders input, including the following:

- Coaching and feedback
- Developing trust and respect
- Inspiring and motivating others
- Building teamwork and collaboration
- Clarify purposes (mission) and direction (vision)

Think of a leader you admire or someone whom you believe is a good leader. Can you think of leaders or leadership situations in which the above leadership practices have been experienced or demonstrated? What worked? What did not work? Why were the leaders effective or ineffective?

According to Blake and Mouton,[21] leadership has a dual focus that emphasizes task orientation or achieving results and developing relationships. **Servant leaders**, as first described by Greenleaf[22] and later Ebener[15] and Keith,[23] are more motivated to serve than to lead. Servant leaders are motivated by missions, visions, and core values, and their heart is at the service of the organization. Servant leaders are at the service of others and are therefore willing to share their power with others.[3,15,22,23]

Leadership is truly about change. What do you want to change as a leader? And more importantly, why? Generally speaking, only babies with wet diapers really thrive on change. As a leader, to empower change, you will need to somehow convince others why a change is needed. How will you facilitate change to occur as a leader? How will you incorporate the leadership qualities and characteristics to more effectively lead as a health care professional?

Did you know that the best test of leadership is not how many followers you lead, but how many leaders you develop? The "Beatitudes of a Leader" are shared here for your reflection, further exemplifying the servant leader concepts[22,23]:

Blessed is the leader who has not sought the high places, but who has been drafted into service because of their ability and willingness to serve.

Blessed is the leader who knows where they are going, how they are going, and how to get there.

Blessed is the leader who knows no discouragement, who presents no alibi.

Blessed is the leader who knows how to lead without being dictatorial; true leaders are humble.

Blessed is the leader who seeks the best for those they serve.

Blessed is the leader who leads for the good of the most concerned and not for the gratification of their own ideas.

Blessed is the leader who develops leaders, while leading.

Blessed is the leader who marches with the group and interprets correctly the signs on the pathway that leads to success.

Blessed is the leader who has their head in the clouds, but their feet on the ground.

Blessed is the leader who considers leadership an important opportunity for service.

LEADERSHIP: FRAMEWORKS AND TEAMING

In *Reframing Organizations, Artistry, Choice and Leadership*, Bolman and Deal[5] described that there are at least 4 frames, or ways of looking at organizations, to help make sense of the organizations within which we work. Bolman and Deal[5] said that the frames help us to see things and look at things differently from before and, therefore, people find them helpful. Typically, the 4 frames are considered to be in a cross shape, as in a window frame. The frames are defined as follows: (1) The Structural Frame is the rationale side of an organization, with a central concept of efficiency; (2) The Human Resource Frame is the people side of an organization, with a central concept of needs, skills, and relationships; (3) The Political Frame is the conflict side of an organization, with a central concept of power and competition; and (4) The Symbolic Frame is the cultural side of an organization, with a central concept of culture and meaning. Each frame is further described with metaphors, values with frameworks, and tools for organizing experiences within the organizations.[5] As a leading choreographer of change, you will conduct in all 4 frames.

Most organizations exhibit at least 1 and often 2 of the frames or depend upon only a few frames for daily operations and function, which are representative of the culture within the organization. A preference is shown for 1 or 2 frames; no one uses only one frame all the time. The idea is that at various times, in order to solve leadership challenges, one may need to reframe the organization (eg, to keep an organization heading in the right direction [Structural Frame] or to keep people involved and informed [Human Resource frame]). Bolman and Deal[5] suggested that in order to not misread things, the correct frame needs to be identified in which to take action, and in order to understand complex problems, leaders need to use multiple lenses, or frames. Learning to use all 4 frames allows leaders to be effective architects, servants, advocates, and prophets. The 4-frame approach deepens the appreciation for and understanding of the organizations within which we lead or serve in health care teams.

Speaking of teams, this chapter would be lacking if we did not also consider how to differentiate how teams are working, or not, in health care. Zenger et al[24] provided excellent team evaluation instruments that you may wish to consider using in your learning and health care teams (Table 10-4). Use the instrument with your team to determine if you are helping to create a team identity, moving the team forward, or making the most of team differences. Part A considers your contributions to the team, and Part B, the teamwork.

TABLE 10-4
ZENGER-MILLER SAMPLE TEAM EVALUATION INSTRUMENTS

Part A: Response choices:

Never (1)   Seldom (2)   Sometimes (3)   Usually (4)   Always (5)

Part A: How often do you make a conscious effort to do the following?
1. Help clarify and reinforce the overall purpose of the team.
2. Help the team set clear, achievable goals.
3. Recognize and celebrate the team's achievements.
4. Treat team members with respect while acknowledging their different motivations, values, work styles, and traditions.
5. Encourage each team members to participate fully.
6. Help the team get unstuck when differences lead to conflict.
7. Keep an open mind about new ways of doing things.
8. Encourage and reward team members who promote innovation.
9. Share new information with the team.

Part B: Response choices:

Strongly   Disagree (2)   Neither   Agree (4)   Strongly
Disagree (1)   Disagree or Agree (3)   Agree (5)

Part B: How well are we working together as a team?
1. The team knows exactly what it has to get done.
2. Team members get a lot of encouragement for new ideas.
3. Team members freely express their real views.
4. Every team member has a clear idea of the team's goals.
5. Everyone is involved in the decisions we have to make.
6. We tell each other how we are feeling.
7. All team members respect each other.
8. The feelings among team members tend to pull us together.
9. Everyone's opinion gets listened to.
10. There is very little bickering among team members.

Are you satisfied or dissatisfied with the way you are working as a team? _____

Why? _____

Identify the item the team needs to work on most when examining your results compared with the teams:

_____

This item needs attention because _____

My best idea for helping the team work better together at this time is: _____

_____

Note: Teamwork is considered strong if the average score is Agree or Strongly Agree; if the average is neither Agree nor Disagree, teamwork is considered healthy, with room for improvement; if the average is Disagree or Strongly Disagree, something is getting in the way of teamwork. Whatever the score, discussing it with the team with an open mind is likely to improve teamwork.

Reprinted with permission from Zenger JH, Musselwhite E, Hurson K, Perrin C. *Leading Teams: Mastering the New Role*. Homewood, IL: Zenger-Miller, Inc, Business One Irwin, 1994. Reproduced with permission of McGraw-Hill Education.

TABLE 10-5
THE 8 ARCHETYPES OF LEADERSHIP
Collaborator: Empathetic, team-building, talent-spotting, coaching-oriented
Energizer: Charismatic, inspiring, connects emotionally, provides meaning
Pilot: Strategic, visionary, adroit at managing complexity, open to input, team-oriented
Provider: Action-oriented, confident in his or her path or methodology, loyal to colleagues, driven to provide for others
Harmonizer: Reliable, quality-driven, execution-focused, creates positive and stable environments, inspires loyalty
Forecaster: Learning-oriented, deeply knowledgeable, visionary, cautious in decision making
Producer: Task-focused, results-oriented, linear thinker, loyal to tradition
Composer: Independent, creative, problem-solving, decisive, self-reliant
Adapted from West K, Stixrud E, Reger B. Assessment: what's your leadership style? *Harvard Business Review.* https://hbr.org/2015/06/assessment-whats-your-leadership-style. Published June 25, 2015. Accessed July 13, 2015.

What Is Your Leadership Signature?

You may be beginning to wonder about your own personal leadership style or questioning how you will be perceived as a leader. In order to better understand how leaders lead, West et al[25] created a psychometric survey to measure the inter-related facets of leadership. Specifically, they did the following:

> *...identified degrees of leadership in (a) a thriving 'mind-set'[26] (including a sense of purpose, deep commitment to learning and conveyed sense of optimism); (b) a combination of self, social and situational awareness; and (c) essential leadership values such as performance orientation, ethical integrity, ability to collaborate and openness to change, among others.*

With more than 1000 research participants, largely US-based executives at companies with more than 250 employees, West et al[25] discovered 8 archetypes of leadership (Table 10-5). They emphasized that there is no right or wrong in these leadership types, but recognizing a person's go-to style may be helpful, just as recognizing your own personal learning style helps you to be a better learner and teacher; knowing your type of leadership approach would benefit your own understanding of leadership and other styles and approaches that could make one a better leader in varying situations that one might encounter. The researchers believe their work is in the early stages, but it has relevance. You may also wish to check out your own leadership archetype results using the leadership inventories resources at the end of the chapter to determine your leadership archetype and/or leadership style.

ADVOCACY IN ACTION

Health care is rapidly evolving. Due to changes in reimbursement and decision making surrounding health care, medical necessity, and the management of care, our roles as health care professionals have had to expand. This is partly due to social and economic change and partly due to having no clearly established meta-paradigm in relation to other professions. We have discovered that economic and social influences contribute to a person's health and disease. Hence, health care professionals have taken on new responsibilities and skills to include much more advocacy work. If we do not take action, the professions that exist today may be gone tomorrow, or they may be assumed by others who may be less expert at providing the rehabilitation care needed. We need to assist others in understanding not only what we do, but also what differences and impacts we have on those we serve in society. Political advocacy is the art of persuading policy makers to change policy; there is often opposition. Just like leadership, advocacy is also an influential process; your attitude toward advocacy and shared experiences can have an impact.

Our national membership organizations help us to accomplish advocacy for those we serve because advocacy is not the work of one, but of many working together to affect a change. Often, our national rehabilitation organizations work collaboratively on issues of mutual import. Most national organizations have things readily set up for you to advocate directly through the professional association resources. Take Action sites are as follows:

- American Physical Therapy Association (APTA): http://www.apta.org/TakeAction/
- American Occupational Therapy Association (AOTA): http://capwiz.com/aota/home/
- American Speech-Language-Hearing Association: http://www.asha.org/advocacy/

Take a look at the website that applies most directly to you and consider the issues that are part of the public policy plan that your professional organization is directly addressing at this time. Consider the following:

1. What is the aim of the proposed policy or bill(s)? What outcomes are desired if the bill would be achieved? What is the problem that is being addressed?

2. Who are the main constituents? Who are the stakeholders?

3. What are the obstacles, if any, regarding the issue? Who might be against the bill? Why?

We will revisit these websites again in the exercises. Advocacy should be considered a core competency for you to be able to speak up on behalf of your patients and act on any of their unmet needs. You may also wish to collaborate with local community-based groups.

Understand that your target audience for advocacy is your elected officials at the state and national levels. To make a difference, you will need to become a constituent who has a relationship with your legislators. To promote a bill or policy change with your elected legislators, they need to know the following 3 things:

1. **Who?** Who you are, what you do for their constituents, and how you serve society; get to know your legislators on a personal level first! What do you have in common with them in your district?

2. **What?** What is the issue you want them to act on (bill numbers), and what are the merits of the bill, as well as the pros/cons, in brief?

3. **Why?** Share your powerful and impacting patient story of why the bill is relevant (or not) and the change the policy would make for others.

To accomplish advocacy, you need to have a practiced and polished "elevator talk" to be able to deliver your messaging in 2 minutes or less because you may not have much time, especially during the legislative sessions; if you get more time, then by all means expand. You may be speaking with a legislative aide who also has much influence, and you should not be disappointed to speak with him or her. Reach out via phone and email and in person when possible. Unfortunately, as we will discuss in Chapter 16, policy does not change rapidly or overnight in most instances. Some legislation has taken decades. (A quick revisit to how a bill becomes a law illustrates the many steps: http://visual.ly/how-does-bill-become-law). There can be many hurdles and detours in committees and subcommittees and unrelated or positive amendments that need to be renegotiated. So, repeat messaging is required, too!

We need you to join the cause and help the effort for our patients! You must be appropriately persistent, and compromise will often need to occur. Money and votes speak to policy makers. Contributing to your membership's political action committee, in any amount, for the cause will help. Advocating to convince your lawmakers that a significant amount of the voting public shall benefit from, care about, and support the cause that a particular bill stands for is most relevant and part of our professional obligation in service to society today. If we don't speak up, who will? We need to develop relationships with our legislators so that we can engage with them regularly and persuade them to cosponsor and sponsor legislation needed by our patients and in many cases to ensure that patients are able to continue to receive needed care. In my experience with advocacy, not only have I been able to expand my scope of influence and help have our patients' needs be better met, I have made new friends and colleagues pulling for the same cause. Our students regularly participate in advocacy days and events at the state and nation's capital, as well as repeatedly via the Take Action sites provided. Spread the word, assist those who cannot always help themselves, get involved today, and always keep the grassroots advocacy going in your local community. We will have the opportunity to further address in Exercise 3.

"Never doubt that a small group of thoughtful, committed citizens can change the world. Indeed, it's the only thing that ever has." –Margaret Mead

LEADERSHIP: TRANSFORMING SOCIETY

In Chapters 7 and 8, we discovered and practiced effective communication and appropriate assertive skills. As leaders, our communication and especially listening and engagement skills are just as important. In a Harris poll of approximately 1000 US workers, the impact of communication was key when it came to pointing out where leaders fell short in being effective. Note that the communication issues that were most often cited as preventing effective leadership included not recognizing others' achievements (63%), not giving clear directions (57%), not taking time to meet with others (52%), taking credit for others' ideas (47%), not offering constructive feedback (39%), not communicating on the phone or in person (34%), and not getting to know your team players (23%).[27] According to Solomon,[27] in order to continue to connect while achieving every day, leaders can easily rectify this by simply asking or saying the following:

- Here's what I appreciate about you or your contribution...
- Thank you (personal and public)
- What do you think?
- Here's what's happening and what you can expect...
- I have some feedback for you...
- Let me tell you about something I learned the hard way...
- Hello [insert the person's name]...

Although leadership is hard and influencing others is also challenging, promoting real change in others is part of what we do as health care professionals. Changing our own and others' paradigms is no easy task (we will practice more in Chapter 15). However, there is great joy in serving as a leader and guiding others to achieve. Some of my greatest leadership successes are when my patients achieve their goals, when my current and former students share their accomplishments, when someone I have mentored achieves their goals, and when an organization or team I have led accomplishes more than they thought possible—these make it all worthwhile! Most of these accomplishments involved transforming society in some manner. Let's look more closely now at the concept of transformation within health care.

One of the many influential leaders in our profession, Shirley Sahrmann, PT, PhD, FAPTA,[28,29] describes **movement** as the core of physical therapy and how we have evolved from technicians to professionals in the evolution of thinking about the **Movement System**. She shared how a team of leaders gathered over decades to continue the ideas of professional identity, integrating the concepts of movement science in professional education, leading up to the new vision for the profession and subsequent ongoing discussions regarding diagnostic dilemmas[28,30] related to the Movement System. The guiding principles in the APTA Vision Statement state that "the physical therapy profession's greatest calling is to maximize function and minimize disability for all people of all ages. Movement is key to optimal living and quality of life for all people of all ages that extends beyond health to every person's ability to participate in and contribute to society."[31,32] Adopted by the APTA's House of Delegates in 2013 was the APTA's Vision Statement for the Physical Therapy Profession: "Transforming society by optimizing movement to improve the human experience."[31,32]

Although this vision is specifically for the physical therapy profession, it may inspire others in society and other disciplines to promote movement and collaborate with physical therapy. I recently asked my student interns how they were serving as leaders in their clinical education experiences to meet the intents of the Vision Statement and its guiding principles for the profession of physical therapy. While on clinical education, you may find the following excerpts of different students' voices inspiring as you reflect on your personal and professional leadership ahead. Figure 10-2 illustrates students' progression from entry into the early phases of classroom learning (see Figure 1-4) to emerging as student health care professionals in hospitals and clinics. Continue to envision your personal progression to successfully becoming a health care professional.

I feel that my job at the cancer center is completely transforming society and the people in it. I have patients who are postsurgery procedures from cancer (eg, total hip and knee replacements due to bone tumor, soft tissue resections, radical mastectomies, etc) who have many limitations. After a few days of working with a patient postoperatively, he or she is walking more than 150 feet with an assistive device. I love to see how much people can improve and in such a short amount of time. At first, the patient is hesitant and scared and feels that he or she may not get better. But with just a few days of physical therapy and teaching them how to ambulate again, strength and mobility comes back. Endurance takes much longer. I also work with many patients with leukemia who come in for bone marrow transplants. Typically, about 1 week after transplant, their white blood cell count and platelets decrease dramatically, so weakness and fatigue are quite common. I always try to remain as positive as possible and let each patient know that I am here for him or her and for his or her recovery. I actually started a new thing—making certificates for patients. I made one called the "marathoner award." It is for patients who are here for a very long time but continue to push through and work as hard as they can every day. I gave it to a man with leukemia who has been here since the day I started at the cancer hospital (about 6 weeks now). He was so happy. It gave him even more motivation to keep trying and working hard. I love seeing people transform themselves and feel better overall. Working with people who have cancer is very inspirational. Each day I go home thinking about the patients I have treated and how lucky I am to have met such amazing people who have such great attitudes, work very hard, and are overall a pleasure to work with, and I have the greatest job to lead them back to health, optimizing their movement to improve their function.

Figure 10-2. Leading the way for health care on clinical education internships: Johnny Gray, SPT, USF, DPT, class of 2016; Dr. Kelly Miller, PT, DPT, Clinical Instructor; and Kristina Terrana, SPT, USF, DPT, class of 2015, Florida Hospital, Connerton, Florida.

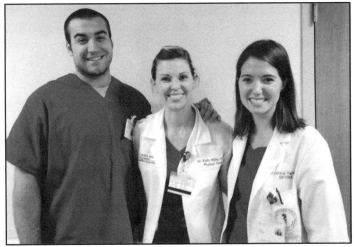

Currently, my caseload has a significant portion of patients with amputations. Every month, the patients get together for an empowerment group. They refer to this as an empowerment group NOT a support group because that's what it is—empowering! The prosthetic empowerment group meetings are all about how they optimize their performance in society; they reach out to each other and discuss the successes and obstacles they have encountered along their paths. Their objective is to work together to become more empowered in the community, and I am pleased to say I will be presenting at their next meeting. I am preparing a presentation on wound care for people with amputations because 75% of people with amputations experience dermatologic issues with their limb, and 65% experience these issues more than once. To further optimize movement and improve the human experience, I am reaching out to this population to further empower them on what they can expect and how they can react when these issues arise. I will be creating a brochure/handout for everyone to take home as well. I am finding out what they know in advance and planning for what new information I can share and the best format.

I am helping society through improving movement and function through building rapport with patients and their caregivers. In my view, no matter how knowledgeable someone is, if he or she cannot build a professional, friendly relationship with a patient, then that patient's optimal human experience through movement will be very difficult to obtain. The pediatric setting is where this applies most because children at young ages will not sit there and comprehend what you as a physical therapist are trying to accomplish. Building rapport, making timid kids open up, and making a majority of treatment interventions into games will help facilitate advancement toward set goals, thus optimizing the human experience via movement. Also, with parents who just see pediatric physical therapy as play, building rapport with them is even more crucial for patient success because the parents/caretakers are the ones ultimately responsible for the child's home exercise program and compliance with therapy. Education and explanation of the rationales for what you, the physical therapist, do for their daily experiences will help caretakers realize that what you're doing with their children has meaning and purpose and why home exercise compliance is so needed! For instance, the children are not just walking upstairs or putting a dinosaur magnet on a board; they are strengthening their entire lower extremity musculature, developing motor planning through the activity, and developing safety and environmental awareness through verbal and tactile cues, all while improving proprioceptive input into their ankle, knee, and hip joints to improve body function and motor control, which decreases their risk for falls and helps them become more independent. Patient/caregiver education is critical to patient success, and without building rapport with patients and their caretakers, it is pretty hard, if not impossible, to improve their livelihood. I lead toward the vision by educating and facilitating movement with children and their caregiving parents or family/support members.

I am transforming society by optimizing movement to improve the human experience by treating the whole patient, not just a body part. In orthopedics, it can be easy to get hung up on the referring diagnosis, such as hip pain, but treating just the hip is not likely going to fix the problem. Educating the patient is an important part of this plan because he or she may wonder why you are working on something such as foot posture when they came in for hip pain. I am presently doing this on my clinical education internship by performing thorough examinations, creating detailed documentation, and educating patients on all of my findings. I treat the deficits that I find and then work toward incorporating functional activities into the treatments that are meaningful to the patient's desires and goals. This mantra should be applied in any setting ("treating the patient, not the disease") because treating the disease or treating just one body part is not going to get the patient back to the functional goals for which he or she is seeking physical therapy.

We have the opportunity to serve and rehabilitate all people from society, regardless of their medical status. I have been mainly treating people within the neurological population, and with them, I am constantly reminded that every day is a gift. I help them learn how to sit, stand, walk, negotiate stairs, and perform any other functional movement—functional activities that "normal" people take for granted every day. Last week, I evaluated an older man who sustained a left-side stroke infarction that left him with right-side hemiparesis and severe expressive and receptive aphasia. He could not follow any commands during the initial evaluation period and required 2 people to perform a sit-to-stand transfer. However, this week, he was fully alert and oriented, only required minimal assistance of one person for sit-to-stand transfers, and now is able to ambulate approximately 60 feet with a rolling walker and minimal assistance of one person for balance and safety. I am blessed to help people rehabilitate to a life that they feel is worth living by optimizing their movement, and it is also my pleasure to be doing a lunch talk for the local Optimist Club, which meets at the hospital, to talk about what physical therapists do and how we impact society.

Now, consider and answer how you will transform society by optimizing movement to improve the human experience. (You may substitute your own profession's vision or that of your organization.)

REFERENCES

1. Covey SR. *The 7 Habits of Highly Effective People: Powerful Lessons in Personal Change*. New York, NY: Simon & Schuster; 2013.
2. Musolino GM. Fostering leadership in entry-level DPT education. Abstract presented at: Annual Conference and Exposition of the American Physical Therapy Association; June 8-11, 2011; National Harbor, MD.
3. Bolman LG, Deal TE. *Leading With Soul: An Uncommon Journey of Spirit*. 3rd ed. San Francisco, CA: Jossey-Bass; 2011.
4. Sackett DL. *Evidence-Based Medicine: How to Practice & Teach Evidence-Based Medicine*. 2nd ed. Philadelphia, PA: Elsevier Health Sciences; 2000.
5. Bolman LG, Deal TE. *Reframing Organizations: Artistry, Choice and Leadership*. 5th ed. San Francisco, CA: Jossey-Bass; 2013.
6. Bolman LG, Deal TE. *The Wizard and the Warrior: Leading with Passion and Power*. San Francisco, CA: Jossey-Bass; 2006.
7. Kouzes JM, Posner BZ. *The Leadership Challenge: How to Make Extraordinary Things Happen in Organizations*. 5th ed. San Francisco, CA: Jossey-Bass; 2012.
8. Mitroff II, Denton EA. A study of spirituality in the workplace. *Massachusetts Institute of Technology Sloan Management Review*. 1999;40;(4):83-92.
9. Goodman MJ, Sands AM, Coley RJ; Educational Testing Service. America's skills challenge: millennials and the future. http://www.ets.org/s/research/30079/asc-millennials-and-the-future.pdf. Published January 2015. Accessed July 7, 2015.
10. Smith A. Americans and text messaging. Pew Research Center. http://pewinternet.org/2011/09/19/americans-and-text-messaging/. Published September 19, 2011. Accessed May 1, 2015.
11. Stahl A. Five reasons why helicopter parents are sabotaging their child's career. *Forbes*. May 27, 2015. http://www.forbes.com/sites/ashleystahl/2015/05/27/5-reasons-why-helicopter-parents-are-sabotaging-their-childs-career/. Accessed June 1, 2015.
12. Vinson KE. Hovering too close: the ramifications of helicopter parenting in higher education. *Georgia State University Law Review*. 2013;29:423-451.
13. Kouzes JM, Posner BZ. *The Leadership Challenge Workbook*. 3rd ed. San Francisco, CA: Jossey-Bass; 2012.
14. Bennis W. *On Becoming a Leader: The Leadership Classic*. 4th ed. New York, NY: Basic Books; 2009.
15. Ebener DR. *Blessings for Leaders: Leadership Wisdom from the Beatitudes*. Collegeville, MN: The Liturgical Press; 2012.
16. Maxwell JC. *The 360 Degree Leader*. Nashville, TN: The Thomas Nelson; 2011.
17. Maxwell JC. *Good Leaders Ask Great Questions: Your Foundation for Successful Leadership*. New York, NY: Center Street Books; 2014.

18. Kotter JP. *Leading Change*. Cambridge, MA: Harvard Business School Press; 2012.

19. Bisognano M, Kenney C. *Pursuing the Triple Aim: Seven Innovators Show the Way to Better Care, Better Health, and Lower Costs*. San Francisco, CA: Jossey-Bass; 2012.

20. Kouzes JM, Posner BZ. *The Truth About Leadership: The No-Fads, Heart-of-the-Matter Facts You Need to Know*. San Francisco, CA: Jossey-Bass; 2010.

21. Blake RR, Mouton JS. *The Managerial Grid: Leadership Styles for Achieving Production Through People*. Houston, TX: Gulf Publishing; 1994.

22. Greenleaf RK. *Servant Leadership: A Journey into the Nature of Legitimate Power and Greatness*. Westfield, IN: Greenleaf Center for Servant Leadership.

23. Keith KM. *The Case for Servant Leadership*. Westfield, IN: Greenleaf Center for Servant Leadership; 2008.

24. Zenger JH, Musselwhite E, Hurson K, Perrin C. *Leading Teams: Mastering the New Role*. Homewood, IL: Irwin Professional; 1994.

25. West K, Stixrud E, Reger B. Assessment: what's your leadership style? *Harvard Business Review*. https://hbr.org/2015/06/assessment-whats-your-leadership-style. Published June 25, 2015. Accessed July 13, 2015.

26. Dweck CS. *Mindset: The New Psychology of Success*. New York, NY: Ballantine Books; 2007.

27. Solomon L. Leadership: the top complaints from employees about their leaders. *Harvard Business Review*. http://hbr.org/2015/06/the-top-complaints-from-employees-about-their-leaders. Published June 24, 2015. Accessed July 13, 2015.

28. Sahrmann SA. The Twenty-Ninth Mary McMillan Lecture: Moving precisely? Or taking the path of least resistance? *Phys Ther*. 1998;78(11):1208-1219.

29. Sahrmann SA. The human movement system: our professional identity. *Phys Ther*. 2014;94(7):1034-1042.

30. Stith JS, Sahrmann SA, Dixon KK, Norton BJ. Curriculum to prepare diagnosticians in physical therapy. *J Phys Ther Educ*. 1995;9(2):46-53.

31. American Physical Therapy Association. Vision statement for the physical therapy profession and guiding principles to achieve the vision. www.apta. org/vision/. Updated September 9, 2015. Accessed July 7, 2015.

32. American Physical Therapy Association. Human movement system. www.apta.org/movementsystem/. Updated November 24, 2015. Accessed December 22, 2015.

SUGGESTED READINGS

Alexander E. *Proof of Heaven: A Neurosurgeon's Journey Into the Afterlife*. New York, NY: Simon & Schuster; 2012.

Aquinas T. *The Summa Theologica of St. Thomas Aquinas*. Vol 1-5. Rev ed. London, UK: Burns, Oates and Washburne; 1920.

Blanchard K, Hodges P. *Lead Like Jesus: Lessons from the Greatest Role Model of All Time*. Nashville, TN: Thomas Nelson; 2008.

Buckingham M, Coffman C. *First, Break All the Rules: What the World's Greatest Managers Do Differently*. New York, NY: Simon & Schuster; 1999.

Cain S. *Quiet: The Power of Introverts in a World That Can't Stop Talking*. New York, NY: Broadway Books; 2013.

Collins J. *Good to Great: Why Some Companies Make the Leap...and Others Don't*. New York, NY: Harper Business; 2001.

Craik RL. Thirty-Sixth McMillan Lecture: Never satisfied. *Phys Ther*. 2005;85:1224-1237.

Delitto A. We are what we do. *Phys Ther*. 2008;88(10):1219-1227.

Divine M. *The Way of the SEAL: Think Like an Elite Warrior to Lead and Succeed*. New York, NY: Reader's Digest; 2013.

Duncan PW. One grip a little stronger. *Phys Ther*. 2003;83(11):1014-1022.

Dunwoody A. *A Higher Standard: Leadership Strategies from America's First Female Four-Star General*. Philadelphia, PA: Da Capo Press; 2015.

Gawande A. *The Checklist Manifesto: How to Get Things Right*. New York, NY: Metropolitan Books; 2009.

Gladwell M. *Outliers: The Story of Success*. Boston, MA: Little Brown and Company; 2011.

Greenleaf RK. *The Servant-Leader Within: A Transformative Path*. Mahwah, NJ: Paulist Press; 2003.

Guccione AA. Destiny is now. *Phys Ther*. 2010;90(11):1678-1690.

Hersey P, Johnson DE, Blanchard KH. *Management of Organizational Behavior: Utilizing Human Resources*. Englewood Cliffs, NJ: Prentice Hall; 1969.

Hislop HJ. Tenth Mary McMillan Lecture: The not-so-impossible dream. *Phys Ther*. 1975;55(10):1069-1080.

Holbeche L. *The Agile Organization: How to Build an Innovative, Sustainable and Resilient Business*. Philadelphia, PA: Kogan Page; 2015.

Jackley J. *Clay Water Brick: Finding Inspiration from Entrepreneurs Who Do the Most with the Least*. New York, NY: Spiegel & Grau; 2015.

Jensen GM. Learning: what matters most. *Phys Ther*. 2011;91(11):1674-1689.

Jette AM. 43rd Mary McMillan Lecture: Face into the storm. *Phys Ther*. 2012;92(9):1221-1229.

Johnson GR. Twentieth Mary McMillan Lecture: Great expectations: a force in growth and change. *Phys Ther*. 1985;65(11):1690-1695.

Karlgaard R, Malone MS. *Team Genius: The New Science of High-Performing Organizations*. New York, NY: Harper Business; 2015.

Kearns Goodwin D. *Team of Rivals: The Political Genius of Abraham Lincoln*. New York, NY: Simon & Schuster; 2006.

Kendall FP. Fifteenth Mary McMillan Lecture: This I believe. *Phys Ther*. 1980;60(11):1437-1443.

Kounios J, Beeman M. *The Eureka Factor: Aha Moments, Creative Insight, and the Brain*. New York, NY: Random House; 2015.

Lencioni P. *Death by Meeting: A Leadership Fable About Solving the Most Painful Problem in Business*. San Francisco, CA: Jossey-Bass; 2010.

Lencioni P. *Overcoming the Five Dysfunctions of a Team: A Field Guide for Leaders, Managers, and Facilitators*. San Francisco, CA: Jossey-Bass; 2010.

Magistro CM. Twenty-Second McMillan Lecture. *Phys Ther*. 1987;67(11):1726-1732.

Markova D, McArthur A. *Collaborative Intelligence: Thinking With People Who Think Differently*. New York, NY: Spiegel & Grau; 2015.

McChrystal S, Collins T, Silverman D, Fussell C. *Team of Teams: New Rules of Engagement for a Complex World*. New York, NY: Portfolio; 2015.

Michels E. Nineteenth Mary McMillan Lecture. *Phys Ther*. 1984;64(11):1697-1704.

Mittroff II, Mittroff D. *Fables and the Arts of Leadership: Applying the Wisdom of Mister Rogers to the Workplace*. New York, NY: Palgrave Macmillan; 2012.

Moffat M. Thirty-Fifth Mary McMillan Lecture: Braving new worlds: to conquer, to endure. *Phys Ther*. 2004;84(11):1056-1086.

Patterson K, Grenny J, McMillan R, Switzler A, Roppe L. *Crucial Conversations: Tools for Talking When the Stakes Are High*. 2nd ed. New York, NY: McGraw Hill Education; 2011.

Phillips DT. *Lincoln on Leadership: Executive Strategies for Tough Times*. New York, NY: Warner Books; 1992.

Pope Francis. *The Church of Mercy*. Chicago, IL: Loyola Press; 2014.

Pope John Paul II. On social concerns. *Population and Development Review*. 1988;14(1):211-217.

Pronovost P, Vohr E. *Safe Patients, Smart Hospitals: How One Doctor's Checklist Can Help Us Change Health Care From the Inside Out*. New York, NY: Plume; 2010.

Purtillo RB. Thirty-First McMillan Lecture: A time to harvest, a time to sow: ethics for a shifting landscape. *Phys Ther*. 2000;80(11):1112-1119.

Rothstein JM. Thirty-Second McMillan Lecture: Journeys beyond the horizon. *Phys Ther*. 2001;81(11):1817-1829.

Shepard KF. Mary McMillan Lecture: Are you waving or drowning? *Phys Ther*. 2007;87(11):1543-1554.

Solomon LM. *Say Something Real: Humanizing Communication Is Today's Best Business Strategy*. Botley, Oxford: SPARK Publications; 2008.

Talgam I. *The Ignorant Maestro: How Great Leaders Inspire Unpredictable Brilliance*. New York, NY: Penguin Publishing; 2015.

Weisinger H, Pawliw-Fry JP. *Performing Under Pressure: The Science of Doing Your Best When It Matters Most*. New York, NY: Crown Publishing; 2015.

Whitehurst J. *The Open Organization: Igniting Passion and Performance*. Boston, MA: Harvard Review Press; 2015.

Winstein CJ. The best is yet to come. *Phys Ther*. 2009;89(11):1236-1249.

Wolf SL. Thirty-third Mary McMillan Lecture: "Look forward, walk tall": exploring our "what if" questions. *Phys Ther*. 2002;82(11):1108-1119.

Wood R. Twenty-third Mary McMillan Lecture: Footprints. *Phys Ther*. 1989;69(11):975-980.

LEADERSHIP STYLE AND SIGNATURE INVENTORIES

Brief assessment. https://hbr.org/2015/06/assessment-whats-your-leadership-style

Galford RM, Maruca RF. Your Leadership Legacy Assessment. http://www.yourleadershiplegacy.com/assessment/assessment.php

Leadership Practice Inventory. www.leadershipchallenge.com/

West KA. What's your leadership signature? http://www.heidrick.com/Knowledge-Center/Article/What-is-your-leadership-signature

ASSOCIATION RESOURCES

American Occupational Therapy Association—Emerging Leaders Development. Program for students and new practitioners that provides training to become leaders. For more information, visit http://www.aota.org/education-careers/advance-career/eldp.aspx

American Physical Therapy Association—Oral Histories. First-person recollections of leaders who have shaped or continue to shape the profession. Audio and video have been recorded since 1980. The APTA provides a listing of more than 110 interviews that are available via http://www.apta.org/History/OralHistories/

Leadership Development Training: APTA—Health Policy and Administration Section—The Catalyst. A specialty component offers Leadership, Administration, Management, and Professionalism Certificate Programs—The Institute for Leadership in Physical Therapy for the development of personal and professional leadership skills. For more information, visit www.aptahpa.org

EXERCISES

POST-EXERCISE 1: REFLECTIONS ON *THE 7 HABITS OF HIGHLY EFFECTIVE PEOPLE: POWERFUL LESSONS IN PERSONAL CHANGE*

In Pre-Exercise 1, through your proactive reading, reflection, and writing exercise, you explored your own personal and professional leadership queries. Now, as you continue your formal and informal leadership and on into clinical education health care teams and in advocacy work for our patients served by the health care professions, you will continue to grow and develop as a leader. Because real-world health care professionals cannot possibly keep current on all evolving concepts in leadership and management, proactive reading and writing is one approach to facilitate critical thinking while consuming contemporary media that may or may not be viable for practice.

Now, in Post-Exercise 1, you are asked to consider peer insights provided in Table 10-6, with excerpts from proactive reflections of key learning by peers who have traveled this journey before you. In Post-Exercise 1, you are simply asked to reflect on the responses provided and link back to your leadership learning (see Pre-Exercise 1). Consider how you will continue to develop and change as a leader.

Take time now to journal about who you are becoming as a leader.

TABLE 10-6

PROACTIVE READING REFLECTION RESPONSES

QUERY	SELECT RESPONSE EXCERPTS
How can I maintain my morals and continue ethical decision making in my daily life?	*By living "proactively" as Covey[1] states, I realize that I am responsible for the choices I make. My favorite Covey[1] quote is "response-ability—the ability to choose your response." As obvious as it may be, people often forget they have a choice. Likewise, if I don't set my values, it will be difficult to make decisions I am happy with.*
How can I practice effectively to ensure I run my practice morally and ethically and challenge myself to stay current in knowledge?	*Far too often, therapists get aggravated with patients for being lazy, but they may not realize what the patient is going through. Covey[1] related, "Breaking deeply embedded habitual tendencies such as procrastination, impatience ... involves more than willpower and a few minor life changes." If I really want to change, I must work on it daily and recognize the need to stay current. Like Eartha Kitt said, "I am learning all the time; the tombstone will be my diploma."*
How can I be a nurturing mother, loving wife, and thriving career woman?	*To "... begin with the end in mind"[1] means to approach my role as a parent, as well as my other life roles, with my values and directions clear. "First seek to understand" the needs of my patients, children, and life partner ... Additional discussion on Quadrant II ("things that are not urgent, but important"[1]). One must identify the key roles and make them the priority while avoiding burnout by trying to accomplish too much, "sharpening the saw," and taking time for rest and relaxation.*
How can I improve my problem-solving skills?	*... 4-step process ... "First see the problem from the other point of view. Really seek to understand"[1] ... through utilizing empathic and reflective listening like we discussed in the Patient Practitioner Interaction workbook. ... Fourth is "new options to achieve results." The topics I picked were based on my clinical education mentoring, and I realized I lacked most in communication in the early weeks and worked on this through the 4-step process, which motivated me to do better. The process is key, and it is good to have for future reference.*
How does leadership content relate to physical therapy practice?	*"... admission to ignorance is often the first step in our education."[1] In physical therapy, we must learn to listen and acquire understanding ... we must build an emotional bank account with our patients and trust is an important part of leadership ... as physical therapists, we must do continuing education to improve knowledge and skills. This helps to earn patient's trust ... If you do not have trust, the patient will doubt your ability to heal and may not value what you have to offer.[5] ... Covey[1] described "diagnose before you prescribe," ... which is so important for professional liability and efficiency and effectiveness[5] in practice ...*
How can I have a successful physical therapy business?	*Covey[1] shed some positive light on this ... unfortunately, many close acquaintances started their own businesses with purely a monetary motivation... Covey[1] described "no commitment, no involvement"; in other words, I need a shared mission statement with those I work with, and it needs to be revised regularly to change with times. There is also a necessary balance to be a manager and a leader at different times.*
How can I prevent becoming complacent as a physical therapist?	*One of the worst downfalls of physical therapy is to become complacent ... it is easy to get overly routine and lose interest in new techniques or learning. I have seen this happen with certain types of patients, and not individualized care. I do not want to fall into this category. "Habits are powerful factors in our lives ... constantly express character and produce effectiveness or ineffectiveness."[1] Covey[1] talked about having knowledge, skill, and desire ... need to fall out of "works for me, so why change?"... think of each patient as unique and always examine the evidence for best practice and continuously be open to learn...*

Note: Excerpts shared anonymously with author permission; with special gratitude and acknowledgment to the University of South Florida School of Physical Therapy & Rehabilitation Sciences, Tampa, FL, classes of 2011 and 2012.

Adapted from Musolino GM. Fostering leadership in entry-level DPT education. Abstract presented at: Annual Conference and Exposition of the American Physical Therapy Association; June 8-11, 2011; National Harbor, MD.

EXERCISE 2: FUTURE LEADERSHIP TRANSFORMATION

The next time you encounter a leadership challenge, ask yourself these questions to assist in guiding you through your leadership challenge:

- Why is there a challenge?
- What am I trying to achieve?
- What am I doing that is working?
- How have I communicated the goal(s)?
- Have I developed and set direction?
- How am I addressing all generations with which I am working through this effort?
- Have I gathered all the information needed to inform the process?
- How am I influencing others to participate (or not)?
- What am I doing that is slowing me down?
- Where in the process did a breakdown occur?
- What can I do to change?
- Is the solution the best or are others possible?
- How can I better incorporate Covey's Habits 4 to 6?
- How can I enable others to act?
- Where is the process stuck and how can I reset the direction?
- Are there or were there missed expectations?
- Am I inspiring others to lead?

Alternatively

Interview a respected leader in your profession about their own leadership challenges and use the previous questions to guide your interview. Summarize their responses and what you learned in 1 to 2 pages.

Alternatively, in 1 to 2 pages, summarize your leadership learning reflections by one of the following:

- Viewing or listening to one of the APTA living history interviews. Available at http://www.apta.org/History/OralHistories/
- Reviewing one of the APTA Mary McMillan Lectures (see Suggested Reading, or available at ptjournal.apta.org).

EXERCISE 3: ADVOCACY IN ACTION

In 2015-2016, in collaboration with the APTA and constituent members, Congressman Gus Bilirakis (R-FL), along with Congressman Ben Luján (D-NM) and Senators Charles Grassley (R-IA) and Bob Casey (D-PA), introduced and sponsored the bipartisan bill Prevent Interruptions in Physical Therapy Act of 2015 (H.R. 556/S. 313) to allow for locum tenens arrangements under Medicare. We are also advocating for the Medicare Access to Rehabilitation Services Act (to permanently repeal the therapy cap on outpatient rehabilitation services, H.R. 775/S. 539) and the Physical Therapist Workforce and Patient Access Act to provide for student loan reimbursement with the National Health Services Corp Loan Repayment Program (H.R. 2342/S. 1426) to assure that rural and underserved areas have access to rehabilitation services.

Discover your local grassroots legislators and your national leaders in Congress; if you do not already know, you can look them up via the League of Woman Voters website (http://lwv.org/); select "Contact Your Local Officials" then "Find Your Elected Officials" by inserting your ZIP code. You are then provided the contact information for those you want to reach out to regarding issues of importance for the patients we serve. You are also able to find additional information on the websites for your state and national legislators on your state and national websites.

- The US House of Representatives: http://www.house.gov/
- The US Senate: http://www.senate.gov/

You may also research on the Library of Congress THOMAS site (in the spirit of Thomas Jefferson; http://thomas.loc.gov/home/thomas.php). Through this website, you can look up any bill being considered by Congress. (Your state website offers similar opportunities.) Plug in your profession (eg, physical therapy or occupational therapy), similar related health care terminology (eg, rehabilitation), or perhaps a disease (eg, Parkinson's or stroke) and see how many bills are in process or under consideration for the current Congressional session. Why do you think these bills are important, timely, and worth consideration to become law?

Now, find out what the key legislative issues are in the current year for the public policy agenda items being considered by your profession for our patients and clients; within your district, region, state; or at the national level. Check with your national and state membership organizations to determine which bills are being worked for cosponsorship or are opposed. Then, do your part and advocate for the health care bills by doing any and all of the following:

1. Contact your national or state membership organizations (APTA, AOTA, etc) to obtain the latest information and talking points regarding bills affecting your patients and profession. Most national organizations have things set up for you to advocate directly through the association resources. Take Action Sites are as follows:

   - APTA: http://www.apta.org/TakeAction/
   - AOTA: http://capwiz.com/aota/home/
   - ASHA: http://www.asha.org/advocacy/

2. Email your Congresspersons directly, provide your reasons why they should support the bill and why it will benefit society and the patients you serve, and share your story. The national Take Action sites are all set up for you to be able to take action directly, without much effort, and you should continue with repeat messaging as the bill goes through multiple committees and until the final bill is acted upon or the session ends. (Then the process starts up all over again in the next session!) Congress listens to constituents!

3. Visit your members of Congress when they are in your district and do the same with your local state representatives. Get to know them in person as their constituent and ask them to visit your practice. Again, don't be shy; this is the time to brag about how you help your patients and how they can help you to better serve society. Have your members of Congress speak with a few of your grateful patients to share firsthand the impact of the work of the profession.

4. Follow the bill, and continue to follow up with your state and national representatives. Have your patients help by showing them how to act, too! APTA offers a specific Take Action Center just for patients. Promoted positively, social media can be a big help in getting messages out and building enthusiasm for the policy agenda.

5. If you enjoy legislative advocacy, get in touch with your state and national membership staff and elected leaders from your APTA, AOTA, ASHA, and other member associations to see how you can further assist in defending occupational therapy, physical therapy, and other health care rehabilitation needs for our patients. You may also find it helpful to partner in the advocacy efforts with local community health organizations, health care centers, and support groups. All politics remain local; hence, it is relevant to connect on the national and local levels at every opportunity. Participate in town halls and other events in your home district and share with others how your profession makes a difference!

"If your actions inspire others to dream more, to learn more, to do more, and to become more, you are a leader."
–John Quincy Adams

EXERCISE 4: STRETCHING—PUTTING IT ALL TOGETHER: PATIENT-FAMILY EDUCATION PLAN

Please complete this exercise once you have completed all the chapters in *Patient Practitioner Interaction*. The exercise is introduced here to begin to stretch you to think about this patient case as you proceed with your additional learning in the upcoming chapters. Then come back to the exercise and put it all together.

Consider a patient, Kim, within a neurorehabilitation unit who is receiving ongoing therapies twice per day. You are going to instruct her parent and the patient in a home educational program for the long weekends and after hours when therapy is not in session. The patient is a 19-year-old female who was traveling with 3 friends back to Florida from Mardi Gras. They were drinking and driving; she was not wearing a seatbelt, but everyone else in the vehicle was. They were involved in a motor vehicle accident, and she was thrown from the car through the window and sustained a traumatic brain injury. Kim had graduated from high school, where she had run track, and has been attending the local community college and working at the Gap. Her mom has a high school education and works part-time as a waitress, and her father completed vocational school and works at the local wheel manufacturing plant. Kim was living at home at the time of the accident. Her parents are Bible Baptist, raised their child in their religion, and were not aware that she consumed alcohol at all. The mother wants her to get rest so that her brain heals more quickly and does not want to cause her further injury, but the father is very worried about the medical bills and wants her to be discharged as soon as possible. Kim was released from the acute care hospital after 5 days and discharged to the neurorehabilitation unit for a potential 30- to 90-day stay.

Currently, Kim requires the assistance of 1 to 2 health care professionals, minimally to moderately, for all of her activities of daily living, including bathing and dressing. Kim is able to ambulate with moderate to maximum assistance of 1 to 2 health care professionals. Her primary problem with upright gait is that she has extreme trunk extension in standing and is therefore unable to maintain her center of gravity within her base of support in upright postures. When ambulating, she tends to lean to the right side, and it becomes more pronounced as she fatigues. However, she is able to sit with the standby assistance of 1 health care professional for short periods of time. She must use a posey vest when seated in the wheelchair, even with the use of the tray table, due to lack of safety recognition and sudden movements.

Kim has a 1- to 2-beat clonus in her right lower extremity and approximately a one-finger-width subluxation at the right glenohumeral joint, with pain with flexion above 90 degrees and beyond 45 degrees of abduction. She tends to hold her arm in a flexed and adducted position across her body, as if it were in a sling. The therapist reported this to the doctor, and a plain x-ray was completed, which ruled out any fracture. The physical and occupational therapists have been doing cotreatments once a day because her endurance for activities is still only about 45 minutes at a time. She is also receiving speech therapy and speaks in a very monotone pattern, without voice inflections. She is having memory problems but is emerging in cognition. She is able to follow 1- to 2-step commands. She is inconsistent in her bowel and bladder control and therefore wears a disposable diaper garment. Kim is able to write her name, but it is micrographic and excessively slanted, not like she used to write at all.

Kim is experiencing some right-side neglect and has netting over her bed, called a full-enclosure bed or posey bed, that is like a canopy with netting/webbing on all 4 sides (to avoid needing night restraints so she does not need to be in posey garments during the night) to keep her from wandering at night or injuring herself or others, along with full bed rails. The nursing staff has video monitoring of the room to ensure that suffocation or entrapment is not a concern, and they do rounds every hour. Kim is eating and drinking well and requires minimal to moderate assist of 1 aide to help with meals due to distractibility and difficulty grasping objects and placing consistently. She has challenges with utensil use and putting on her makeup. She can brush her hair but tends to ignore the right side. We are trying to determine if she might have a hemianopia. She is unable to stand and balance on 1 leg without maximum assistance from 1 health care professional and has trouble maintaining middle line with stationary standing, even in the parallel bars with cueing and the use of a mirror for feedback.

- Glasgow Coma Scale: Eye Opening, 4; Verbal Response, 3; Motor Response, 6
- Rancho Los Amigos Scale: Level V and Level VI (fluctuating)

Develop a measurable education goal (in the ABCD format) for the patient with traumatic brain injury's parent(s), and expand the plan to include the educational elements provided by the Sluijs checklist (see Table 15-4). Consider in your educational plan the learning style of the family member(s), cultural elements, active teaching strategies, leadership principles, the potential need for conflict resolution, generational differences, effective communication, aspects of interpersonal interactions, the FOG and Flesch formulas, the stage of change determinations, and any need for consultation or referrals. Prepare your educational plan based on the goal, following the checklist, as applicable related to your selected goal, and be prepared to implement it in a class session designated by your instructor. Don't forget to use peer and self-assessment of your developed patient education plan. Please consider safety aspects related to Kim's emerging coma status.

> **The exercises at the end of this chapter are also available online.**
> **Please refer to the sticker in the front of the book and enter the access code provided.**

COMMUNICATING TO ESTABLISH RAPPORT AND REDUCE NEGATIVITY

Helen L. Masin, PT, PhD

OBJECTIVES

- To appreciate the importance of developing rapport in effective communication.
- To recognize principles of neurolinguistic psychology (NLP) to assist health care professionals (HCPs) in developing effective verbal and nonverbal communication skills.
- To compare and contrast NLP, primary representational systems, and the impact on effective communication skills.
- To distinguish generational differences in communication styles.
- To realize the impact of digital applications in communication.
- To discover and practice mindfulness principles to reduce health care professional stress and enhance patient-practitioner interactions (PPIs).
- To understand principles of positive psychology, which recognize human strengths and promote resilience and resourcefulness in ourselves and in our patients.
- To learn principles of nonverbal communication for enhancing PPIs.
- To acquire the problem-solving approach of "MYOUR" as used in NLP as a model for enhancing effective communication skills.

The importance of rapport has long been recognized in health care; it is commonly referred to as *bedside manner*. Exactly what constitutes appropriate bedside manner? A patient can easily tell you when it is present and when it is not present, although the patient may not be able to describe specifically what characteristics exemplify good PPI. If a health care professional has good rapport, the patient may perceive that health care professional as warm and caring. However, if the health care professional has poor rapport, the patient may perceive that health care professional as cold and distant. The purpose of this chapter is to help you recognize rapport and develop skills in using rapport to enhance your therapeutic presence for best practice with PPI.

Stop now and think of a time when you went into a health care professional's office for the initial visit. In your mind's eye, envision this experience from beginning to end before reading this chapter.

If you felt comfortable with the health care professional, you may have decided to use his or her services again. If you did not feel comfortable, you probably decided to find another health care professional. Take a moment to list the factors

Davis CM, Musolino GM. *Patient Practitioner Interaction: An Experiential Manual for Developing the Art of Health Care, Sixth Edition* (pp 181-198).
© 2016 SLACK Incorporated.

TABLE 11-1
PROFESSIONAL BEHAVIORS FOR THE 21ST CENTURY
Critical thinking—The ability to question logically; identify, generate, and evaluate elements of logical argument; recognize and differentiate facts, appropriate or faulty inferences, and assumptions; and distinguish relevant from irrelevant information. The ability to appropriately utilize, analyze, and critically evaluate scientific evidence to develop a logical argument, and to identify and determine the impact of bias on the decision-making process.
Communication—The ability to communicate effectively (ie, verbal, nonverbal, reading, writing, and listening) for varied audiences and purposes.
Problem solving—The ability to recognize and define problems, analyze data, develop and implement solutions, and evaluate outcomes.
Interpersonal skills—The ability to interact effectively with patients, families, colleagues, other health care professionals, and the community in a culturally aware manner.
Responsibility—The ability to be accountable for the outcomes of personal and professional actions and to follow through on commitments that encompass the profession within the scope of work, community, and social responsibilities.
Professionalism—The ability to exhibit appropriate professional conduct and to represent the profession effectively while promoting the growth/development of the physical therapy profession.
Use of constructive feedback—The ability to seek out and identify quality sources of feedback reflect on and integrate the feedback and provide meaningful feedback to others.
Effective use of time and resources—The ability to manage time and resources effectively to obtain the maximum possible benefit.
Stress management—The ability to identify sources of stress and to develop and implement effective coping behaviors; this applies for interactions for self, patients/clients and their families, members of the health care team, and in work/life scenarios.
Commitment to learning—The ability to self-direct learning to include the identification of needs and sources of learning and to continually seek and apply new knowledge, behaviors, and skills.
Reprinted with permission from Kontney L, May W, Iglarsh A. *Professional Behaviors for the 21st Century, 2009-2010.* Marquette University College of Health Sciences–Physical Therapy. http://www.marquette.edu/physical-therapy/documents/ProfessionalBehaviors.pdf.

that made your experience comfortable or not very comfortable. Specifically, what were some of the health care professional's behaviors that you identified? What were some of your responses to those behaviors? Finally, focus on what role verbal and nonverbal communication played in your interpretation of the behaviors.

To be effective, health care requires interaction with people who often are not functioning at top levels. Increasingly, health care professionals are bombarded with information regarding the importance of effective communication skills. In 1995, May et al[1] identified 10 generic abilities that clinicians determined were essential for success as a physical therapy professional. One was communication skills, or the ability to communicate effectively (speaking, body language, reading, writing, listening) for varied audiences and purposes. A second was interpersonal skills, including the ability to interact effectively with patients, families, colleagues, other health care professionals, and the community and to deal effectively with cultural and ethnic diversity issues. A third was use of constructive feedback, which involves the ability to identify sources of feedback, seek out feedback, and effectively use and provide feedback for improving personal interactions.

Kontney et al[2] updated their research on professional behaviors to address the Millennials (born 1982 to 2000), who are now the largest share of the United States workforce. In keeping with changes in the profession of physical therapy, with the move to a doctoring profession, Kontney et al[2] updated the former generic abilities using focus groups and input of all stakeholders, which resulted in the *Professional Behaviors for the 21st Century, 2009-2010* (Table 11-1) and the Professional Behaviors Assessment Tool. The research identified the same 10 behaviors identified in the original work; however, the rank order for the items changed, with critical thinking abilities moving up due to the doctoring profession. Communication and interpersonal skills and use of constructive feedback are still identified by professionals as essential professional behaviors for health care professionals.[2] Schmoll[3] reinforced the need for responsive PPIs by saying,

"Increasingly, our professional role will encompass that of an educator. If I treat you, it's for today. If I teach you, it's for a lifetime." In classical Latin, *doctor*, from "docere," means just that—to teach.

An essential component for success in the managed care environment is to listen to the customer (patient/client).[4] By listening carefully to your customers (patients/clients), you will find that the things that satisfy them are not the costly things that you do.[4] Be sure that what you are doing has demonstrated value to your customer (patient/client). All of the interactive processes are critical to the rendering of effective health care.

As discussed in Chapter 6, professional knowledge and skill are critical to health care professionals, but we also need to be able to interact in healing ways. Indeed, "[h]ow we approach patients, speak to them, touch them, and listen to them has as much, or more of an impact on healing, than do knowledge and skills of our professional preparation."[5] For health care professionals, the ability to communicate with patients is a critical component to being successful in therapy with patients. To be successful in these therapeutic processes, we must understand the nature of communication, the nature of therapeutic relationships, and the context in which this communication takes place (see Chapter 12).

COMMUNICATION FROM A QUANTUM PERSPECTIVE

Because so much of what we know about the process of interpersonal interaction involves nonverbal communication, or energetic vibration (we even refer to the "vibes" someone is sending), it is important to take a closer look at the concept of energy exchange as an important process in interaction and communication.

Current research in quantum physics supports a view that acknowledges the importance of relationships. In the quantum world, relationships are not just interesting. To many physicists, relationships are all there is to reality.[6] The physics of our universe is revealing the primacy of relationships. As we let go of our Cartesian, linear, and mechanistic models of the world, we begin to step back and see ourselves in new ways, to appreciate our wholeness.[6] We are observing in ourselves, as well as in all living entities, boundaries that preserve us from and connect us to the infinite complexity of the outside world. Jantch[7] stated that, "in life, the issue is not control but dynamic interconnectedness." None of us exists independent of our relationships with others. If this is true, then all of us need to develop better skills in communicating in all of our relationships.

The developments in quantum physics present us with a dramatic paradigm shift regarding what we perceive as real. Newtonian physics taught us that the basic elements of nature were small, solid, indestructible objects. However, quantum physics teaches us that atoms, the building blocks of all matter, actually consist of vast regions of space in which very small particles move. Depending on how these small particles are observed or considered, they may behave as particles or as waves. Given this quantum interpretation, solid objects are no longer perceived as solid. Even though our 5 senses tell us that we are made up of solid matter, we are probably more like a mass of energy set in constant motion. This energy is constantly breaking itself down and building itself back up. Research in psychoneuroimmunology addresses this "energy flow" as a force that responds to our own inner chemistry. Mind and body are united in a whole nurtured by the flow of vital energy, or chi.[8]

This paradigm shift is important for health care professionals to understand in facilitating the healing process. Many of the integrative therapies in rehabilitation, such as reflexology, craniosacral therapy, and acupuncture, address the concept of energy flow in the therapeutic process.[8] What this chapter means to emphasize is that all interaction is, at its essence, vibrational. Therefore, sensitivity to one's own energy (vibration) and the energy of others helps a great deal to clarify and improve the effectiveness of our communication.

In quantum physics, relational holism demonstrates how whole systems are created among subatomic particles. Through this interaction of particles, parts of the whole are changed, drawn together by a process of internal connectedness. Electrons are drawn into intimate relations as their wave aspects interfere with one another, overlapping and merging; their own qualities of mass, charge, spin, position, and momentum become indistinguishable from one another. According to Zohar,[9] it is no longer meaningful to talk of the constituent electrons' individual properties because these continually change to meet the requirements of the whole. If we apply this microcosmic model from quantum physics to the macrocosmic model of human communication, then we have a dynamic paradigm for communication that reflects the interactive processes that occur with each communication encounter.

Remember from Chapter 6 that the process of empathy as described by Stein[10] and Davis[11] includes self-transposal, followed by a "crossing over" or shared moment of meaning, followed by sympathy. This unique form of intersubjectivity illustrates the dynamic interactive aspect of communication and introduces this idea that energy, as meaning, can cross over and be exchanged in meaningful interaction.

Slight Adjustments Can Make Large Differences

Another fascinating finding from the research in quantum physics indicates that a very small change may have an impact far beyond what could have been predicted. Until recently, observations from empirical research that fell outside the predicted, linear, hierarchical model were generally discounted or explained away. For example, we were trained to believe that small differences averaged out, that slight variances converged toward a point, and that approximations would give us a fairly accurate picture of what could happen. However, the research in chaos theory has changed these beliefs; when we view the world as a dynamic, changing system, the slightest variation can have explosive results.[6] If we were to create a difference in 2 values as small as rounding them off to the 31st decimal place after 100 iterations or repetitions of the values, the whole calculation would be skewed. Scientists now find that the very small differences at the beginning of a system's evolution may make prediction impossible, referred to as "sensitive dependence on initial conditions."[6] Iteration or repetition creates powerful and unpredictable effects in nonlinear systems. For example, in the first 6 months of human pregnancy, the embryo may experience a change that will significantly modify the outcome of the newborn infant, such as a cleft lip or palate, or even a tumor that will not manifest until much later in life (eg, schwannoma, acoustic neuroma).

In complex ways that we do not understand, the system feeds back on itself, enfolding all that has happened, magnifying slight variances, and encoding it in the system's memory. In this way, prediction is prohibited. If we apply this concept to communications models, slight variations in communication patterns may produce dynamic changes in communicative interactions. As stated in Chapter 7, therapeutic communication requires learning new skills, as well as unlearning habitual, nonhelpful ways of interacting. The purpose of using effective communication is to improve one's therapeutic presence with patients. By communicating in ways that help to solve problems while simultaneously respecting and honoring the human being, practitioners can facilitate the healing process. In sum, practitioners can use the patient-practitioner relationship itself, so important in the nonlinear quantum model, for therapeutic intervention.

Neurolinguistic Psychology

The utilization of NLP has been reported to enhance communication effectiveness in health care settings.[12-14] Laborde[15] defined NLP as a discipline based on the idea that neurology, language, and behavior are interrelated and can be changed by specific interventions. The theoretical basis for NLP emerged from studies of the work of masters in several fields.[15] O'Connor[16] defined NLP as the art and science of excellence, derived from studying how top people in different fields obtained their outstanding results. He described NLP as a practical set of models, skills, and techniques for thinking and acting effectively in the world. Bandler and Grinder[17] believed that by identifying excellence, one could analyze it, model it, and use it. Their initial work studied 3 outstanding communicators: Perls,[18] founder of Gestalt therapy; Satir,[19] founder of family therapy; and Erickson, psychiatrist and hypnotherapist.[20] Grinder and Bandler[17] were also strongly influenced by the work of Bateson,[21] a British anthropologist who wrote on communication and systems theory.

The basic framework for NLP comes from the awareness that our neurological processes are sensory based and that we use linguistics, or language, to order thought and behavior and to communicate with others. In our roles as health care professionals, we are constantly challenged to communicate effectively with our patients, their families, our colleagues, and our support staff. NLP gives us the tools and skills to assist us in enhancing our verbal and nonverbal skills. In NLP terms, the meaning of communication is based on the response that you get. As health care professionals, this puts a great deal of responsibility on the provider to use forms of communication to which the patient can respond. Research conducted by Mehrabian and Ferris[22] using the word *maybe* has shown that communication has multiple aspects. Asking the listener how he or she interpreted what the communicator meant by *maybe*, the interpretation by the listener was 55% from body language (including posture, gesture, and eye contact), 38% from tone of voice, and 7% from the verbal content of the message. Because the study only used one word, it is difficult to generalize the findings to multiple word communications. However, the study raises awareness that the process of our communication may be even more important to the message than the content of our communication.

Rapport

In order to effectively communicate, we must first establish rapport with our client, creating an atmosphere of trust and confidence. Rapport also helps to solidify the participation within which people can respond freely. Think back to your opening visualization at the beginning of this chapter. What were the behaviors that you identified in the scenario with the health care professional that helped establish rapport? What were the behaviors that broke rapport with the health care professional in the PPI?

When 2 people in conversation are in rapport, communication seems to flow. Body language and voice tonality flow together; bodies and words match each other. What is said can create or break rapport, but remember that verbal communication is only part of the total communication. People in rapport tend to match each other's posture, gestures, and eye contact. When rapport is established, people mirror each other, and their body language is complementary.[16] At its best, rapport flows into a focus of concentration that takes on a life of its own, and for a few moments, time is forgotten. Rosenzweig[12] stated that rapport implies a working relationship between 2 people. The patient and practitioner recognize each other's needs, share information, and set common goals. Rapport implies mutuality, collaboration, and respect; however, rapport results from more than just good intentions. Words and actions must be carefully and sensitively chosen in PPIs.

The presence of rapport helps to diminish illness, enhances satisfaction and compliance, and prevents malpractice litigation.[12] Egbert et al[23] described a special therapeutic rapport that was established with an experimental group of patients undergoing elective laparotomy; these patients received extra reassurance and information. As you might expect, postoperatively, the patients needed only half as many analgesics and were discharged almost 3 days earlier than the control patients. Another study by Inui et al[24] found that enhanced communication skills of physicians resulted in clinically significant improvement in the patients' blood pressure control.

Studies of mothers' compliance with physicians' recommendations were reported by Korsch et al[25] and found that mothers' satisfaction and compliance with treatment depended on whether the doctor was perceived as friendly and on how well the physician conveyed information. Finally, malpractice specialists reported that poor rapport between the physician and patient might be the single most common cause of malpractice suits. The risk of litigation increases when patients experience the physician as uncaring, when they fail to discuss or disclose, or when patients are left with unrealistic expectations.[12]

Neurolinguistic Psychology and Rapport

NLP provides a framework that may assist health care professionals in establishing rapport with their clients. The 3 key steps in establishing rapport are matching, pacing, and leading.[16] Matching a person's body language with sensitivity and respect helps to build a bridge between the practitioner and the patient's model of the world. The premise is based on the idea that when people are like each other in body language, they will be more easily connected and in sync. In a sense, the practitioner is matching the patient's explanatory model as described by Kleinman[26] through matching the patient's body language (see Chapter 12).

Matching

Matching is very different from mimicry. Matching involves the subtle modeling of others' movements by small hand movements, body movements, and head movements. It also involves matching distribution of body weight and basic posture. Matching breathing and voice matching are other ways to develop rapport. Matching can occur with voice tonality, speed, volume, and rhythm of speech. Vocabulary and voice matching can be used in telephone conversations as well as in face-to-face encounters.[16]

For some people, matching another initially may feel uncomfortable or unnatural. For others, it may happen naturally. Notice your reactions when you are matching or when you are being matched. If you want to establish rapport and the person has fidgety movements, you may want to cross-match by subtly swaying your body or moving subtly without actually fidgeting yourself. It is not necessary to like the person to establish rapport. You are using this skill to better understand the person and thus develop a working relationship with him or her.[16] Try it with someone you have difficulty understanding. Matching his or her body posture and movements may help you grasp his or her point of view. In some situations, by matching the other person's body language, you may experience what he or she is feeling in your own body and thus better appreciate his or her nonverbal communication with you.

In some cases, you may choose not to establish rapport. For example, in a situation in which the other person appears hostile, you may choose to break rapport. You can break rapport by mismatching body language, tonality, speed, volume, or rhythm of speech. If you are seated, you may stand up to indicate nonverbally that the interaction is over. If you need to continue the communication at a later time, you can suggest another time to meet once the person has had some time to calm down. You might ask the person to write down his or her concerns to bring to your subsequent meeting. By writing down his or her concerns, he or she may release some of the tension that caused you to end the initial meeting. If you sense that you are still unable to resolve the issue at your rescheduled meeting, you may wish to ask another colleague to be present for your meeting.

> Tim and Chris were trying to decide whether to spend the evening going to a movie or studying for an exam they had coming up next week. Chris really wanted to go to the movie and was angry with Tim for "never wanting to have any fun." Chris was disappointed that Tim was not interested in going to the movie with her. However, she decided to see the situation from Tim's perspective. She matched his posture and his tone of voice and suddenly she remembered that he had barely passed the last exam and was worried that he might not pass this course. As she matched his voice and posture, she felt his fear and vulnerability and suggested that they both study alone for a while and then quiz each other later. Tim breathed a sigh of relief and suggested that if they got enough accomplished, they might go out for a while later.

A good example of a time when you would want to break rapport would be when a patient was acting inappropriately, such as in a sexual manner.

> Judy, a physical therapist, was treating a man with cervical disk herniation with manual therapy while he lay supine on the treatment table. She was seated at his head and was gently mobilizing his very tense neck muscles when he asked her out of the blue, "Are you turned on when you do this?" She responded, directly but not unkindly, that she was thinking about his neck pathology and that sexuality was not at all a part of her concern. Besides that, she was happily married and wanted to keep the relationship with her patients on a strictly professional level. Not to be put off, her patient replied, "Well, does your husband make you happy in bed?"
>
> At that point, Judy knew she had to break rapport. She stood up, looked her patient in the eye and said firmly, "This treatment is over. As I said, it is very important that we keep a professional relationship between us. If you cannot do that, I will have to refer you to another therapist. Please make a follow-up appointment for next week, but recognize that I will not see you if you continue to be inappropriate with me."

Pacing and Leading

Once you have established rapport with someone, you can change your behavior, and he or she is likely to follow you. This is referred to in NLP as *pacing and leading*, and it consists of the use of rapport, developing respect for the other person's world view, and assuming a positive intention. To pace and lead successfully, one must pay attention to the other person and be flexible enough in one's own behavior to respond to what one sees, hears, and feels.[16] Superior teachers do this intuitively. First, they establish rapport with their students, enter the students' world, and then pace the students to move into the subject or skill that is being taught; health care professionals can do the same thing with practice.

Pacing or matching behavior creates the bridge through rapport and respect. When leading, you change your behavior so that the other person can follow. However, one must have rapport before one can pace and lead. When the health care professional is pacing the patient, the health care professional matches the patient's posture, verbal tonality, and speed of speaking to establish rapport. When the health care professional recognizes that he or she has matched the patient's pace and that he or she has rapport with the patient, he or she introduces a change in posture, verbal tonality, and speed of speaking, and the patient then follows the health care professional's lead. This only occurs once the health care professional has established rapport with the patient by first matching and pacing the patient on several levels of communication (eg, posture, tonality, speed). Rapport is a critical skill in intercultural communication, as will be discussed in Chapter 12. Without rapport, intercultural communication may be doomed from the start. Because much of communication is perceived nonverbally, there is a chance to establish rapport even though there are verbal language differences.

Nonverbal communication is the language of culture. Through the development of rapport, the health care professional matches the patient's body language, tonality, speed, volume, and rhythm of speech.[16] If the dialogue is between a low-context (individualistic) and a high-context (collectivistic) individual, the practitioner can take nonverbal cues from the patient that will assist in establishing rapport, even if the practitioner does not speak the language of the patient. The person from a low-context (individualistic) culture will generally rely heavily on the spoken word and demonstrate little gesturing or touching in the communication interaction. The person from the high-context (collectivistic) culture will generally rely less on spoken words but will use more gesturing or touch in the communication interaction.

When using a medical interpreter, the health care professional can match the body language and tonality of the patient while listening to the medical interpreter. Thus, at the unconscious level, the therapist is establishing rapport nonverbally with the client, while listening to the words of the medical interpreter.[27]

Pacing is especially helpful in dealing with intense emotions in communications. If someone is angry, you must first match his or her anger at a lower intensity. This will keep the anger from escalating. Once you have matched, you gradually reduce the intensity of your own behavior to lead the person to a calmer state. If someone approaches you with a sense of urgency, you can match him or her by speaking a little louder and quicker than usual and then pace the person to a softer and slower speed.[16] When lack of pacing and leading occurs, the PPI can escalate or the other person may sense a lack of understanding. The nuances of PPI require much practice and attentiveness. Try videotaping yourself practicing pacing and leading with the simple scenarios described and review to learn how you are progressing.

PREFERRED REPRESENTATIONAL SYSTEMS—PREDICATES

As human beings, we are all capable of thinking. However, we tend to think about **what** we are thinking about rather than **how** we think. Because of this, we often believe that other people think in the same manner we do. This often causes difficulty in communications with people who have different ways of thinking. In NLP, these patterns or ways of thinking are called *representational systems*. They are another tool in NLP that may assist health care professionals in communicating with patients.

Representational systems are the ways in which we take in, store, and code information in our minds through seeing, hearing, feeling, tasting, and smelling. Thought patterns have direct physical effects on the mind and body. For example, think about eating your favorite food. Although the food may be imaginary, your production of saliva is measurable. This Pavlovian conditioned reflex is a good example of the influence of the mind on the body. We use the same neurological paths to envision or represent experience inwardly as we do to experience it outwardly or directly. These same neurons generate electrochemical charges that can be measured by electromyography readings. We use our sensory systems (sight, touch, hearing, smell, and taste) to perceive the world, and then we inwardly represent the world in our minds.[16]

According to O'Connor,[16] visual (V), auditory (A), and kinesthetic (K) systems are the primary representational systems in Western cultures. In NLP, the senses of taste and smell are often included with the kinesthetic sense. People from Western cultures generally use all 3 of these primary systems all the time, but they are not equally aware of them, tending to favor some over the others. The visual system has external (E) representations when one is looking at the outside world (VE) and internal (I) representations when one is mentally visualizing (VI). The auditory system is divided into hearing external sounds (AE) and internal sounds (AI). The auditory system of internal sounds includes the internal voices and dialogue of the individual.[16] For example, the health care professional may be hearing the client say "good morning" in the external environment of the clinic and, at the same time, he or she may be having an internal dialogue about why he or she got a speeding ticket on the way to work. Remember from Chapter 2 that the way we view ourselves and the world is directly influenced by the internal sounds of the voices of our parents that we have interjected or incorporated, usually not on purpose.

The kinesthetic system includes the feelings that accompany tactile sensations such as touch, temperature, and moisture (KE) and internal feelings (KI) of remembered sensations; emotions; and inner feelings of balance, body awareness, and proprioception. Human behavior is based on a mixture of these internal and external sensory experiences. If a person uses one internal sense habitually, it is called his or her *preferred representational system (PRS)*. The words that a person uses in conversation indicate his or her PRS, and thus yield important clues for establishing rapport.[16] For example, we all know some people who constantly respond, "Oh, I see," and others who reply, "I hear you."

According to Jepson,[13] the visual PRS is found in about 60% of the population. People who are organized, appearance oriented, and observant tend to fall into this category. They are good spellers and memorize in their mind's eye. They are distracted by noise but often have difficulty following verbal instructions. They prefer reading for themselves rather than hearing the words (auditory). They become distracted if they are given too much verbal information.[13] Stop and think—are you a person who will read the written instructions first before attempting to put a new purchase together out of the box?

People with auditory PRS account for about 30% of the population. They are experts at matching pitch, accents, timbre, and tones. When reading silently, they may move their lips. They may have a tendency to talk out loud to themselves. They are good listeners and can follow verbal instructions easily.[13] Stop and think—would you rather have someone verbally teach you a new theory than read about it?

The remaining 10% of people have a kinesthetic PRS. They enjoy hands-on experiences and prefer to learn by doing. They are generally physically oriented and physically demonstrative. They may tend to appear restless. They may live in a disorganized environment.[12] Stop and think—do you want to put that new purchase together from the box without reading the directions first?

Figure 11-1. This illustration shows what you see when looking at another person.

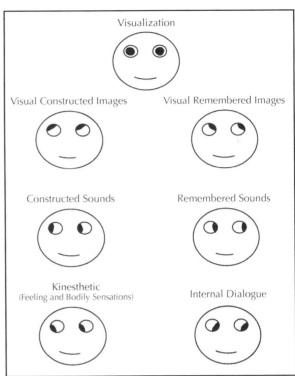

Remember that to build rapport, the listener matches the speaker. As a practitioner, one can listen for the language that a person uses to find out whether someone's PRS is visual, auditory, or kinesthetic. Because language communicates our thoughts, words will reflect the PRS that we prefer using. For example, 3 people with different PRSs may read the same book. The visual individual might say that he or she **saw eye-to-eye** with the author's premise. The auditory person might say that the author's message **sounded clear as a bell** to him or her. Someone who is primarily kinesthetic might say that he or she had a **solid grasp** of the author's premise. Although all 3 read the same book, they all responded differently. One was thinking in pictures (visual), one in sounds (auditory), and one tactilely (kinesthetic).

In NLP terms, these sensory-based words (verbs, adjectives, and adverbs) are called *predicates*. Understanding the use of predicates enables a practitioner to match predicates with the patient as another means of gaining rapport. When working with a patient who is nonverbal, it is a good idea to use a mixture of visual, auditory, and kinesthetic predicates to optimize the communication because the person's PRS cannot be elicited verbally. It is also important to use a mix of predicates when addressing a large group of people to engage all 3 PRS styles.[16]

DISCOVERING PREFERRED REPRESENTATIONAL SYSTEMS: OBSERVING EYE MOVEMENTS

Another important tool in NLP is the observation of what is termed *eye accessing*. Dilts[28] discovered visible behavioral changes that signaled neurophysiological outputs that were clues to PRSs, including eye movements made during accessing of memory, breathing changes, skin color changes, and body postural changes. Neurological studies have shown that eye movement laterally and vertically appears to be associated with activation of different parts of the brain. It is useful to observe eye movements in someone to better understand that person's experience as we are communicating with others. There appears to be some common neurological connection between eye movements and PRS because the same patterns are found worldwide (except for the Basque region of Spain).[16] When patients visualize from the past, they tend to move their eyes up and to the left. When they construct a picture or imagine something they have never seen, they tend to move their eyes up and to the right.

Defocusing the eyes or looking straight ahead is another way to know if the speaker is using visualization. The speaker will appear to be looking beyond the listener as if watching an imaginary movie picture. The eyes tend to move to the left for remembered sounds and across to the right for constructed sounds. When the eyes go down and to the right, the patient is usually accessing kinesthetic PRS. When the patient talks to him- or herself, the observer will see the eyes go down to the left (Figure 11-1).[16] Eye accessing cues occur quickly, so the observer needs to watch the patient closely. In some cases, the eye accessing directions may be reversed. The person observing needs to ask several questions to determine whether the patient may have a reverse eye accessing pattern. Reverse eye accessing is sometimes seen in individuals who are left-handed, but it may occur in anyone.

POSITIVE DESCRIPTIVE STATEMENTS

The NLP tool of using positive descriptive statements is useful in communicating with patients. A *positive descriptive statement* is a statement describing the behavior that you want the patient to do, rather than the behavior that you do not want. For example, if a child is told, "Don't spill the milk," he or she first has to visualize spilling the milk in order to not spill it. If an adult is told, "Don't cross your legs" as a hip precaution, he or she first visualizes crossing his or her legs in order to not cross them. The health care professional might want to instead say, "Keep your legs parallel" or "Keep your feet pointing straight ahead" so that the person can visualize only the outcome that is being recommended. The health care professional is then reinforcing the preferred visual image to support the physical movement desired.

When working with children, elderly patients, or patients who are easily confused, the use of positive descriptive statements make a big difference in the patient's understanding of your directions. When writing home programs for patients, using positive descriptive statements is extremely helpful in assisting the patients to understand the exercise you want them to practice. However, health care professionals should be careful not to bombard a patient with overstimulation or redundant repetition within any PRS realm. The patient may stop listening, tune out, or be overwhelmed with too much stimuli, resulting in the opposite desired effect. Less is more in most situations, and allowing time for processing is imperative to successful PPIs, especially when the movement systems are affected by disease processes.

GENERATIONAL DIFFERENCES IN COMMUNICATION

Generational differences may also impact communication in unexpected ways. Expectations regarding feedback in communication vary across generations. Traditionalists born before 1946 feel that "no news is good news." Baby Boomers, born from 1946 to 1964, feel that feedback is best once a year whether it is needed or not. Generation X-ers, born 1965 to 1981, frequently ask, "How am I doing?" Millennials, born 1982 to 2000, prefer feedback from a "virtual coach" at the push of button.[29] Technology has impacted our communication dramatically. Computers, Internet, and email have made instant communication possible, but the expectations of appropriate communication vary across the generations.

Many Traditionalists and Baby Boomers use more formal written communication and prefer that titles be used in oral and written communication. Many Gen X-ers and Millennials are more informal and prefer not to use titles in oral and written communication. Because of these differences, conflicts may arise between individuals of different generations in educational settings and clinical settings. For example, a Baby Boomer faculty member may be offended by a Millennial student who not only does not use the formal title in oral or written communication but greets him by his first name. In the clinic, a Traditionalist patient may be offended by a Gen-X physical therapist who calls her by her first name instead of addressing her by her title and surname. As valuable as it is to recognize and honor these important generational differences in style, the fact remains that it is important for health care professionals to value and demonstrate respect for the older client or faculty member if the student wishes to build rapport and enhance communication across the generations. Respect and rapport across these generations begin with the use of a title or surname.

DIGITAL COMMUNICATION AND PROFESSIONAL BEHAVIOR

Gen X-ers and Millennials have been described as "digital natives," and Traditionalists and Baby Boomers have been described as "digital immigrants."[30] Because Gen X-ers and Millennials have grown up with digital communication, they are generally more comfortable with email, texting, social networking, and blogging compared with Traditionalists and Baby Boomers. Because of the popularity of these applications among today's students, educators have little evidence or guidance about preventing misuse and ensuring standards for professional conduct.[31] The digital applications can be a blessing and a curse. As a blessing, they can facilitate communication across time and distance and promote interaction. As a curse, they can create communication glitches because expectations differ regarding the appropriate use of digital communication. Because emailing and texting are 2-dimensional communications, the reader only gets part of the message. The nonverbal, energetic elements of tonality, facial expression, gesture, pitch, pacing, and environmental context are all missing. Can you think of a time when you sent an email to someone and his or her interpretation was totally different from what you had intended? Without the nonverbal cues, email can easily be misinterpreted.

Faculty who are Traditionalists and Baby Boomers may be uncomfortable with the informal tone of emails and texts from students. For example, difficulties may arise when a student sends an email or text in which the salutation uses the faculty member's last name without the title. Sometimes a distressed student may send an emotionally charged email to a faculty member rather than speaking to the faculty member in person. Finally, legal challenges have arisen because the email or text was inadvertently forwarded to someone who found it offensive. In these situations, it is critical for educational institutions to develop policies regarding the appropriate use of digital communication and to address unprofessional digital behaviors as soon as they arise.[32] Respect for others is the key moral component in this discussion. One medical school advises students to "think before you post."[31] We advise students not to send an email unless they are sure that they could comfortably say the precise content of the message to the person, face-to-face and in a respectful manner.

What are your thoughts about policies and procedures regulating email or text conversation between students and faculty? Can you imagine as a student receiving an email or text from a faculty member that offended you and that you wish would not have been sent? What would it contain? Why would it offend you?

Likewise, as a student, can you imagine sending an email or text to a faculty member that might be offensive? What would the circumstances be? How could it be misinterpreted?

Health professional organizations and health care companies are proactively addressing the need for policies related to digital communications. The American Physical Therapy Association Position, Standards of Conduct in the Use of Social Media from the House of Delegates, is one example (http://www.apta.org/uploadedFiles/APTAorg/About_Us/Policies/Ethics/StandrdsConductSocialMedia.pdf). Please review the national governance position and consider the impact on your use of social media as a health care professional. You may also wish to review social media tips and policies within other health professions to determine the similarities or differences and how you shall proceed in your day-to-day use of social media with your patients/clients, peers, and colleagues as we enter a new era with telehealth PPIs.

One final comment: Recent research has indicated that we cannot truly multitask the way that our technology leads us to believe that we can.[30] The mental balancing required to multitask has been shown to shortchange some of the areas of the brain related to memory and learning.[33] Research is revealing that our use of digital technology has begun to alter our attention span. We are beginning to rewire our brains for speed rather than mindfulness. In the health care professions, we must be cognizant of how digital technology impacts us and our patients in positive and negative ways. Then we must make every effort to ensure that we use it for the highest good of all concerned.

Mindfulness in Practice

Mindfulness-Based Stress Reduction (MBSR) is recognized in the health literature of the past 30 years as a helpful tool for individuals coping with clinical and nonclinical problems. These groups have included clients experiencing pain, cancer, heart disease, depression, and anxiety.[34] In addition, MBSR is also helpful in stress management with healthy subjects.[35] MBSR helped to decrease ruminative thinking and anxiety in healthy subjects while increasing empathy and self-compassion. Mindfulness is the practice of cultivating nonjudgmental awareness of each moment in our day-to-day lives.

Originally developed by Zinn at the University of Massachusetts Stress Reduction Clinic, the MBSR is a basic 8-week training that includes formal and informal meditation and yoga practices, which are designed to promote moment-to-moment awareness in participants. Research on the usefulness of MBSR continues in a variety of disciplines, including health care, law, psychology, and education.[36,37] Willgens and Sharf[38] described how mindfulness meditation was taught to physical therapy graduate students as a means of promoting intrapersonal awareness for students who face challenges in their clinical education experiences. Learning mindfulness meditation appears to be a potentially powerful tool for assisting health care professional students who face challenges in integrating effective skills in the clinical setting.

Positive Psychology and E.M.P.A.T.H.Y.

Another helpful tool for health care professionals is the utilization of *positive psychology*. Positive psychology evolved out of humanistic psychology and promotes using the scientific method to understand the positive, adaptive, creative, and emotionally fulfilling aspects of human behavior.[39] Positive psychology examines how different cultural groups experience well-being, including positive human traits, such as kindness, curiosity, and the ability to work on teams, as well as human values, interests, talents, and abilities. All of these positive human characteristics in clinicians contribute to one's therapeutic presence as a health care professional. Health care professionals can benefit from applying positive psychology strategies for themselves, using this chapter's exercises for promoting one's own well-being. Huta and Hawley[40] found that positive emotions can help to fight psychological disorders, such as depression. Compton and Hoffman[39] discovered that a greater capacity for empathy correlates with higher life satisfaction and more positive relationships. Contemporary research in medical education has focused on teaching health care professionals PPI through nonverbal detection techniques and expressions of empathy, including assessing the nonverbal behaviors that are described in the acronym E.M.P.A.T.H.Y.[41]:

- E—eye contact
- M—muscles of facial expression
- P—posture
- A—affect
- T—tone of voice
- H—hearing the whole patient
- Y—your response

More attention is now being focused on nonverbal displays to ensure effective PPI in health professions curricula. Empathy is essential for detection of emotions in patients. If there is a mismatch between verbal cues and nonverbal cues, there may be a lack of congruence in the patient's communication about their condition. In order to better understand the patient's perspective, it is vitally important for the clinician to recognize and address any incongruences during PPIs.

In addition to recognizing nonverbal cues in their patients, health care professionals need to be aware of their own nonverbal cues and how they are being interpreted by the patient and other staff members. The E.M.P.A.T.H.Y. behaviors can be included in assessment tools for evaluating students' interpersonal and communication skills in patient care and team building.[41] Prior to clinical experiences, students may not have received specific feedback on their nonverbal behavior and its impact on patients and colleagues. By bringing nonverbal behaviors to the student's conscious attention, the student has an opportunity to change the behavior to promote better communication. Students sometimes feel that "this is just the way I have always been." As a student develops as a health care professional, his or her behaviors must change to reflect professionalism in all of his or her interactions.[42,43]

Another important aspect of positive psychology is resilience. It has been defined as the ability to adapt positively to a challenge, risk, adversity, or negative event. The American Psychological Association has identified factors that promote the development of resilience, as follows[44]:

- Making connections with family, friends, or community
- Avoiding seeing crises as insurmountable problems
- Accepting that change is part of living
- Moving toward one's goals
- Taking decisive action
- Looking for opportunities for self-discovery
- Nurturing a positive view of oneself
- Keeping events in perspective
- Maintaining a hopeful outlook
- Taking care of oneself by attending to one's own needs and feelings

Through combining NLP skills, positive psychological attitudes and behaviors, E.M.P.A.T.H.Y. behaviors, and mindfulness strategies in communication, the health care professional enhances the ability to be a therapeutic presence in the health care environment. By integrating the skills for one's own well-being, the clinician is better equipped to be a therapeutic presence for clients, families, and coworkers. By cultivating these skills and developing resilience, you shall enhance the development of your own professionalism and optimal communication skills. Now that the Millennials surpass Gen X-ers as the largest labor force in the United States and we have 5 generations represented in health care teams and patients, communicating to reduce negativity has become even more relevant today.[45]

THE MAP VERSUS THE TERRITORY DESCRIBED BY THE MAP

A final critical concept in NLP is that the map is not the territory it describes. The map is a symbol for the territory but it is not the territory itself. Each individual has a perception of the world from his or her point of view, such as the generational differences described. The perceptual filter is our bias with which we experience the world around us. As health care professionals, we must be mindful of our bias, lest it become prejudice. Conflicts may occur between us because we have different maps of reality, as described in the digital miscommunications. Each of us has personal models of the world (explanatory models as will be described in Chapter 12) with our own sets of filters that may include visual, auditory, or kinesthetic PRSs, as well as ways of sorting or categorizing stimuli in the environment. For example, one individual may observe a glass as half full and another individual may observe the same glass as half empty. The glass is exactly the same, but each individual perceives it according to his or her own sorting style. Different sorting styles also act as filters for how the individual perceives a situation in the environment. Another example might be a patient who perceives exercise as an unpleasant requirement in the recovery process, whereas another patient might perceive it as a blessing in his or her recovery process.[16]

If we choose to be successful in our communications with our patients, families, colleagues, and support staff, we must recognize that each person has a different map (or explanatory model) and different filters for the territory in which we all find ourselves. Through the use of NLP, we can learn to respect and appreciate the different maps and filters. Laborde[15] suggested using the acronym "MYOUR" as a way to remember and summarize the communication skills in NLP. "MY" is what I want, "YOUR" is what you want, and "OUR" is making sure everyone gets it. Once we appreciate the different maps and filters that we all have, we are in a better position to work together toward common goals.

CONCLUSION

It is important to remember that NLP, positive psychology, E.M.P.A.T.H.Y, and mindfulness provide us with tools for helping us to connect with our patients, their families, and our colleagues. As health care professionals, we must be willing to be sensitive and flexible to match, pace, and lead for the benefit of others. Whether our patient prefers visual, auditory, or kinesthetic cues, there is no one approach. The health care professional who is able to understand and adapt to the patient's/client's way of thinking and receiving will have much better results with PPI. The health care professional's task is to make the therapeutic relationships as smooth, helpful, and free from conflict as possible. By practicing the basic NLP principles and techniques, positive psychology strategies, E.M.P.A.T.H.Y, and mindfulness, you will be greatly equipped for building your PPI rapport, calming negative PPIs, and promoting well-being in yourself and in your patients/clients. The exercises that follow will give you a start in the process.

REFERENCES

1. May W, Morgan B, Lemke JC, et al. Model for ability-based assessment in physical therapy education. *J Phys Ther Ed.* 1995;9:3-6.
2. Kontney L, May W, Iglarsh A. Professional behaviors for the 21st century, 2009-2010. http://www.marquette.edu/physical-therapy/documents/ProfessionalBehaviors.pdf. Accessed April 19, 2015.
3. Schmoll B. Physical therapy today and in the twenty-first century. In: Scully RM, Barnes MR, eds. *Physical Therapy.* Philadelphia, PA: Lippincott Raven; 1989.
4. Ketter P. Understanding driving forces behind managed care is crucial for survival. *Phys Ther Bull.* 1997;12(29):6-7.
5. Davis CM, Musolino GM. *Patient Practitioner Interaction: Instructor's Manual.* 6th ed. Thorofare, NJ: SLACK Incorporated; 2015.
6. Wheatley MJ. *Leadership and the New Science: Discovering Order in a Chaotic World.* 3rd ed. San Francisco, CA: Berrett-Koehler Publishers; 2006.
7. Jantsch E. *The Self-Organizing Universe: Scientific and Human Implications of the Emerging Paradigm of Evolution.* Philadelphia, PA: Elsevier Science & Technology Books; 1980.
8. Davis C. *Integrative Therapies in Rehabilitation.* Thorofare, NJ: SLACK Incorporated; 2016.
9. Zohar D. *The Quantum Self: Human Nature and Consciousness Defined by the New Physics.* New York, NY: Harper Collins Publishers; 1991.
10. Stein E. *On the Problem of Empathy.* 3rd ed. The Hague, The Netherlands: Martinus Nijhoff; ICS Publications; 1989.
11. Davis CM. *A Phenomenological Description of Empathy as It Occurs Within Physical Therapists for Their Patients* [dissertation]. Boston, MA: Boston University; 1982.
12. Rosenzweig S. Emergency rapport. *J Emerg Med.* 1993;11(6):775-776.
13. Jepson CH. Neurolinguistic programming in dentistry. *J Calif Dent Assoc.* 1992;20(3):28-32.
14. Konefal J. *Chronic Disease and Stress Management.* Denver, CO: NLP Comprehensive International Conference; 1992.
15. Laborde G. *Fine Tune Your Brain.* Palo Alto, CA: Syntony; 1989.
16. O'Connor S. *Introducing NLP.* San Francisco, CA: Conari Press; 2011.
17. Bandler R, Grinder J. *The Structure of Magic.* Palo Alto, CA: Science and Behavior Books; 2005.
18. Perls FS. *Gestalt Therapy Verbatim.* Gouldsboro, ME: Gestalt Journal Press; 1992.
19. Satir V. *The New Peoplemaking.* Palo Alto, CA: Science and Behavior Books; 1988.
20. Gordon D, Meyers-Anderson M. *Phoenix: Therapeutic Patterns of Milton H. Erickson.* Cupertino, CA: Meta Publications; 1981.

21. Bateson G. *Steps to an Ecology of Mind*. University of Chicago Press; 1999.

22. Mehrabian A, Ferris S. Decoding of inconsistent communications. *J Pers Soc Psychol*. 1967;6:109-114.

23. Egbert LD, Battit GE, Welch CE, Bartlett MK. Reduction of postoperative pain by encouragement and instruction of patients: a study of doctor-patient rapport. *N Engl J Med*. 1964;270:825-827.

24. Inui TS, Yourtee EL, Williamson JW. Improved outcomes in hypertension after physician tutorials: a controlled trial. *Ann Intern Med*. 1976;84(6):646-651.

25. Korsch BM, Gozzi EK, Francis V. Gaps in doctor-patient communication: 1. Doctor-patient interaction and patient satisfaction. *Pediatrics*. 1968;42(5):855-871.

26. Kleinman A. Concepts and a model for the comparison of medical systems as cultural systems. *Soc Sci Med*. 1976;12:85-93.

27. Lattanzi JB, Masin HL, Phillips A. Translation and interpretation services for the physical therapist. *HPA Resour*. 2006;6(4).

28. Dilts R. Roots of neuro-linguistic programming part II (the experiment). 1983. In: Jepson C. Neurolinguistic programming in dentistry. *CDA J*. 1992;20(3):30-31.

29. Lancaster LC, Stillman D. *When Generations Collide: Who They Are. Why They Clash. How to Solve the Generational Puzzle at Work*. New York, NY: Harper Business; 2003.

30. Life on the virtual frontier: distracted by everything. Frontline, Digital Nation. www.pbs.org/wgbh/pages/frontline/digitalnation/view/?utmcampaign=viewpage&utm_medium=grid&utm_source=grid. Accessed April 24, 2015.

31. Farnan JM, Paro JA, Higa JT, Reddy ST, Humphrey HJ, Arora VM. Commentary: the relationship status of digital media and professionalism: it's complicated. *Acad Med*. 2009;84(11):1479-1481.

32. Hickson GB, Pichert JW, Webb LE, Gabbe SG. A complementary approach to promoting professionalism: identifying, measuring, and addressing unprofessional behaviors. *Acad Med*. 2007;82(11):1040-1048.

33. Freeman J. *The Tyranny of Email*. New York, NY: Scribner; 2009.

34. Grossman P, Niemann L, Schmidt S, Walach H. Mindfulness-based stress reduction and health benefits: a meta-analysis. *J Psychosom Res*. 2004;57(1):35-43.

35. Chiesa A, Serretti A. Mindfulness-based stress reduction for stress management in healthy people: a review and meta-analysis. *J Altern Complement Med*. 2009;15(5):593-600.

36. Rogers SL, Jacobowitz JL. *Mindfulness and Professional Responsibility*. Miami, FL: Mindful Living Press; 2012.

37. Scholeberlein D. *Mindful Teaching and Teaching Mindfulness*. Boston, MA: Wisdom Publications; 2009.

38. Willgens AM, Sharf R. Failure in clinical education: using mindfulness as a conceptual framework to explore the lived experiences of 8 physical therapists. *J Phys Ther Educ*. 2015;29(1)70-80.

39. Compton WC, Hoffman E. *Positive Psychology: the Science of Happiness and Flourishing*. Belmont, CA: Wadsworth, Cengage Learning; 2012.

40. Huta V, Hawley L. Psychological strengths and cognitive vulnerabilities: are they two ends of the same continuum or do they have independent relationship with well-being and ill being? *J Happiness Stud*. 2010;11(1):71-93.

41. Riess H, Kraft-Todd G. E.M.P.A.T.H.Y.: A tool to enhance nonverbal communications between clinicians and their patients. *Acad Med*. 2014;89(8):1108-1112.

42. Masin HL. Education in the affective domain: a method/model for teaching professional behaviors in the classroom and during advisory sessions. *J Phys Ther Educ*. 2002;16(1):37-45.

43. Masin HL. Integrating the use of the generic abilities, clinical performance instrument, and neurolinguistic psychology processes for clinical education intervention. *Phys Ther Case Rep*. 2000;3(6):258-266.

44. American Psychological Association. The road to resilience. http://www.apa.org/helpcenter/road-resilience.aspx. Accessed April 24, 2015.

45. Fry R. Millennials surpass Gen Xers as the largest generation in US labor force. Pew Research Center. http://www.pewresearch.org/fact-tank/2015/05/11/millennials-surpass-gen-xers-as-the-largest-generation-in-u-s-labor-force/. Published May 11, 2015. Accessed August 27, 2015.

EXERCISES

EXERCISE 1: CLINICAL ENCOUNTERS

1. Sit across from someone in your class. One person will role-play the therapist and one person the client. Role-play a situation that you remember from a patient-therapist interaction that you have observed. Talk to the patient as you normally would without paying any special attention to matching or mirroring.

    a. What do you experience as the therapist?

    b. What do you experience as the patient?

    c. Do you experience rapport with each other? Why or why not?

2. Sit across from another person in your class. Again, one person is the therapist and one person is the client. Role-play the same situation that you recall from a patient-therapist interaction that you have observed. This time, the therapist will subtly match the body posture, gesture, hand movements, and breathing of the patient.

    a. What do you experience as the therapist?

    b. What do you experience as the patient?

    c. Do you experience rapport with each other? Why or why not?

EXERCISE 2: UNDERSTANDING PREFERRED REPRESENTATIONAL SYSTEMS—PREDICATES

1. Sit across from another person in your class. One person tells a story about his or her favorite vacation. The other person listens to the story and responds as he or she normally would.

   a. What do you experience as the storyteller?

   b. What do you experience as the listener?

   c. Did you experience rapport? Why or why not?

2. Sit across from another person in your class. One person tells a story about a favorite vacation. The other person listens to the story and pays close attention to predicates—the use of visual, auditory, or kinesthetic words and phrases. The listener responds by matching the PRS of the storyteller.

   a. What is the PRS of the storyteller? How do you know?

   b. What is the PRS of the listener? How do you know?

   c. Did you experience rapport? Why or why not?

   d. Describe a clinical situation where use of predicates may be helpful to establish rapport.

EXERCISE 3: EYE ACCESSING ACTIVITY

1. Get together with someone in your class. Ask that person the following questions and record his or her eye movements below. The person responding to the questions can have the eye motion chart on his or her lap facing the person asking the questions so that the person asking the questions can more readily identify what each eye accessing movement indicates. The thought process and the eye accessing are what you want to understand in this exercise. The verbal responses are not important.

    a. What color is the couch in your living room?

    b. What did you see on your way to class?

    c. What would your ideal house look like?

    d. What would you look like with pink hair?

    e. What is the sound of a busy signal on the telephone?

    f. How would your voice sound underwater?

    g. Recite a nursery rhyme in your head.

    h. How does silk feel next to your skin?

2. What did you discover about eye accessing with your partner?

3. How might you use eye accessing in a clinical situation to enhance rapport?

EXERCISE 4: ENHANCING ONE'S OWN WELL-BEING

Imagine several evidence-based strategies, described below, that have been shown to be effective in promoting one's own well-being. Choose one different activity to practice each week during this class. Journal about your experience implementing that strategy; continue as you enter the real world as a health care professional during your internship, clinical, or field work experiences.

1. Savoring—Practice savoring something good that has happened to you by sharing your positive experience with others while it is happening or afterwards. Create a symbol of the event to remind you of the positive experience such as a photo or souvenir of the experience.

2. Gratitude—Write a letter of gratitude to someone who has impacted your life in a positive way and explain why you are grateful to that person. If possible, deliver it in person. If not, mail or fax the letter and follow-up with a phone call.

3. Three good things—Reflect on the positive events you experience each day by writing them in a journal each day followed by your explanation for why this good thing happened.

4. Ways to increase positive emotions:

    a. Become kinder—practice random acts of kindness.

    b. Find healthy distractions to keep you mind off your troubles (eg, joy of a simple walk).

    c. Enjoy natural settings nearby—notice the details in nature.

    d. Be sociable with strangers and acquaintances.

    e. Apply your strengths and virtues in your daily habits.

    f. Practice mindfulness by reaching your highest potential—strive for the best, not mediocre.

    g. Meditation—take a quick but relevant 5 minutes or a deeper 30 minutes.

    h. Help others—anticipate other's needs, open doors, pick up dropped items, let someone in your lane.

    i. Practice gratitude—express your thankfulness to others daily.

    j. Savor positive feelings—write them down, place them in a positive jar, and pull them out when you are feeling bad; reflect on the positive when experiencing the negative.

    k. Visualize your future—tomorrow, next week, next month, 6 months, 1 year, 2 years, 5 years—who are you becoming and how are you developing as a professional? Where are you going? What shall you plan to accomplish? Envision your successful and preferred futures.

EXERCISE 5: MINDFUL EATING

1. Turn off all distractions, including your phone, Facebook, and Internet.

2. Put a raisin in your hand.

3. Focus on the raisin as if you have never seen one before. Imagine that you have just arrived from another planet and you have been given some raisins. Notice how the raisins look and feel in your hand. Notice the textures and colors of the raisins.

4. Bring a raisin to your nose and smell it. Notice if you have thoughts like, "What is the purpose of this strange exercise?" or "I hate raisins." When you have these thoughts, just acknowledge them and bring your awareness back to the raisin.

5. Bring the raisin to your ear and squeeze it and roll it around. Notice if you hear anything.

6. Bring the raisin slowly to your mouth and notice if your mouth begins to water.

7. Slowly put the raisin in your mouth and move it gently around with your tongue.

8. When you are ready, intentionally bite down on the raisin and notice where it goes in your mouth. Notice how it tastes.

9. Slowly chew the raisin and notice how its consistency changes as you chew.

10. When you are ready to swallow, notice your intention to swallow and then track the sensations of the raisin as it moves from your mouth to your esophagus and into your stomach.

11. Take a moment to congratulate yourself for taking this time to experience mindful eating.

12. How might the present moment awareness that you have experienced in this mindful eating experience be useful to you in your patient interactions?

The exercises at the end of this chapter are also available online.
Please refer to the sticker in the front of the book and enter the access code provided.

12

COMMUNICATING WITH CULTURAL SENSITIVITY

Helen L. Masin, PT, PhD

"Of all the forms of inequality, injustice in health care is the most shocking and inhumane." –Dr. Martin Luther King Jr

OBJECTIVES

- To examine the impact of culture and population trends on the delivery of health care.
- To explore and appreciate one's own and other's cultural heritage.
- To recognize the National Standards for Culturally and Linguistically Appropriate Services (CLAS) in health and health care.
- To value the utilization of trained medical interpreters.
- To distinguish the impact of spiritual beliefs, as cultural constructs, effecting health outcomes.
- To examine intercultural communication and issues of cultural competence research.
- To acquire a problem-solving approach that assists health care professionals (HCPs) in enhancing intercultural communication skills.
- To compare and contrast the influence of the health care delivery system environments with respect to communication and culture.
- To identify resources that describe the lives and culture shifts of individuals living with disabilities and/or the lives of their families and friends.

Have you ever experienced culture shock? How did you know? With the ever-increasing options for travel and information exchange via the Internet and other technologies, people who come from different cultures are meeting through work, play, travel, and shared interests. Because of the increasing exposure to different cultures, it has become extremely important to develop an appreciation of, and respect for, people whose culture differs from one's own. To be effective health care professionals, developing professionals and health care professionals must learn to communicate with cultural sensitivity and to work effectively with patients, families, colleagues, staff, and support personnel.

Davis CM, Musolino GM. *Patient Practitioner Interaction: An Experiential Manual for Developing the Art of Health Care, Sixth Edition* (pp 199-222).
© 2016 SLACK Incorporated.

CULTURE SHOCK—WHAT IS IT?

Culture shock has been defined as the stress experienced when individuals cannot meet their everyday needs as they would in their own culture. They may have difficulty communicating, making themselves understood, or figuring out why the locals are behaving in a certain way. In response to the stress of culture shock, one may feel a sense of loss and a sense of shock that others behave so differently and seem to have such a different world view.[1]

When culture shock occurs, familiar ways of behaving that you learn through socialization in your own culture do not work in the new culture. Culture shock may occur when you visit another country; when you move from one type of climate to another; when you talk with people who are members of a different generation from yours; when you meet people who have a different sexual orientation from yours; when you meet people who have a disability; or when you meet people who have a different race, religion, or political view from your own. Culture has the broadest connotation when viewed in this way. If these differences pose challenges to communication among people in daily life, you can imagine the impact of these differences in patient care.

As health care professionals, we are committed to putting the needs of our patients first. In order to do this effectively, the health care professional must be aware of and appreciate the cultural mores and expectations of the individual from the world view of that person. Once the other person's world view is understood, it may be easier to establish a therapeutic relationship. The goal of this chapter is to introduce you to intercultural communication in health care to assist you in developing awareness and skills to work effectively in our increasingly diverse communities.

A Personal Experience

One of my first challenges as a new therapist working in an early intervention program for infants and toddlers with disabilities in Miami, Florida, was to develop a feeding and eating program. I had been involved with a feeding and eating program in the public school system in Maryland, where I had worked prior to moving to Miami. The program had been quite successful in Maryland, and I was delighted to share my experiences with my colleagues in my new setting. I suggested that the classroom teachers begin the feeding program with a food-play activity. The therapeutic objective was to encourage the children to play with the food on their tray. Through play, it has been shown that children will eventually want to bring the food to their mouths to explore it, laying the foundation for the hand-to-mouth feeding behavior essential for self-feeding.

Based on my previous success with this approach in Maryland, I enthusiastically asked the nutritionist at the program to give me several jars of baby food to use for the food-play activity. Many of the children in the program were former premature infants who were generally extremely tactile defensive around their mouths and often resistant to eating food other than in a bottle. The nutritionist gave me the food, and I poured out the jar on the tray of the corner chair of one of the toddlers. The child enthusiastically placed both hands into the food and smeared it all over the tray and all over himself and eventually brought his hands to his mouth to taste the food. Of course, I felt extremely pleased that he had been so engaged in the activity and that he had indeed brought his hands to his mouth and tasted the food as I had hoped. Because this child had a history of tactile defensiveness, this was an excellent response—a real success. The next day I hoped to use the food-play activity with several of the other children in the program.

When I went to work the following day, I suggested that the preschool teachers might want to join me to help introduce the activity with several of the other children with tactile defensiveness. As the teachers politely declined, one by one, I wondered why they were not enthusiastic about my suggestion. I proceeded to work with another child and was again delighted to see that the food play also helped him develop the hand-to-mouth skill. After several more successful days with the food-play activity, I was hopeful that the preschool teachers would finally join in the activity. Because they still politely declined, I decided to ask them whether they had any concerns about the activity. They all said that it made them feel extremely uncomfortable. When I asked them what caused them to feel uncomfortable with the activity, they responded that you are viewed as a bad mother in their culture (Cuban) if you have a messy child. The food-play activity was simply too threatening to them because it challenged their cultural norms about what was acceptable behavior for good mothers with their children.

Once I understood the cultural origins of the issue, I had a much better understanding of the teachers' and parents' concerns. I politely explained to the teachers that my intention had not been to offend them or the mothers, and I asked whether there might be an alternative way that we could address the problem. After talking with them, we decided to implement a solution that addressed my concerns, as well as the mothers' concerns. We decided that we would have the children in diapers for the food-play activity. That way, we could bathe them after the activity and then put their clean clothes back on them. Thus, the children had the benefit of the food play without the messiness. The teachers, parents, children, and I were all pleased. If we had not taken the time to understand the cultural norms involved in this situation, the teachers and families might have been labeled as noncompliant and the children would not have had the benefit of the food-play learning experience that was so valuable for the development of their independent feeding skills.

As a new therapist in Miami, I quickly realized that I wanted to learn as much as I could about the cultures of the children and families with whom I was working. I began a pilot study to investigate maternal perceptions and knowledge about physical therapy in an early intervention program.[2] Through my reading and research, considering matters of diversity, population trends,[3] and the Miami-Cuban culture and values specifically, I learned a great deal, which enabled me to provide more culturally competent care to my patients and their families.

CULTURAL DIVERSITY IN THE UNITED STATES

Christensen's[4] research with clinical professionals pointed out that the ability to work effectively with culturally diverse families requires health care professionals to acknowledge their own cultural backgrounds and to develop a general understanding of specific cultures. Cultural background can be a powerful force in the relationship between health care professionals and the families they serve.[4] As we have learned in most of the chapters in this text, relationships are critical to the therapeutic use of oneself in health care or therapeutic presence.

To understand the need for competent care in health care, one must first recognize the increasing diversity that is developing in the United States. According to the 2014 US Census Bureau data, the percentage of the total population distribution was as follows[3]:

- 63% White alone, non-Hispanic
- 17% Hispanic (any race)
- 13% Black or African American alone
- 5.1% Asian alone
- 1.2% American Indian or Alaska Native
- 0.2% Native Hawaiian and Other Pacific Islanders
- 2.4% two or more races

Some respondents identified with more than one classification due to being multiracial. The United States is projected to become a majority-minority nation for the first time in 2043.[3] Based upon the 2043 projection, the White (non-Hispanic) population will remain the largest single group; however, no group will make up a majority. Further projections from the US Census Bureau predict for the year 2060 that the population distribution in the United States shall increase from 319 million to 417 million, reaching 400 million by 2051.[3] By 2030, 1 in 5 Americans is projected to be 65 years of age or older. By 2056, for the first time, the older population is projected to outnumber those younger than 18 years.[3] The US Census Bureau further projected that the working-age population (18 to 64 years) is expected to increase by 42 million between 2012 and 2060, from 197 million to 239 million; whereas its share of the total population will decline from 62.7% to 56.9%.[3] The shifts in population distribution and diversity are notable for the impacts for health care professionals, especially in regions of nonpluralism of health care professionals, as compared with those served. Aging societies may have fewer working aged health care professionals available to serve, and the number of health care professionals are not yet meeting today's societal needs, especially in rural regions.

CULTURE AND RELATIONSHIPS

According to Wheatley,[5] the quantum physics of our universe is revealing the primacy of relationships. In other words, each aspect of the universe is affected by its relationship to every other aspect of the universe. In quantum physics, nothing exists independent of its relationship with something else, which challenges our traditional Cartesian models of a linear, quantifiable universe.

For example, in organizations, we may ask which is most important—the system or the individual. The quantum physicist will answer, "It depends." It is not an either/or question. It is not important to decide between the 2, but rather to recognize the relationship that exists between the person and the setting. Relationships will always be different and will generate different responses depending on the person at that moment in time. People, like quantum particles, are "fuzzy." They may go from being predictable to being surprising, just as wave packets of matter include potentialities for both forms—particles and waves. If we can appreciate both the "waveness" and the "particleness" in ourselves as well as others, we have a better chance of developing the potential in all of us.

The potential for being a wave or a particle depends on the environment, culture, and context. If we can understand our own environment/culture/context and that of our clients, we have a better chance of developing the therapeutic relationship. Given this quantum physics paradigm of the primacy of relationships and the fuzziness of people, we have more appreciation for our own culture and the cultures of our patients and clients. With this paradigm perspective, we have better chances of developing effective therapeutic relationships within the health care professional's patient-practitioner interactions (PPIs).

The importance of understanding one's cultural world view was emphasized when the US government mandated that care for children be delivered in a culturally competent manner. The federal legislation that began with Pub L No. 94-142 in 1975 required that public school education be provided for all children from 6 to 21 years of age, regardless of handicapping condition. This law was modified as Pub L No. 94-457 (Education of the Handicapped Act of 1986) to include public school education for all children aged 3 to 21 years, regardless of handicapping condition. The law specified that ancillary health services, including physical and occupational therapy (among others), should be provided for all children in a "culturally competent" manner. In 1991, the 2 laws were subsequently reauthorized as Pub L No. 101-119 Individuals With Disabilities Education Act (IDEA), which also specified that these services be delivered in a culturally competent way. The most recent amendments by Congress were passed in December 2004, with final regulations published in August 2006 for school-aged children and September 2011 for babies and toddlers. The current law in effect is the Individuals With Disabilities Education Improvement Act (IDEIA) of 2004, PL No. 108-446.[6] The current law ensures that all children with disabilities receive services and governs how states and public agencies provide for early intervention, special education, and related services, such as evaluations, re-evaluations, and individualized education programs. We are now going to focus on the aspects related to cultural competence; however, you may be interested to know that additional training and resource information on IDEA is available through the US Department of Education website (http://idea.ed.gov/).

CULTURAL COMPETENCE

What constitutes cultural competence? Cross et al[7] defined cultural competence as "the set of congruent behaviors, attitudes, and policies that come together in a system, agency, or among professionals to work effectively in cross-cultural situations." This type of health care professional service recognizes and incorporates the importance of culture, assessment of cross-cultural relations, understanding dynamics of cultural differences, expanses of cultural knowledge, and modification of services to meet culturally unique needs.

The concept of cultural competence is also referred to as *cultural sensitivity* or *intercultural communication*. The term *cross-cultural* refers to comparative studies in multiple cultures. The study of people from different cultures interacting together is called *intercultural communication*. This chapter highlights results of cultural competence research, including cross-cultural and intercultural communication, as they relate to enhancing one's therapeutic effectiveness as a health care professional.

IMPACT OF CULTURE ON THERAPEUTIC EFFECTIVENESS

Given the continuing increase in diversity of the population of the United States in the 21st century, the ability to successfully communicate in culturally diverse settings is essential for all health care professionals. Training in cross-cultural communication enhances the effectiveness of therapists working with clients whose cultures differ from their own.[8] In order to appreciate the importance of developing skill in intercultural encounters, one must first understand the nature of culture itself.

Anderson and Fenichel[9] defined culture as the specific framework of meanings within which a population, individually and as a group, shares its lifeways. Margaret Mead (1901-1978),[10] an American cultural anthropologist, curator of ethnology at the American Museum of Natural History, and prolific author, conducted expeditions to Samoa and New Guinea, with 24 field trips to 6 South Pacific peoples, defined culture as follows:

> *Abstractions from the body of learned behavior which a group of people who share the same traditions transmit to their children and, in part, to adult immigrants who become members of the society. It covers not only the arts and sciences, religion and philosophies to which the world culture has historically applied, but also the system of technology, the political practices, the small intimate habits of daily life, such as the way of preparing or eating food, or of hushing a child to sleep, as well as the method of electing a prime minister or changing the constitution.*

Given these definitions, you can begin to grasp how culture is a critical element in understanding how someone responds to illness or disability. According to Brislin,[11] cross-cultural research shows that complex concepts do not have the same meaning in all cultures. For example, good health to someone in the United States may mean an absence of bacteria or viruses. To someone in China, good health may mean harmony between yin and yang. Therefore, health care professionals must understand general and specific components of complex health concepts.

Culture-general concepts are concepts that are applicable across all cultures. Culture-specific concepts are concepts that are unique to a particular group. People learn to express symptoms of distress in ways that are acceptable to others in the same culture. For example, in India, stress-related disorders are often suspected when the patient is suffering from an upset stomach. In the United States, stress-related disorders are often associated with painful headaches. Compared with other countries, there is a notable difference that shows in the widespread advertising of painkillers in the United States.[11]

As part of the socialization in one's own culture, one learns that certain complaints about distress are acceptable and elicit understanding, whereas other complaints are unacceptable. Understanding the cultural basis for the client's symptoms becomes more critical to accurate evaluation of the presenting problem, leading to an accurate clinical diagnosis. The majority of all United States health care professionals are White Americans. To examine one profession more closely, as of 2012-2013, just more than 80% of physical therapy students are White, whereas 19.9% are from all other ethnicities combined and are represented as follows: 6.1% Asian, 3.2% Black, 3.9% Hispanic/Latino, 1% representing 2 or more races, 0.4% each American Indian/Alaskan Native and Native Hawaiian/Other Pacific Islander, and 4.1% unknown.[12] As the populations served by physical therapists become increasingly diverse, it is essential that health care professionals become skilled in cultural competence and the ability to communicate with clients and families from cultures different from their own. The American Physical Therapy Association's (APTA) Department of Minority/International Affairs is dedicated to increasing the presence of minorities in the profession, as well as educating the current membership regarding intercultural issues. Similar ethnic homogeneity and racial uniformity exists for health care professionals in medicine, nursing, occupational therapy, and speech language pathology. Professional organizations for health care professionals continue to work to address issues of diversity and cultural competence. Later in the chapter, specific guidance shall assist you in assessing and beginning your personal efforts toward cultural competence.

CULTURE AND BELIEF SYSTEMS

In order to understand the ramifications of culture in health care, one must also understand the relationship among beliefs, attitudes, and behavior. According to Dillman,[13] beliefs are what people think is true, attitudes are how people feel about something, and behaviors are what people do. Because culture impacts all 3 of these areas, health care professionals must be sensitive to clients' beliefs, attitudes, and behaviors regarding their illness, injury, or disability as important components of evidence-based practice. When the health care professional understands what the client is experiencing, the client is more likely to feel that he or she can be helped. Belief in the possibility of positive outcomes is central to the delivery of and acceptance of health services.[14] In order for health care professionals to understand the belief systems of their clients, they must first understand the explanatory model of the client.

Kleinman[15] first described the explanatory model as the explanations that are offered for the etiology, onset of symptoms, pathophysiology, course of sickness, and treatment for the particular problem being addressed. On the cultural level, there may be differences between the explanatory model of the family and the explanatory model of the health care professional. These differences can hamper effective delivery of health care. However, by respecting the explanatory model of the client, the health care professional PPI may be enhanced. For optimal healing to occur, there must be a fit between the expectations, beliefs, behaviors, and evaluation of the outcome between the client and the health care professional.

RESEARCH IN INTERCULTURAL COMMUNICATION

Desantis's[16] and Harwood's[17] transcultural studies in medicine and nursing demonstrated that understanding cultural variables is critical to working effectively with different ethnic groups. Jackson[18] discovered that the amount of time spent with the client affected patient satisfaction with medical care for the Black American population receiving treatment for hypertension. DeSantis[16] detected an increased compliance with nursing interventions with Hispanic and Haitian mothers when clients' belief systems were explored and respected by the professional. Harwood[17] stated that ethnic differences appeared to be important determinants of observed differences in health behavior. He found that ethnicity was shown to be particularly relevant to what an individual believes and how he or she behaves with regard to various health practices.

CULTURE AND HEALTH CARE

Cultural differences in relation to health care are reflected in many facets of daily life. Next, we shall examine some of the critical cultural issues that may assist health care professionals in better understanding their clients, including the following:

(1) understanding the characteristics of collectivistic (high-context) cultures and individualistic (low-context) cultures; (2) understanding Eastern and Western perceptions of locus of control and how they differ; (3) the concept of face, heard so often in discussions of Asian cultures; (4) nonverbal intercultural communication patterns; (5) personalismo, a concept critical to understanding expectations of Hispanic culture; and (6) somatization.

In addition to exploring these differences, health care professionals must understand differences related to disability, racism, ageism, sexism, sexual orientation, and intergenerational expectations. Provided at the end of the chapter are numerous resources chronicling the life experiences of individuals and their families living with disabilities, medical conditions, and diseases and/or those affected by race, class status, or aspects of culture and ethnicity. The shared lived experiences provide insight into the challenges faced by persons with disabilities, their altered status in society or culture, and the effects on the lives of their families, caregivers, and friends. Environmental conditions, such as poverty, homelessness, and minimal formal education, are variables that transcend all cultures.

HIGH-CONTEXT AND LOW-CONTEXT CULTURES

First, let's examine the difference between high- and low-context cultures. Cultures that are usually associated with individualism (low-context) include North America (the United States is considered the most individualistic), Western Europe, Australia, and New Zealand. Cultures that are usually associated with collectivism (high-context) include Asia, Africa, Central and South America, and Pacific Island societies.[11]

In order for health care professionals to understand the meaning of these cultural distinctions, they must first be cognizant of their own culture. Saunders's[19] classic works identified numerous characteristics of the Anglo-European culture and/or Western medical culture that may impact the patient-practitioner relationship. Because the majority of health care professionals currently are from Anglo-European roots, it is helpful to understand those values that impact health care, which include the need for personal control over the environment, need for change, time dominance, human equality, individualism, privacy, self-help, competition, future orientation, action/goal/work, openness/honesty, practicality/efficiency, and materialism.[20] These values may conflict with other cultures that may espouse collectivistic beliefs, attitudes, and behaviors.

Collectivistic cultures differ from individualistic cultures in critical ways. Collectivism refers to the tendencies of a system that emphasizes the importance of the "we" identity over the "I" identity, group rights over individual rights, and in-group–oriented needs over individual wants and desires. Individualism refers to the tendencies of a system in emphasizing the importance of individual needs over group needs. The Western Cartesian (individualistic) tradition tends to perceive the self in opposing dualistic terms, whereas the Eastern (collectivistic) tradition tends to perceive the self in a complementary, relational, whole perspective.[21] Differences in world views create very different perceptions for the people who are members of these cultures.

In cross-cultural interactions, low- and high-context cultures reveal marked differences. Graham and Miller[22] stated that low-context cultures, such as most North American and Northern European societies, place emphasis on individualism and individual goals, facts, the management of time, nonverbal communication, privacy, and compartmentalization. Essentially task oriented, they focus on data to provide the answers to living well. Progress is measured in acquiring tangibles or material goods, and goals are action oriented and geared to produce short-term material profits. The driving force of low-context cultures is work. The usual place in which a person is honored is at work. Low-context societies are structured to honor individuals who are financially successful. Emotions may be considered inappropriate in most social and work settings.[22]

Low-context individuals, such as chief executive officers (CEOs) of major corporations in America, are often highly individualistic, directive, and dominating. CEOs tend to be results oriented, independent, strong willed, and quick to make decisions. CEOs may also be impatient, time conscious, solution oriented, and self-contained. They may have a high need to be recognized for performance. When working in groups, low-context individuals need less time to develop relationships in the group, so new and progressive programs can be changed easily and quickly. However, these individuals may create less cohesion and stability in the group and are less committed to group agreements or planned actions. Individualists find that clearing their plans with others may interfere too much with their desire to do their own thing.[22]

In contrast, Tirandis[23] stated that collectivistic or high-context cultures and peoples place emphasis on relationships, group goals, the process, and surrounding circumstances, with time as a natural progression, verbal communication, communal space, and interrelationships. The high-context norms are primarily group oriented. High-context cultures place the relationships of the cultural group before that of an out-group, such as a university, company, or country. The ties to family and community are strong. In general, feelings and emotions are valued, and expression of feelings is encouraged. Religious and spiritual beliefs are highly valued. Behavior is perceived in a complex way. Nuances of meaning are important in nonverbal communication cues, and the status of others is viewed in context.

To reiterate, Asian cultural norms are considered high-context. The personal characteristics that are valued are being indirect, highly affiliative and team oriented, systematic, steady, and quiet. The person is expected to be patient, loyal, dependable, sharing, and respectful; generally slow in making decisions; and a good listener. A longer amount of time is needed for individuals to become acquainted with and trusting of each other, but once the trust is established, the communication is fast. In general, the culture has strong links to the past and is slow to change. The society is highly stable and works as a unified group. The group members feel comfortable with the constant psychological presence of a group. The members are loyal to the group. They demonstrate cooperation and contribution to the group without the expectation of immediate reciprocity and show public modesty about individual abilities.[23] Individuals are more committed to group agreements and planned actions.

The critical importance of understanding the cultural beliefs and norms of clients became apparent while providing physical therapy at a preschool for a 2-year-old boy with cerebral palsy and with a history of grand mal seizures. His family had recently immigrated to Miami from Haiti. All of the professional staff were extremely concerned about him because he was having grand mal seizures at the preschool. The staff contacted the mother to determine whether she was giving him the phenobarbital that had been prescribed by the neurologist. She assured the staff that she was giving her son the medication. When the seizures continued, the staff called the mother again and had a Creole translator speak with her about the phenobarbital. However, the boy still continued to have the seizures at school. Extremely concerned about him, his mother was invited to school and asked to demonstrate how she was administering the phenobarbital. This turned out to be the critical question that had not been initially asked. His mother demonstrated that she administered the phenobarbital to him by bathing him in the medication. No one had even considered that the medicine would be given in any way other than by mouth. An assumption was made based on the Western medical model of oral administration of the medication. Fortunately, after explaining that the medicine had to be administered orally to be effective, once the mother understood this, she followed through with the oral administration. She explained that in the part of Haiti where she had lived, medicine was administered by bathing in it. The practice of oral administration was as strange to her as bathing was to Americans. According to Brislin,[11] whenever people have experiences during which they have to make adjustments, they learn that culture is much more than an abstraction.

Whenever a client is not responding in the way one would have anticipated, it is important to ask whether cultural differences might be causing the difficulty. Health care professionals may ask, "Which of these symptoms is familiar to me, given my own cultural background, and which seem strange?" The symptoms will seem strange if the health care professional has not encountered them in his or her own socialization. According to Turner,[24] there are 3 questions that a health care professional should ask when working with clients to avoid potential biases:

1. How is this client like all human beings?

2. How is this client like some human beings?

3. How is this client like no other human being?

By asking these 3 questions, the health care professional can avoid stereotypes and generalizations and move toward the person's unique problems, needs, and resources.

THE CONCEPT OF FACE

The concept of face, regarded as a universal construct, refers to the sense of self-respect or self-esteem that people demonstrate in communicating with each other. The management of face differs from one culture to the next. According to Ting-Toomey,[21] managing face involves maintaining a claimed sense of self-dignity or regulating a claimed sense of self-humility in interaction. Three possible issues related to face communication include dignity-humility, respect-deference, and imposition-nonimposition. As anyone who has ever done business in the East will tell you, if one wishes to be successful in keeping face, one must understand the cultural background of face work issues, as well as the norms and boundaries inherent in face work negotiation.[21]

According to Haglund et al,[25] the issue of face dialectics proved to be critical to one hospital's retention of Asian nurses. In reviewing the employment records of the Asian nurses, the administration learned that the Asian nurses were leaving after only 90 days of employment. The hospital policy required that all employees receive performance evaluations after 90 days of employment. The Asian nurses were not accustomed to receiving negative feedback face-to-face, which is a Western norm. As a result, the nurses would immediately quit their jobs after the performance evaluation rather than lose face. Misunderstandings are likely to occur more frequently, with increasing diversity in the health care workforce, unless education in intercultural communication becomes a part of pre-employment and ongoing in-service education training for all health care professionals and support staff.

What ideas can you think of that might solve this problem to avoid the loss of face yet still provide adequate feedback to the Asian nurses? In general, one can predict that in individualistic cultures, individual pride is more likely to be overtly expressed, whereas individual shame is more likely to be demonstrated through other ego-based emotional reactions, such as anger, frustration, or guilt. In contrast, in collectivistic cultures, relational shame or face loss, such as face embarrassment or face humiliation, is more likely to be experienced, and individual-based pride is more likely to be suppressed. Overall, the individualistic cultures stress ego-based emotional expressions and individual self-esteem, whereas collectivistic cultures value other focused emotions management and protection of collective self-esteem.

Belenky et al,[26] through gender-based research, indicated that Euro-American males tended to engage in the "morality of justice," whereas Euro-American females tended to engage in the "morality of caring." The ego-based emotions are associated with morality of justice, whereas the other focused emotions are associated with the morality of caring. In other words, in a moral dilemma between doing the right thing vs doing the caring thing, people from individualistic cultures will choose the right action over the caring action. Doing the caring action is more reflective of the high-context or collectivistic world view.

Numerous scholars have noted that individualists in Western cultures tend to perceive emotion, cognition, and motivation as located in the mind, whereas collectivists in Eastern cultures tend to perceive these 3 constructs as stemming primarily from the heart.[27] Western vocabularies tend to emphasize the relationship between self-conception and cognition, whereas Eastern vocabularies and metaphors tend to emphasize self-conception and emotional harmony.[27]

CULTURAL ISSUES OF TIME, SPACE, AND ENVIRONMENTS

Hall and Hall[28] identified time and space as factors of "context" that are universal in all cultures. They distinguished between *monochronic time* and *polychronic time*. In low-context cultures, monochronic time is used. The individual pays attention to time and does only one thing at a time. Time is used to compartmentalize events, functions, people, communication, and information flow.

In high-context cultures, polychronic time is used. In this paradigm, many things may happen or get attention at the same time (multitasking). There is more involvement with people and events. People take precedence over time and schedules. Emphasis is placed on completing human interactions. In low-context perception of monochronic time, information flow and communication are restricted. Meetings and communication in low-context cultures are used to pass on information and/or determine information from which to evaluate and make decisions. In the high-context perception of polychronic time, information flows freely among all participants. Because the information is available to everyone, it is expected that people will use intuition and understand automatically. In high-context cultures, meetings are held to reach a consensus about what is already known. Each person has invisible boundaries of personal space or territory, which often implies ownership or power when linked to physical location. Spatial changes influence and give meaning to human interaction, even more so than the spoken word. Spatial cues, such as distance between the speaker and listener, are perceived by all the senses. Cultures may vary as to which senses are most attuned to spatial cues. For example, appropriate distance between speaker and listener in Anglo cultures is about 2.5 to 3 feet. In Middle Eastern cultures, it is about 2 to 2.5 feet. A popular example of this norm in North American culture is shown when the speaker expresses annoyance that someone is "in my face." However, the Middle Eastern speaker may be confused as to why the North American listener keeps moving away from him or her in conversation.

In some cultures, spatial cues may be primarily perceived by vision, hearing, touch, or kinesthetic prompts. Vision, hearing, and kinesthetic cues are important components of health care professional communication, as described in Chapter 11.

For low-context, monochronic societies and individuals, personal space is perceived as private, controlled, and often large. For high-context polychronic societies or individuals, space is frequently shared with subordinates and centralized or shared in an information network. Time and space are closely linked because access to individuals is often determined by location and timing.[22] Correspondingly, one finds in athletic events on the international scale, such as with the World Cup Soccer games, crowds and teams maintain highly close contact at all times, whereas North American soccer events generally present with greater personal space maintained by all participants. You may also have some experience within time and space cultural differences with "Southern hospitality" or "Cuban time." With Southern charmers, you may always be welcome to come over anytime and stay indefinitely. In Cuban time, if you arrive too early, it may be considered rude, and it is better to arrive an hour or more late. The majority of US health care facilities maintain strict time schedules with precise adherence to time and specific planned utilization of space and equipment. Hence, these approaches to time and space may be problematic and lead to cultural clashes with health care professionals and their patients or coworkers.

However, some regions experience therapy as a shared cultural experience vs a singular experience. A student of clinical education, while participating in outpatient services in Hawaii, was surprised to experience "island time" in which participants attend therapy during the day (scheduled at any time), make an event of the therapy sessions, and everyone brings nourishment to the clinic for all to partake in throughout the day. It is a shared cultural experience vs a singular experience. Certain patient units are also geared toward more inclusive participation by the families, such as joint camps for pre- and postoperative joint replacement rehabilitation. At joint camp units, patients are allowed and encouraged to designate and bring a family member to participate directly in their care on a regular basis, and the patients participate in group rehab sessions, along with the individual care. Group therapy fosters support and a culture of shared experiences in a formal networking process, with the opportunity for informal interactions during meal breaks and planned recreational therapy. Many support groups for specific conditions and diseases benefit from group approaches to coping, management, and recreational and conditioning activities. Families and patients benefit from the collective experiences of all participants sharing and exchanging thoughts, ideas, and strategies.

In addition, variations in the types of setting in which one works may have an impact on your concentration and that of your patients' abilities and stressors. For example, the Neonatal Intensive Care Unit and the Intensive Care Unit (ICU) are very fast-paced and involve caring for critically ill patients with life-sustaining measures, with multiple lines, tubes, and patient-monitoring devices. ICUs, while hectic, also strive to reduce the negative environmental impacts on the patients. Patients desire to move on from the intensive setting quickly but are unable to do so until they are stable (Table 12-1). The acute care setting is somewhat fast-paced and moves patients toward discharge quickly due to the high cost of services in the more acute settings, and the patients are less ill in acute care than the patients in the ICUs. The goal in acute care is discharge to the next level of care or return to home. The rehabilitation and long-term care settings are more moderately paced and involve longer stays for the patients, with less focus on life-sustaining measures and more focus on function and daily living skills. As you look back on the reflections in Chapter 10 of how developing health care professionals are transforming society, you will note variations in the lived experiences of the students in the various types of health care settings, along their professional development journies.

The goal in a rehabilitation unit is to provide more intensive rehabilitation therapies, typically for several hours each day, to improve the patient's ability for daily function and sustained quality movement. Subacute rehabilitation may be in a specialty hospital that may provide acute and long-term rehabilitation services. Extended care or skilled nursing facilities provide for therapies, predominantly for elderly patients who require longer-term nursing care, rehabilitation, and other services. The pace of inpatient facilities is often census driven and based upon the fragility of the patients receiving services. The pace may fluctuate from fast to moderate to slow, depending upon admissions, support staff, and diagnoses being treated. The outpatient setting is fast paced to very fast paced; however, the patients are able to self-mobilize, in general, and commute to attend therapy. Generally, outpatient services address predominantly musculoskeletal and neuromuscular injuries and impairments that may be limiting a person's life function or role in society. Those receiving outpatient rehabilitation services generally attend therapy sessions in less frequent bouts (2 to 3 times a week or several times a month) depending upon the conditions and impairments and functional limitations being addressed. Some patients/clients also receive outpatient services for ongoing alterations in movement abilities and function due to chronic disease processes and the impact on the movement systems.

Rehabilitation services, as mentioned previously in the chapter when discussing IDEIA,[6] are also provided in the school and preschool settings. The educational environment is the setting for preschool, elementary, and secondary education facilities and is coordinated with families and teachers.[6] In traditional home health settings, rehab services are provided in the patient's residence. Traditional home health may serve the elderly and children who are unable to otherwise attend therapy in outpatient or school-based services.[6] Home health may also occur in the patient's room within a care facility, group home, or elsewhere in the community. In today's society of accessibility, home care is also provided in the home at the convenience, preference, or request for the patient, with outpatient therapy services provided in the home as a service option. Home care involves the added stressor of travel between locations for the health care professional (rather than the patient) daily, with one-to-one therapy within the home that may involve the family unit. In-home, outpatient therapy services are particularly popular with aging populations, who are less safe to drive and rural populations where travel is not possible or resourced. Hospice care provides for therapy services in the final phase of disease for functional abilities and pain management. The pace is highly variable in home care environments and the context variable.

Rehabilitation services may also be provided for in industries or occupational work environments; through local, state, and federal government agencies, such as Veterans Health and Indian Health Services (IHS); and in research centers with private or government funding. Each setting has its own culture and expectations for care by the professional staff members. Veterans often present with complex and multi-systems concerns and with multiple conditions, and they may be impacted heavily by psychological concerns such as posttraumatic stress disorder (PTSD) and/or concussive syndromes. Rehabilitation centers with IHS may not be fully resourced with needed health care professionals, and patients may receive

TABLE 12-1

OVERVIEW COMPARISON OF TREATMENT SETTINGS

SETTING CRITERIA	GENERAL ACUTE AND/OR INTENSIVE	REHAB HOSPITAL	SNF/ SUBACUTE REHAB	HHA/ALF	LT ACUTE CARE	OUTPATIENT	SCHOOL BASED	HOSPICE	PUBLIC HEALTH IHS/GOV VISN	INDUSTRY
Patient audience	Captive	Captive	Captive	Earned/ captive	Captive	Earned	Captive	Captive	Earned/captive	Earned/ captive
Patient expectations	○ Save my life ○ Get me well	○ Get me well ○ Help me function at maximum capacity	○ Get me well ○ Take care of me with dignity ○ Help me reach my goals	○ Get me well ○ Teach me to manage myself in my home environment	○ Save my life ○ Get me better ○ Help me reach greater function while addressing my serious condition(s) with longer time, patience	○ Get me well ○ Get me ready to get back to work/sports ○ Help me function at maximum capacity ○ Don't keep me waiting	○ Help me reduce my physical limitation in order to maximize my ability to learn ○ Help me play	○ Control my pain ○ Take care of me with dignity until it is my time to die ○ Caring attitude any environment	Get me well but keep me in harmony with my values and beliefs	○ Get me well ○ Get me ready to go back to work safely
Primary services provided	○ Life-sustaining services ○ Medical stabilization ○ Diagnostic Services	Intensive team-oriented rehab ≥6 hours/day	○ Primarily geriatrics ○ Maybe life-sustaining subacute unit/beds	Primarily geriatrics rehab	○ Acute care, LT, avg >25 days transferred from ICU/CCU; longer inpatient stay ○ Movement and function	○ Acute to subacute ○ Diagnostic and minor surgical ○ Movement and function for chronic diseases	Developmental peds rehab	Palliative care	Same as with acute, OP, and home health, et al	○ Primarily orthopedics, some neuro, cardio ○ Burns/falls/ traumas
Role of PT	○ Early mobilization ○ Pain control ○ Wound care ○ Consult/ screening	○ Functional mobility: return to life/ community ○ Work with rehab team	○ Functional mobility ○ Establish patient movement programs for nursing/ care providers	○ Functional mobility in home environment ○ Patient movement program family/ caregiver involvement	○ Improvements of function and mobility ○ Work with rehab team and very closely with nursing	○ Manager of PT department ○ Direct/ primary hands-on ○ OP may be offered in homes	Direct hands-on, then consult/ advise teachers/ aides and parents/ caregivers	○ Some direct hands-on ○ Some consulting	○ Direct/ hands-on ○ Medical missionaries ○ Often primary	○ Direct/ hands-on ○ Consultation/ screenings

(continued)

TABLE 12-1 (CONTINUED)

OVERVIEW COMPARISON OF TREATMENT SETTINGS

SETTING CRITERIA	GENERAL ACUTE AND/OR INTENSIVE	REHAB HOSPITAL	SNF/ SUBACUTE REHAB	HHA/ALF	LT ACUTE CARE	OUTPATIENT	SCHOOL BASED	HOSPICE	PUBLIC HEALTH IHS/GOV VISN	INDUSTRY
Availability of support staff	Excellent, especially for life-sustaining activities	Excellent for broad spectrum of team members	Fair/adequate	You may be sole provider	○ Excellent to good ○ Similar to inpatient hospital with longer stays, 3 to 6 concurrent diagnoses, comorbidities	Could be sole practitioner or broad spectrum of disciplines	Sole practitioners with non-professional staff within earshot or aides	○ Nursing support ○ Support staff varies ○ Home services: sole	As with acute, OP and home health, et al	○ Usually sole practitioner/employer ○ Consults
Discharge criteria	When medically stable	Depends on payer source, usually 20 to 60 days max	○ Medicare ○ Managed care when can be handled at home	○ When no longer homebound ○ When reached max potentials ○ When functional goals met or fluctuating	○ Ready to return to home or stable to LT care if still requiring custodial care with feeding and dressing or assisted living ○ Pain managed	○ Payer source often determines ○ Medicare: when reached max potential ○ RTW ○ Managed care: contract ○ Commercial: highly variable	○ Usually continues through public school education ○ Public Law 94-142 requires	○ When pain is controlled ○ Comatose/deceased	When goals are met or patient refuses	○ With successful RTW FT, part-time ○ Disability determination ○ Functional Capacity Evaluation ○ Alternate duty determined

ALF = assisted living facility; CCU = critical care unit; FT = full-time; GOV = government; HHA = home health agency; ICU = intensive care unit; IHS = Indian Health Service; LT = long-term; OP = outpatient; PT = physical therapy; RTW = return to work; SNF = skilled nursing facility; VISN = Veteran's Integrated Health Service.

infrequent care; therefore, one may encounter more chronic conditions that have not been addressed in early phases or may serve as the primary provider. Health care professionals may also need to consider greater efforts toward primary prevention to assist in the potential gaps in care. Physical and occupational therapy rehabilitation services have been provided in the IHS only since the late 1950s and early 1960s. Today, all rehab services continue to expand in tribal programs and cultural appreciation is key as an IHS health care professional. Patients/clients want to get well but in harmony with their values and beliefs (see Table 12-1). IHS offers services addressing patients with diabetes; pediatric, cardiopulmonary, mental health, and orthopedic conditions; specialty hand and foot care; wound care; health promotion; neurological rehabilitation; prosthetics/orthotics clinics; gender-health programs; and others. A strong generalist with the ability to provide community outreach and preventative education is needed in IHS. Sometimes, student loan repayment opportunities for a dedicated service and time commitment are available for service in remote and rural areas for health care professionals to address the underserved needs (visit the www.va.gov and www.ihs.gov websites to learn more about these unique cultural settings and practice opportunities). As you can see, a wide variety of practice environments exist for health care professionals in rehabilitation services. While during your training you shall focus on the skills to enter into practice in a variety of settings initially, your preferences for the setting type, cultural exchanges, context, time, and environmental influences may further guide your decision making in your preferred practice setting. In any event, as a health care professional one must acculturate to the people we serve to effect a change within the health care professional PPI.

In the exercises at the end of the chapter, you will further explore a patient's journey through the health care system. For now, so that you may begin to understand the patient's perspectives, in the context and cultures of the health care environment, select a few videos from the John Hopkins website that explore what it is like to experience being a patient in an ICU setting (http://www.hopkinsmedicine.org/pulmonary/research/outcomes_after_critical_illness_surgery/oacis_videos_news.html). After reviewing, share and discuss with your classmates what you learned, how it will change your communication approach, and how you felt after viewing.

Hidden Dimensions or Implicit Meanings in Culture

In order to understand the complete or true meanings in intercultural communication, one must understand the multiple hidden dimensions of unconscious culture. Hall and Hall[28] stated that context will largely determine the message that the person receives. In collectivistic, high-context communication, the vast majority of the information is already understood, either internalized in the individual or in the physical context of the situation. Only a small amount of the meaning is in the explicit transmission or coding of the message. For example, in high-context cultures, the mere presence of an official representative at a meeting, regardless of whether something is said by the official, indicates that the meeting is understood to be important by all those present. In contrast, in low-context, individualistic communication, the majority of information is in the explicit coding of the message, rather than within the individual or the situational (context).

According to Hall and Hall,[28] it is up to each person to perform the critical function of correcting for distortions or omissions, in the messages he or she receives. To be truly effective in intercultural communication, one must know the degree of information or context that has to be supplied in order to correctly interpret another individual's verbal and nonverbal behavior. The context or the information surrounding the event that gives it meaning will vary from culture to culture, and it is often the critical factor in determining whether individuals from different cultures will communicate effectively with one another.

For the Anglo-American health care professional working with Native American clients, understanding the context of the situation is critical to effective intercultural communication. For example, Brislin[11] described the very different cultural interpretations of silence in Native American communication compared with Anglo-American communication. For the Native American, silence is a culturally acceptable response to ambiguity. For the Anglo-American, small talk is a culturally acceptable response to ambiguity. For the Anglo-American health care professional who does not understand the Native American context of silence, the client's silence may be perceived as disinterest or noncompliance with the health care professional's recommendations.

Nonverbal Communication

Nonverbal communication refers to information exchange (or difficulties in such an exchange) that does not require oral or written forms of language. These include gestures, positioning of the body, and tenseness of the facial expressions (see Chapter 11 on rapport using neurolinguistic psychology). Unfortunately, there are few cultural universals, except the recognition that all cultures use both verbal and nonverbal means and that people should avoid drawing any conclusions regarding nonverbal behaviors without a great deal of knowledge. Such knowledge involves developing understanding of specific gestures, expressions, and uses of the body, as well as a full grasp of the context of the communication. For example, the distance that people keep from each other is a potent means of nonverbal communication.

In the United States, when a man and woman meet each other for the first time, they usually stand about 2.5 to 3 feet apart. If they stand closer, it may be interpreted as a sign of more than casual interest in each other. However, in Latin America, the typical distance people stand from each other while conversing is about 2 feet. Reduced distance does not convey a special message of "desire for more interaction in the future."[28] For health care professionals working with clients from Latin America, this information is critical to understanding the context of the intercultural communication.

PERSONALISMO

As a new therapist working in Miami, I was initially very surprised to receive invitations to attend celebrations at the homes of the children I treated. I was also confused when the parents of the children I treated asked me questions regarding my parents, marital status, and siblings. Fortunately, I was able to ask my colleagues at the preschool, who served as my cultural informants, why the families were so interested in my personal life. They politely informed me that the families wanted to get to know me as a person as well as a professional. I later learned through my research that this is the concept of *personalismo* in the Hispanic culture and that it is very important in establishing rapport with the families. Once I understood the cultural context of the communication, I felt much more at ease.

SOMATIZATION

Somatization, a behavior more common among Asians, Africans, and Latin Americans than North Americans, refers to the tendency to report physical symptoms when a person is experiencing psychological distress. The patient does not present any identifiable organic causes for the problem but experiences symptoms that are real and troublesome. Somatization is seen more frequently in cultures where complaints about anxiety, worries, and depression are perceived as signs of weakness. In many cultures, people have much less tolerance for mental illness than for physical illness. Therefore, the context of the communication must be understood by the health care professional to have effective intercultural communication. For non-Hispanic health care professionals, the concepts of *nervios* and *ataques de nervios* may present with symptoms of heart palpitations, sleep disorders, and generalized body pains. These somatic symptoms may reflect chronic feelings of stress that are related to various life challenges.

SIX UNIVERSAL ASPECTS OF HEALTH CARE IN ALL CULTURES

Scholars have examined interactions between health care professionals and people seeking help in different parts of the world.[8,11,14] Health care professionals include people with advanced degrees in highly industrialized nations and native healers, shamans, and herbalists in less industrialized nations. Six universal concepts in the delivery of health care were identified:

1. The health care specialist applies a name to a problem.
2. The qualities of the health care professional are important.[14] The health care professionals must be perceived by clients to be caring, competent, approachable, and concerned with identifying and finding solutions to the problem. (With minority groups in the United States, health care professionals must communicate a sense of credibility that they can be of help. In addition, they should be able to offer health-related benefits of some kind as soon as possible. If they do not, the client is not likely to return for an appointment.)
3. The health care professional must establish credibility through the use of symbols and trappings of status that are familiar in the culture.
4. The health care professional places the client's problems in a familiar framework (this implies recognition of the client's explanatory model by the practitioner).
5. The health care professional applies a set of techniques meant to bring relief (this implies recognition of the client's explanatory model).
6. Interactions between the clients and the practitioners occur at a special time and place (this implies recognition of the client's explanatory model).

In order to achieve these 6 universal requirements in the intercultural environment, health care professionals must be educated about their own culture as well as the cultures of the clients, families, colleagues, and support staff with whom they work. Many researchers recommend training in cultural sensitivity to provide optimal care through application of knowledge of culture and cultural differences. Research has indicated that counselors trained in cultural sensitivity were rated higher in the dimensions of expertise, trustworthiness, ability to show positive regard, and empathy compared with counselors not trained in cultural sensitivity.[11] There is a difference between the pseudotolerance that results from "putting the lid on" one's intolerance and the genuine tolerance that stems from developing an open, courageous, and loving heart. Intolerance comes from fear. Knowledge and sensitivity training go a long way to quell the fear of what is different and to yield true tolerance for and enjoyment of the differences among us. The health care professional must demonstrate willingness to bring knowledge to interactions with different clients and be able to take culture into account when discussing important topics related to alleviating pain and stress.

CULTURALLY AND LINGUISTICALLY APPROPRIATE SERVICES STANDARDS

CLAS standards have been mandated by the Office of Minority Health of the US Department of Health and Human Services since 2001.[29] These services include 15 mandates that are organized by theme. CLAS standards address the following key areas: culturally competent care; communication and language assistance; organizational governance; and workforce supports for cultural competence, including standards for engagement, continuous improvement, and accountability. One standard specifically mandates that health care organizations must provide language assistance services in the patients preferred language in writing and verbally and offer language assistance services at no cost to each patient consumer with limited English proficiency.[29] Modern technology has enhanced translation capabilities through the use of language applications, such as Babbel, MediBabbel, Canopy Medical Translator, MedSpeak Translator, Duolingo, Memrise, Busuu, Google Translate, Livemocha, Living Language, Foreign Services Institute, and BBC languages; apps have dramatically reduced the need to rely too heavily on human interpreters. However, the responsibilities and accountabilities for translation for health care professionals and cultural nuances may not be obvious with all technological applications. You might wish to check out a few of the language apps to begin your exploration for those patients you will serve with limited English proficiencies.

A recent study by Clark[30] found that using professional interpreter services dramatically increased satisfaction with patient-provider communication in emergency room visits for patients and providers. Quoting Clark,[30] a senior editor and California correspondent for Health Leaders Media Online said the following:

> *Language and cultural barriers between patients and providers are an increasing concern, as evidenced by the decision by the Joint Commission to release new standards for patient–provider communication, effective January 1, 2011. Several interpreter certification programs are now in development to accredit and/or train would-be interpreters to work in health care settings. The idea is that medical interpreters should have proficiency standards much like those required of court reporters, sign language interpreters, and others who convey essential information. All too often, many hospital officials have acknowledged, children are being used to interpret medical care issues on behalf of their parents. Instructions for taking medication, conversations with family members, and information on diagnoses and prognosis may get muddled when interpreters are not properly trained or sensitive to cultural fears and values. Failure to effectively communicate can also drum up health costs, for example, if a patient has already undergone a test but is unable to convey … Likewise, the inability of a provider to relay the importance of a follow-up visit, or compliance with a medication regimen, can result in avoidable progression of disease or hospitalization.*

Several excellent apps are available today to assist in translation services, where resources may not be as readily available. For example, MediBabble (NiteFloat, Inc) is a professional-grade medical translator application tool that is freely available via www.medibabble.com; most search engines offer translation services in which you can type in the English word and translate to another specified language. If you commonly work with non-English-speaking persons, or those with limited English proficiency, as many of us do in certain parts of the country that are more multilingual and multicultural, you will likely need to become more proficient in languages such as Spanish, Chinese, Tagalog, Creole, French, Farsi, German, Korean, Arabic, Russian, and Italian because these are some of the non-English languages most frequently spoken in the United States according to the US English Foundation, Inc.[31] There are several counties in the United States where more than 100 languages are spoken (in California, Washington, Arizona, Illinois, and New York). Becoming proficient in American Sign Language is also a helpful skill. Take advantage of Spanish courses for medical professionals. Two-way communication is needed with patient care, and this can only happen if we are speaking our patients' preferred language or one that they understand and doing so in an equitable manner, regardless of individual differences. Health care professionals must take reasonable steps to provide meaningful access for those who have limited English proficiency (Federal Law, Civil Rights Act of 1964, Title VI, prohibits discrimination based upon race, color or national origin).

SPIRITUALITY AS CULTURE AND HEALTH CARE

As you will read in Chapter 14, current descriptive literature suggests that spirituality and/or religion are linked with health outcomes. Koenig et al[32] reviewed 1600 studies and found that better health outcomes over time were associated with individuals who had a religious or spiritual practice compared with controls. Health care professionals can conduct cultural/spiritual screenings with their patients to ascertain whether they have a religious/spiritual practice. Four questions to ask include the following:

1. What are your sources of health, strength, comfort, and peace?
2. Are you part of a religious or spiritual community?
3. What spiritual practices do you find most helpful to you personally?
4. Are there any specific practices or restrictions I should know about in providing your care?

Spirituality is a basic human experience. Spirituality exists in our connection to other humans, our environment, and the unfolding universe and the transcendent. Health care professionals can have an impact on the patient's health and healing if they acknowledge and address the patient's spirituality as part of their assessment.[33] Numerous assessment tools are available, including the One-Minute Health Assessment and the Berg Cultural/Spiritual Assessment Tool (http://www.csh.umn.edu/Integrativehealingpractices/culture/tool/tl04.html).

Through the use of assessment tools, the health care professional can learn how the belief system of the patient may impact how the patient deals with his or her illness or disorder.[33]

RESOURCES AND TOOLS—PROMOTING AND VALUING CULTURALLY COMPETENT CARE FOR HEALTH CARE PROFESSIONALS

New tools have been developed to assess and promote cultural competence in educational programs for health care professionals. The Provider's Guide to Quality and Culture Quiz enables learners to self-assess their cultural knowledge and competency.[34] The Quality and Culture Quiz provides learners with an online opportunity to assess their cultural knowledge. It provides immediate feedback with the correct answers and a narrative explanation of why they are correct. By completing the quiz and discussing the answers, deliberations can begin in class about the topics covered in the quiz. Some topics considered include ethnic-, geographic-, spiritual-, and gender-based differences that may occur in health care communications in diverse communities. First, take the 23-question quiz (http://erc.msh.org/mainpage.cfm?file=1.0 .htm&module=provider&language=English).[34]

Following the review and discussion of the quiz, review the related learning modules for PPIs: health disparities, cultural groups, culturally competent organizations, and additional resource links provided. You may discuss and share some of the activities during your in-class sessions, and you shall find many of the resources helpful to refer back to as you transition from classroom to clinical realms. Feel free to explore the website further following your Quality and Culture Quiz.

The Global Health Special Interest Group (GHSIG) within the Health Policy & Administration (HPA) section of the APTA provides educational programming at national conferences and offers other resources related to a wide variety of topics, including global health issues, health disparities, cultural competence, disability issues, service-learning, pro bono clinics, and ethical practice in resource-limited settings domestically and internationally.[35] As members of the HPA Section, GHSIG members may access all section resources, including the GHSIG listserv. The GHSIG listserv and Facebook page allow members to network and share information about global health-related educational, work, volunteer, and research opportunities.

In a more recent 3-year investigation, Musolino et al[36,37] demonstrated that the utilization of interprofessional educational modules for cultural competence and mutual respect produced measurable gains in cultural competence for interprofessional health professions students enrolled in the modules at the University of Utah, Salt Lake City, Utah. The participating students were from physical therapy, medicine, pharmacy, and nursing disciplines. The students enrolled in the modules demonstrated significant progression on comparative postscores in the cultural constructs of attitudes, knowledge, and skills, but not in encounters and desires. Researchers recommend that efforts be made to introduce more culturally competent interactive practice opportunities in health care settings and the cultural competence and mutual respect interprofessional education modules to reduce health care disparities and medical errors for clinicians working in diverse communities.

Another study by Musolino and Feehan[38] demonstrated that service-learning opportunities also promoted the development of cultural competence in students who worked in community-based facilities for school-aged children from 7 to 13 years old from Hispanic migrant farm worker families and low-income Black communities in Southwest Florida. In addition, 31% of the participating children were deaf or hard of hearing or had physical and/or mental disabilities. The physical therapy students were involved in teams whose goals were to increase awareness of the physical therapy profession in diverse communities. Health care professional students developed and implemented interactive learning opportunities to educate the school children about the various aspects of the profession of physical therapy. The physical therapy student projects enhanced their personal development as self-reflective and more culturally aware physical therapy professionals. In addition, the physical therapy students were recognized with the National Student Assembly award Student Outreach for Cultural Diversity Awareness. There are also many books, research articles, and media resources describing the personal experiences of individuals living with disabilities[39-41]; a representative sample of multimedia resources is provided at the end of the chapter.

CONCLUSION

The 21st century offers health care professionals challenges and opportunities. *Ethnocentrism*, the belief that one's own culture is the best, will be challenged, and people will need to expand their thinking to become tolerant of differences and ambiguity. Intercultural researchers are challenged to provide practical applications from their findings. Researchers are challenged to develop the best culturally appropriate intervention programs in the areas of health, education, and worker productivity while addressing ways to reduce stressors related to health care professional intercultural interactions.

Basic information regarding the benefits and pitfalls of intercultural interactions will be widely discussed, just as preventive health behaviors are discussed today.[11] Opportunities will abound as discussions regarding tolerance, understanding, and mutual enrichment evolve and are disseminated. Women will continue to have increasing choices in their lives, and people will analyze the role that culture and cultural differences play in their lives and in the policies of their societies, and especially with health care policy. If health care professionals put time and effort into understanding cultural influences on their own behavior and the behavior of others, they will no doubt enjoy the challenges and the stimulation that intercultural interactions can bring.[11]

If we adopt the quantum physics paradigm regarding the primacy of relationships and their fuzziness, we have a new model to assist us in appreciating and valuing our diversity. With our new awareness of, and appreciation for, our relationships to one another, we can introduce unconditional compassion, or love, into our organizations. According to Wheatley,[5] Chopra,[42] and many very wise people from the beginning of time, love in the broadest sense is the most potent source of power that we have available to us. Love, including respect and caring, is most thwarted when we emphasize how different we are from one another. Knowledge and sensitivity to cultural differences will facilitate our therapeutic presence and our sense of oneness with those fellow human beings who are our patients, their families and caregivers, and our health care colleagues. Finally, a few guided exercises follow to help you on your way to greater self-awareness and cultural sensitivity today!

REFERENCES

1. Solomon S, Greenberg J, Pyszczynski T. A terror management theory of social beahavior: on the psychological functions of self-esteem and cultural worldviews. In Zanna MP, ed. *Advances in Experimental Social Psychology*. Vol 24. San Diego, CA: Academic Press; 1991:93-159.
2. Masin HL. *Parental Attitudes Toward Physical Therapy Services at the Debbie School Early Intervention Program*. Miami, FL: University of Miami, Department of Pediatrics; 1991.
3. Colby SL, Ortman JM. *Projections of the Size and Composition of the US Population: 2014 to 2060*. Current Population Reports. Washington, DC: US Census Bureau; 2014:25-1143.
4. Christensen C. Multicultural competencies in early intervention: training professionals for pluralistic society. *Infants Young Child*. 1992;4(3):49-63.
5. Wheatley MJ. *Leadership and the New Science*. San Francisco, CA: Berrett-Koehler Publishers; 2010.
6. Individuals With Disabilities Education Improvement Act Amendments of 2004 (Pub Law No. 108-446, Federal Register Vol 71, No 156).

7. Cross TL, Bazron BJ, Dennis KW, Isaacs MR. *Towards a Culturally Competent System of Care: A Monograph on Effective Services for Minority Children Who Are Severely Emotionally Disturbed*. Washington, DC: Georgetown University; 1989.

8. Sue S, McKinney, H. Asian-Americans in the community mental health care system. *American Journal of Orthopsychiatry*. 1975;45:11-18.

9. Anderson PP, Fenichel ES. *Serving Culturally Diverse Families of Infants and Toddlers With Disabilities*. Washington, DC: National Center for Clinical Infant Programs; 1989.

10. Mead M. Cultural problems and technical change in United Nations Educations Scientific and Cultural Organization, Paris. In: Saunders L, ed. *Cultural Differences and Medical Care*. New York, NY: Russell Sage Foundation; 1954:247-248.

11. Brislin RW. *Understanding Culture's Influence on Behavior*. 2nd ed. Independence, KY: Cengage Learning; 2000.

12. Commission on Accreditation of Physical Therapy Education. *2012-2013 Fact Sheet, Physical Therapist Education Programs*. Alexandria, VA: American Physical Therapy Association; 2014.

13. Dillman DA. *Mail and Telephone Surveys: The Total Design Method*. New York, NY: Wiley; 1978.

14. Sue S, Zane N, Nagayama Hall GC, Berger LK. The case for cultural competency in psychotherapeutic interventions. *Annu Rev Psychol*. 2009;60:525-548.

15. Kleinman A. Concepts and a model for the comparison of medical systems as cultural systems. *Soc Sci Med*. 1978;12(2B):85-93.

16. DeSantis L. Health care orientations of Cuban and Haitian immigrant mothers: implications for health care professionals. *Med Anthropol*. 1989;12(1):69-89.

17. Harwood A. *Ethnicity and Medical Care*. Cambridge, MA: Harvard University Press; 1982.

18. Jackson J. Urban Black Americans. In: Harwood A, ed. *Ethnicity and Medical Care*. Cambridge, MA: Harvard University Press; 1982:36-129.

19. Saunders L. *Cultural Differences and Medical Care*. New York, NY: Russell Sage Foundation; 1954.

20. Shilling B, Branan E. *Cross-Cultural Counseling: A Guide for Nutrition and Health Counselors*. Washington, DC: US Department of Agriculture and United States Department of Health and Human Services; 1989.

21. Ting-Toomey S. Intercultural conflicts: a face-negotiation theory. In: Kim Y, Gudykunst W, eds. *Theories in Intercultural Communication*. Newbury Park, CA: Sage; 1988:213-238.

22. Graham M, Miller D. *The 1995 Annual: Volume 1, Training*. San Diego, CA: Pfeiffer and Co; 1995.

23. Tirandis HC. In: Graham M, Miller D, Eds. *The 1995 Annual: Volume 1, Training*. San Diego, CA: Pfeiffer and Co; 1995.

24. Turner H. Interacting successfully with people from other cultures. In: Brislin RW, ed. *Understanding Culture's Influence on Behavior*. Fort Worth, TX: Harcourt Brace Jovanovich; 1993:325.

25. Hagland MM, Sabatino F, Sherer JL. New waves. Hospitals struggle to meet the challenge of multiculturalism now—and in the next generation. *Hospital*. 1993;67(10):22-25,28-31.

26. Belenky M, Clinchy B, Goldberg N, Tarul J. *Women's Ways of Knowing: The Development of Self, Voice, and Mind*. New York, NY: Basic Books; 1978.

27. Wiesman R, Koester J, eds. *Intercultural Communication Competence*. Newbury Park, CA: Sage; 1993.

28. Hall ET, Hall MR. *The Dance of Life: The Other Dimension of Time*. Sioux City, IA: Anchor Publications; 1984.

29. US Department of Health & Human Services, Office of Minority Health, National Standards for Culturally and Linguistically Appropriate Services in Health and Health Care (National CLAS Standards), Think cultural health. https://www.thinkcultural-health.hhs.gov/Content/clas.asp#clas_standards. Accessed April 19, 2015.

30. Clark C. Trained interpreters improve patient and provider satisfaction, says study. Health Leaders Media, March 1, 2010. www.healthleadersmedia.com/print/PHY-247284/Trained-Interpreters-Improve-Patient-and-Provider-Satisfaction-Says-Study. Accessed April 5, 2015.

31. Many Languages, One America. US English Foundation, Inc. http://usefoundation.org/view/29. Accessed June 13, 2015.

32. Koenig HG, McCullough ME, Larson DB. *Handbook of Religion and Health*. 2nd ed. New York, NY: Oxford University Press; 2012.

33. Center for Spirituality and Healing. Cultural competency tools. http://www.csh.umn.edu/Integrativehealingpractices/culture/tool/tl04.html. Accessed April 19, 2015.

34. Management Sciences for Health. The provider's guide to quality and culture. http://erc.msh.org/mainpage.cfm?file=1.0.htm&module=provider&language=English. Accessed May 1, 2015.

35. American Physical Therapy Association. Health Policy & Administration Section—The Catalyst, Global Health Special Interest Group. www.aptahpa.org. Accessed March 13, 2015.

36. Musolino GM, Torres Burkhalter S, Crookston B, Harris RM, Chase-Cantarini S, Babitz M. Understanding and eliminating disparities in health care: development and assessment of cultural competence for interdisciplinary health professional at the University of Utah: a 3-year investigation. *J Phys Ther Educ*. 2010:24(1):25-36.

37. Musolino GM, Babitz M, Burkhalter ST, et al. Mutual respect in healthcare: assessing cultural competence for the University of Utah Interdisciplinary Health Sciences. *J Allied Health*. 2009;38(2):e54-e62.

38. Musolino GM, Feehan P. Enhancing diversity through mentorship: the nurturing potential of service learning. *J Phys Ther Educ*. 2004;18(1):29-42.

39. Galanti GA. *Caring for Patients From Different Cultures*. 5th ed. Philadelphia, PA: University of Pennsylvania Press: 2015.

40. Campinha-Bacote J. Cultural desire: the key to unlocking cultural competence. *J Nurs Educ*. 2003;42(6):239-240.

41. Campinha-Bacote J. The process of cultural competence in the delivery of healthcare services. In Douglas M, Pacquiao D, eds. Core Curriculum in Transcultural Nursing and Health Care. *Journal of Transcultural Nursing*. 2010:21 Suppl 1:119S-127S.

42. Chopra D. *The Path to Love*. New York, NY: Random House; 1997.

SUGGESTED READINGS

Albom M. *Tuesdays With Morrie*. New York, NY: Doubleday; 1997. A journalist interviews an older man who had been his college professor; shares his experiences living with and dying from amyotropic lateral sclerosis (ALS).

Ambrose SE. *Band of Brothers: E Company, 506th Regiment, 101st Airborne from Normandy to Hitler's Eagle's Nest*. 2nd ed. New York, NY: Simon & Schuster; 2001. Follows Easy Company of the US Army 101st Airborne Division's mission in WWII Europe, from Operation Overload through VJ Day, exploring the trials of service and resulting PTSD and disabilities.

Beck M. *Expecting Adam: A True Story of Birth, Rebirth, and Everyday Magic*. New York, NY: Times Books; 1999. A PhD candidate shares her pregnancy and life as mother of a child with Down syndrome.

Cahalan S. *Brain on Fire: My Month of Madness*. New York, NY; Simon and Schuster; 2012. The author describes her truly terrifying bout with and eventual recovery from encephalitis.

Cohen RM. *Blindsided: Lifting a Life Above Illness*. New York, NY; HarperCollins; 2005. Richard is television writer who develops multiple sclerosis, affecting his vision and balance, followed by a diagnosis of cancer.

Crimmins CE. *Where Is the Mango Princess?: A Journey Back From Brain Injury*. New York, NY; Vintage Books; 2001. Written by a woman whose husband sustains a severe traumatic brain injury (TBI) in a boating accident; follows his acute rehabilitation and living with the residual deficits.

Coughlin R. *Grieving: A Love Story*. New York, NY; Random House; 1993. A widow tells the story of her husband's death from cancer.

Galli R. *Rescuing Jeffrey*. Chapel Hill, NC: Algonquin Books; 2000. A father's story of his high school son's spinal cord injury (SCI) due to a diving accident.

Gerlach H. *Happily Ever After: My Journey With Guillain-Barré Syndrome and How I Got My Life Back*. Bloomington, IN: Trafford Publishing; 2012. Just 3 weeks after giving birth, young Holly notices her fingertips are numb and her legs weak. She was paralyzed, admitted to the ICU, and placed on a ventilator; she could not speak, move, or hold her daughter. Was her life over? Explores her intensive physiotherapy and recovery.

Graboys T. *Life in the Balance: A Physician's Memoir of Life, Love, and Loss With Parkinson's Disease and Dementia*. New York, NY: Union Square Press; 2008. Dr. Graboys, a successful cardiologist, musician, athlete, husband, and father affected by Parkinson's disease and Lewy body disorder, describes his descent into immobility and dementia.

Grealey L. *Autobiography of a Face*. Boston, MA: Houghton Mifflin; 1994. After undergoing five years of treatment for cancer, a woman is left with facial disfigurement and subsequent reconstructive surgeries.

Halpin B. *It Takes a Worried Man: A Memoir*. Manhattan Beach, CA: Open Road Distribution; 2015. One father's raw account of his experiences after his young wife is diagnosed with breast cancer.

Heffernan DD. *An Arrow Through the Heart: One Woman's Story of Life, Love, and Surviving a Near-Fatal Heart Attack*. New York, NY: Free Press; 2002. One woman's story of life, love, and surviving a near-fatal heart attack.

Hornbacker M. *Wasted*. New York, NY: Harper Perennial; 1998. A young woman with both anorexia and bulimia, further complicated by substance abuse.

Housden M. *Hannah's Gift: Lessons From a Life Fully Lived*. New York, NY; Bantam Books; 2002. A mother tells the story of her three-year old daughter's struggle and death from cancer.

Knapp C. *Drinking: A Love Story*. New York, Bantam Dell Doubleday Publishing, 1996. The author describes her 20-year struggle with alcoholism, rehabilitation, and recovery.

Kyle C, McEwen S, DeFelice J. *American Sniper: The Autobiography of the Most Lethal Sniper in U.S. Military History*. New York, NY; Morrow: Harper Collins Publishers; 2014. Explores the intense life of a US Navy Seal sniper serving in battle and its PTSD effects.

Lydon J. *Daughter of the Queen of Sheba: A Memoir*. Boston, MA: Houghton Mifflin; 1997. NPR reporter writes a memoir of growing up with a mentally ill mother and providing her care.

Parker S. *Tumbling After: Pedaling Like Crazy After Life Goes Downhill*. New York, NY: Crown Publishers; 2002. A wife copes after her husband sustains a C4 SCI after a bicycle accident.

Redfield Jamison K. *An Unquiet Mind: A Memoir of Moods and Madness*. New York, NY; Alfred A. Knopf, Doubleday Publishing Group; 1997. A renowned psychologist describes mercurial living with bipolar disorder and her support system; explores from both the healer and healed perspectives and related struggles.

Rothenberg L. *Breathing for a Living: A Memoir*. New York, NY; Hyperion Books; 2003. A 19-year-old college student with cystic fibrosis shares her memoir, a moving account that follows through her double lung transplant and rehabilitation.

Schlosser E. *Fast Food Nation: The Dark Side of the All-American Meal*. New York, NY: Mifflin Harcourt Publishing; 2001. Explores the fast food industry, related cultural perspectives, and the dark side of the industry related to immigration and the modern tale of Upton Sinclair's *The Jungle* (1906), which exposed the poor conditions in the meat-packing industry.

Sheff D. *Beautiful Boy: A Father's Journey Through His Son's Addiction*. Boston, MA; Houghton Mifflin Company; 2008. A father tells the story of his journey through his son's methamphetamine addiction.

Skloot R. *The Immortal Life of Henrietta Lacks*. New York, NY; Crown Publishing, Random House; 2010. Engaging reading about the immortal cellular line of Henrietta Lacks from her cervical cancer cells in 1951, and the many ethical, racial, and class issues that emerged; considers matters of informed consent.

Simon C. *Mad House: Growing Up in the Shadow of Mentally Ill Siblings*. New York, NY: Penguin; 1998. Part memoir, part practical guide, a reporter describes growing up with 2 schizophrenic siblings.

Suskind R. *A Hope in the Unseen: An American Odyssey From the Inner City to the Ivy League.* New York, NY: Broadway Books, Random House; 1999. Follows Cedric Jennings, a young black teen from the disadvantaged Southside DC district with a single mother, as he traverses high school to the Ivy League and emerges a man.

Suskind R. *Life, Animated: A Story of Sidekicks, Heroes, and Autism.* Glendale, CA: Kingswell; 2014. Follows the life of the author's son, Owen Suskin, afflicted with autism, and how Ron and his wife, Cornelia, communicated with Disney characters as a vehicle for enhanced understandings.

Wilde Hawking J. *Traveling to Infinity: My Life With Stephen.* Surrey, United Kingdom: Alma Books, Ltd.; 2010. Shared by Hawking's wife, Stephen Hawking's (renowned astrophysicist) courage and determination in the face of a crippling motor neuron disease; relevance of assistive and rehabilitation technologies.

Suggested Viewing

American Sniper. Warner Bros. 2014.

Band of Brothers. HBO. 2001.

Body and Soul: Dianna & Kathy. New Day Digital. 2007. Two women with significant disabilities live together and take care of each other so they are able to live independently; demonstrates the use of assistive technology and a symbiotic culture.

The Collector of Bedford Street. New Day Digital. 2005. Adult with developmental disabilities lives on his own and struggles with independence.

Darius Goes West: The Roll of His Life. Indie Film. 2006. A teenager with Duchenne muscular dystrophy goes on a cross-country trip, leaving home for the first time, with his eleven best friends; MTV hosts to find someone to "pimp" his chair.

Emmanuel's Gift. First Look Home Entertainment. 2005. Young African man with a congenital deformity advocates for disability rights biking in Africa.

Fast Food Nation: The Dark Side of the All-American Meal. 20th Century Fox Home Entertainment. 2007.

Including Samuel. Institute on Disability, University of New Hampshire. 2009. School inclusion issues for a child with cerebral palsy.

McFarland, USA. Walt Disney Pictures. 2015. Inspired by a 1987 true story, follows novice runners from a socioeconomically deprived, predominantly Latino high school; considers matters of ethnicity, class, and culture.

My Angel My Hero: Dancing With Parkinson's. 3-Dimensions Films. 2013. Filmed over 6 days, shares the beat of a teenager's life in his fight against Parkinson's disease.

So Much, So Fast. Indie Films. 2006. Chronicles a young husband and father's struggles with ALS and his devoted family support.

The Soldier's Heart. PBS Frontline. 2005. Explores the psychological impact of combat; Iraq/Afghanistan veterans and PTSD.

The Theory of Everything. Working Title Films. 2014.

Through Deaf Eyes. PBS. 2007. Explores the 200-year history of the deaf community in America.

You're Not You. Entertainment One. 2015. A classical pianist's journey coping with ALS with the support of her home care assistant.

EXERCISES

EXERCISE 1: CULTURE SHOCK ACTIVITY

1. Have you personally experienced culture shock? Write a brief description of what you experienced. What did you see, hear, and feel? What was the context of the situation that shocked you?

2. Ask someone you know and admire whether he or she has ever experienced culture shock. Write a brief description of what he or she experienced.

3. List similarities and differences in what you and your colleague or friend described.

4. What are the implications of culture shock for individuals of non–North American cultures when they immigrate to your state? What provisions does your state make for immigrants requiring government support?

EXERCISE 2: WHAT IS YOUR CULTURE/ETHNICITY?

1. Would you describe your culture as primarily individualistic (low-context) or primarily collectivistic (high-context)? Write out 2 examples from your daily life that indicate which context best describes your perception of your culture.

    a.

    b.

2. Describe the culture of someone you know whose culture is different from yours. Write out 2 examples from your observations of that person that validate your perception of that individual's culture as high or low context.

    a.

    b.

3. What did you learn from this activity? What did you take for granted before that has become more apparent through this activity?

4. What implications does this have for your clinical practice? What do you expect will be the nature of your patients' cultural backgrounds?

EXERCISE 3: CLINICAL DILEMMA

1. You are a therapist from an Anglo-European background working in an outpatient clinic that serves a primarily Hispanic patient population. You notice that your clients are frequently late for their appointments. Based on your knowledge of high- and low-context cultural differences, what might be the possible reasons for the lateness?

2. What strategies can you use to address these differences?

    a. What is the worst thing you can do? Why?

    b. What is the wisest thing you can do? Why?

3. What challenges and opportunities are presented to you personally in this clinical dilemma?

Exercise 4: Phyllis Travels to the Long-Term Acute Care Center

The patient you are about to view is Phyllis, a 73-year-old woman with necrotizing, mulilobar pneumonia; septic shock; and atrial fibrillation, with resulting profound muscle weakness due to the prolonged bed rest. She required 5 days of vasopressors, a tracheostomy (respiratory failure), and percutaneous endoscopic gastrostomy. She was ventilator dependent initially. Phyllis was in the ICU for a total of 6 weeks and then was able to move on to acute, long-term rehabilitation care. Following weeks of long-term acute care rehabilitation center therapies, she went home. Phyllis was in the long-term acute care hospital for a total of 10 weeks from her date of admission to final discharge.

View the YouTube video showing Phyllis as she travels through the health care system from the ICU to acute, long-term care and outpatient rehabilitation services (https://www.youtube.com/watch?v=rAEjjcjob-Y). The video is also available on the Hopkins website reviewed earlier in the chapter (http://www.hopkinsmedicine.org/pulmonary/research/outcomes_after_critical_illness_surgery/oacis_videos_news.html). The video is provided with permission for educational instruction purposes by Darin Trees, PT, DPT, CWS with Solara Rehabilitation Hospital, LTAC, Conroe, TX.

Reflect on your impressions:

1. How was the health care professional communication adjusted in the varying settings Phyllis went through in her recovery?

2. How were her family members supportive in the process?

3. What surprised you?

4. What did you consider about cultural context and pace in each setting?

5. What did you find perplexing, confounding, or impressive?

Here is another YouTube link to a short video that you might also find informative: Holly Gerlach's Journey: From Guillain-Barré Syndrome to Happily Ever After (https://www.youtube.com/watch?feature=player_detailpage&v=VwQzjj9aQnQ).

EXERCISE 5: REFLECTIONS AND RUMINATIONS FOLLOWING MULTIMEDIA READING/VIEWING

Choose one book and/or multimedia resource to review from the additional resources provided at the end of the chapter.

1. What did you learn about the situation described?

2. What did you learn that you were not previously aware of regarding the condition?

3. How did you feel after reading/viewing the book/media resource? Remember that feelings are expressed in one word.

4. What would you like to share with your classmates as a result of reading/viewing this book/media resource?

5. How will what you learned from this book/media resource impact your interactions with individuals and their families in your future practice as a health care professional?

6. What is one thing you will change in your approach to patient care as a result of the learning in this resource?

The exercises at the end of this chapter are also available online.
Please refer to the sticker in the front of the book and enter the access code provided.

The Helping Interview

Carol M. Davis, DPT, EdD, MS, FAPTA and
Gina Maria Musolino, PT, MSEd, EdD

"A little bit of mercy makes the world less cold and more just." –Pope Francis

Objectives

- To emphasize the importance of communicating well in the initial stages of the relationship with the patient.
- To describe the characteristics of a helping interview compared with a nonhelping interview.
- To demonstrate the essential skills of the helping interview.
- To explain key points necessary for the successful interview for persons of all ages.
- To portray the qualities of a helpful interviewer.
- To provide the opportunity to begin developing and practicing one's interviewing skills.
- To apply the skills of peer and self-assessment for professional development, working toward reflective, mindful practice.
- To appreciate the impact of communication skills and cultural influences during the helping interview process.

Artful Patient-Practitioner Interactions

This chapter focuses on another specific application of communication skills: the art of establishing a relationship with our patients and gleaning from them the information we need to be of most help. First impressions often count, and the importance of obtaining the patient's trust from the outset of our interaction together is invaluable to the healing process. Interviewing is much more than obtaining a patient history. The interview serves as the cornerstone for the structure of care we give. Patients come to us worried and often in pain. They feel vulnerable and in need of our help and understanding. They want, often desperately, to put this problem behind them and get on with their lives, and they know they cannot do it themselves. They come to us hoping that we will listen carefully, that we will know something about their problem, and that we will be able to help alleviate their worries. Patients sincerely want to trust that they have made a wise decision in coming to us. Not only do they want physical and psychological comfort, they want another human being to resonate

Davis CM, Musolino GM. *Patient Practitioner Interaction: An Experiential*
Manual for Developing the Art of Health Care, Sixth Edition (pp 223-242).
© 2016 SLACK Incorporated.

with their distress.[1] All of this emotion, in varying degrees of intensity depending on the patient and the problem, is presented to us upon our initial contact with the patient. However, most people will utilize maximum coping skills, and few will fully reveal the extent of their feelings about their problem.

Most adults will convey varying degrees of ability to remain in control in an environment that appears at best strange and at worst hostile. As health care professionals (HCPs), the burden is on us to recognize that the patient feels at a distinct disadvantage and to reassure and support even those who convey a remarkable sense of confidence and comfort. At this initial meeting, interest, genuineness, acceptance, and unconditional positive regard are critical to establishing a healing relationship in the health care professional patient-practitioner interaction (PPI). As we have said many times before, the nature of the relationship we have with our patients is critical to the helping process.

HELPFUL ATTITUDE AND SKILLFUL QUESTIONING

Not only is it important to convey a healing attitude for our patients at the outset in the interview, it is imperative that the patient feel listened to and understood so that all of the information can surface that will lead to the most adequate and complete description of the problem. Thus, pragmatically, effective clinical decision making depends on skillful interviewing, which begins with a healing attitude and proceeds with artful questioning. Let's take a closer look at both.

THE HEALING ATTITUDE OF THE INTERVIEW

A good interview depends on appropriate attitude, good timing, and artful phrasing.[2] The nature of the questions and the process of the interview session will flow out of the beliefs that the questioner holds about such things as one's self-esteem, the appropriate nature of one's role in healing, and what patients are like as people. Let's take a look at some ideas, beliefs, and attitudes that facilitate a healing interview.

Positive self-esteem helps one assume a stance of "I'm okay and so are you. Neither of us is perfect, but each of us, I choose to believe, is doing the best we can to move forward in this world, and I want to help you get back to the business of life as soon as possible." This attitude fosters a healthy, collegial relationship with the patient and keeps the locus of control within the patient. Likewise, it hinders any tendency on the health care professional's part to lay blame on the patient for behavior that might have contributed to the problem that he or she comes to us with in the rehabilitation process.

A helpful belief of the nature of one's role in healing is to assist the person needing help to identify and cope with his or her problems quickly and return to a feeling of being in control of his or her life as soon as possible. Patients are simply people who have a problem that they would solve by themselves if they could, but they need our professional help to identify the problem, clarify the nature and cause of the problem, and solve their problem and get on with living.

OBSTACLES TO CONVEYING A HEALING ATTITUDE

People who have an attitude that facilitates healing are able to accept their patients just as they are without judging them. These health care professionals will often have identified and dealt with biases and prejudices about certain behaviors, such as alcohol abuse, laziness, smoking, use of profanity, and obesity. They will have reconciled their abhorrence of some behaviors, such as rape and murder, and are willing to be therapeutically present to people accused of such behaviors. As much as possible, they will be aware of and willing to underplay and/or eliminate deeply held prejudices about race, culture, gender, age, or sexual orientation.

How does all this happen? Obviously not overnight. The previous paragraph describes a mature person whose ego is not bound by the fear that emanates from immature judgmental and dualistic thinking. Behavior that is accepting is nonjudgmental or nonblaming in nature. As much as we might abhor a person's behavior, it is helpful to believe that the person would have acted differently if he or she had more information, had felt less helpless, and had been less impulsive.

Remember from Chapter 2 that many of the immature judgments and prejudices we continue to carry as adults stem from fear that we developed as children from the messages we heard from adults around us. As adults, we must confront the inappropriateness and negativity of these judgments and work to establish more whole, accepting, self-affirming beliefs.

One of the purposes of this text is to assist you in this maturation process by helping you to identify harmful attitudes and behaviors that would interfere with the healing nature of the interview. Practicing our active listening skills and assertiveness skills helps in an interview. True active listening and speaking out of an awareness of your own rights helps one to diminish a tendency to project one's own weaknesses and to minimize a judgmental attitude.

INTERVIEWING ADOLESCENTS

More than 2 million teenagers in the United States have chronic illnesses and disabilities. They are a diverse group, but at this developmental stage, adolescents share some behavioral similarities that are important to understand and be sensitive to during the interview and during treatment.[3] Teenagers are preoccupied with their bodies and peer acceptance and may be embarrassed by certain questions or feel that some questions are trivial or none of the business of the health care professional.

> *The willingness of a teenager to share personal or intimate information depends on the perceived receptiveness of the provider. … It is usually not difficult for patients and providers to discuss routine chronic medical conditions such as diabetes and asthma. Control of these conditions in some teenagers, however, may be related more to dietary indiscretions and marijuana or cigarette consumption, respectively, than to insulin or inhaler use. Such health-compromising behaviors must be identified before they can be dealt with; comments, facial expressions, or body language indicating disapproval can undermine the patient's willingness to disclose confidential behavior.[3]*

Remember from Chapter 11 that practicing the principles of neurolinguistic psychology will assist you in matching, leading, and pacing the patient to help solidify trust.

A nonjudgmental and supportive attitude toward lesbian, gay, bisexual, and transgendered youth (and adults) can help cushion the stigma they may perceive from family and peers. Likewise, teenagers who are depressed usually suffer from fear of exposure and the stigma of having a mental illness and need the support of the health care professional. Sleep disturbance, decreased appetite, hopelessness, lethargy, continual thoughts about suicide, illogical thoughts, and/or hallucinations are signs that the patient has an undiagnosed depression and should be referred for medical follow-up immediately, with the support of the parents or guardians. However, with questioning in the interview, these symptoms may be determined to be contextual—that is, the teen may have no energy to do homework, exercise, or house chores but have unlimited energy to attend concerts, participate in flash mobs, go to the mall with friends, play video games, use social media, and/or party. Likewise, these symptoms may also be secondary to an undiagnosed substance abuse problem, and further follow-up is required. Reassure adolescents that the information they provide will be kept confidential, unless the threat of harm to the patient or others is revealed. Discussions about sex, their bodies, or use of substances should always take place in a private area. If the patient is accompanied by an adult, first solicit appropriate information from the adult, but then request that the adult leave the room for the remainder of the interview.

With regard to compliance with a treatment plan, recognition of a parental problem is important. Teenagers need the support of parents to meet goals set in therapy. Adolescence is a time of testing boundaries. Chronically ill teenagers are often nonadherent with their therapy secondary to a need to feel in control and test limits. The struggle for independence clashes with the need to follow a routine to improve or maintain health.[3] Local peer support groups can help, as can an open and trusting communication with the health care professional. Emphasize the positive outcomes of adherence to quality of life and have patients actively participate in developing a realistic treatment program.[3]

INTERVIEWING OLDER PATIENTS

Patients in their 80s, 90s, and older (the "old-old"—in contrast to the "young-old" in their 60s and 70s) are products of a traditional upbringing (Traditionalists and Boomers) and respond most positively to certain respectful behaviors that may seem trivial to younger clinicians (see Chapter 11). They often respond best if the health care professional addresses them by their last names, shakes hands warmly, establishes good eye contact, walks with them to the treatment area, and makes small talk about family and the weather before starting the interview. Many old-old patients are concerned that any new thing wrong with them may spell the initiation of a downward slope toward death, so they will be looking for reassurance and information about the nature of the illness or disability that is limiting them and will want a realistic perspective about a return to their previous level of function.

Once as a new health care professional, I had established great rapport with Mr. Moe, who was progressing along quite nicely in his outpatient rehabilitation. The Catholic Health Services, hospital-based rehab department, and outpatient services were informal for the most part, and everyone went by first names. One day, Mr. Moe, a conservative Catholic, was sharing his World War II stories; he had not previously talked at all about any of these experiences. He related these stories as we were working on his exercises for his low back pain from a rotated innominate with muscle imbalances. As he was lying supine looking at the ceiling and I was monitoring the quality of his movement performance, it must have struck a memory for him. He shared some unfortunate and moving details related to his time as a Naval air pilot in the bombardment squadron in the South Pacific. I would not be surprised if this may even have been one of the few and only times he talked about his veteran experiences. Unfortunately, I, being clueless and a novice health care professional, made the mistake of interpreting this disclosure as meaning I could now be more informal with him in terms of his namesake. I called him Archie, his first name, as he was departing therapy. Mind you, this gentleman came dressed in his seersucker suit and jacket to therapy daily; the only thing informal was that he did not always wear a tie, making him seem a bit more approachable. He took great pride in his appearance, health, and service to society. He also would walk the 2 miles to the hospital and back to his home each session, no matter the weather. As I called him Archie as he was putting on his hat, luckily I noticed him raise his eyebrows at me and wrinkle his forehead slightly in utter dismay and appeared quite startled as his eyes enlarged (almost as if I had assaulted him!). If I had not been watching his nonverbal communication through his facial expressions, I may have completely missed that I had offended him greatly. I immediately restated and said, "I'm very sorry, I mean Mr. Moe," which quickly brought a gleam back to his eye, and he tipped his hat back to me and said, "Thank you and see you on Friday." He seemed quite relieved the next visit that I continued to refer to him as Mr. Moe! We were back in sync in our health care professional PPI. I also discovered, after his death many years later, that he was one of the sustainers of the hospital and quietly served on the Board of Directors and in many realms of community service as a silent partner. He made a fortune as a founder of a thermoplastics company that made foam air packaging, was very well off, and never let anyone really know his wealth status—a true Traditionalist of the more silent Greatest Generation. I was very relieved that I was able to reestablish the appropriate therapeutic relationship in this health care professional PPI and continue his care. And if you were wondering, he fully recovered from his low back pain.

Older persons often suffer from hearing loss (or other diminished senses, such as depth perception or vision changes) but do not appreciate being shouted at or patronized as if they are stupid. Do not speak louder than is appropriate; speaking more slowly, clearly, and in a moderate tone is more helpful. Ask how you can best communicate if the patient is having difficulty hearing you; you may need to be in a quiet area when doing your intake or ongoing work with the elderly. Taking the time to get a thorough and true interview at the outset will pay off in the long run. Careful questioning about previous illnesses, medications, and comorbid conditions is critical to making an accurate diagnosis and planning an effective treatment. Likewise, a good understanding about support at home is critical to planning an effective treatment.

In sum, interviewing old-old patients takes longer, but a thorough interview that establishes trust and rapport is absolutely necessary for successful treatment and recovery. Older patients may need a break, and ensure that they are hydrating during the interview process to help sustain them (unless they are on fluid restrictions for some reason). Some older patients will be very difficult to communicate with, especially if they have held the identity of victim all their lives and want you to fix all their problems for them. They can be quite demanding, and it is important to set clear limits of what is possible in treatment. Explain your role in the health care professional PPI relationship and not only what you are willing to do, but also what the patient must do for a successful recovery. Rehabilitation is a partnership and requires trust, unconditional positive regard, and a commitment by patient and provider, hopefully with supportive family members and/or caregivers. Perhaps you will find a certain deep pleasure in getting to know other older patients because many enjoy a wisdom and humor that can be the high point of your day. We learn much from our patients who have traveled the journey of life before us, and the geriatric population has many lessons to share. Older persons shall amaze you with their resilience and can often be a pure joy! Most love to share their life stories and teach you, too.

The Interview

Good Timing

With regard to timing, an effective interviewer avoids interruption (which often reveals an underlying harmful attitude of "this person is not very important to me") and listens carefully, effectively using silence. Those who are uncomfortable with silence will miss much of what a person will say when given a chance to pause and reflect. Time is positively manipulated to indicate a seriousness of attention and level of involvement. A specific uninterrupted amount of time is set to spend listening to the patient carefully as he or she tells you the story of the problem.

Artful Phrasing

Artful phrasing, a skill that is learned over time, involves using the right kind of question (open vs closed, direct vs indirect) at the right time; avoiding jargon, slang, and dialect; and tuning one's words and gestures to reassure the patient that he or she is being attended to at a serious and thoughtful level.[2] The patient shall tell you everything you need to know if only you ask! Be careful not to end before you begin…lots of practice is needed to perfect this important skill for best health care professional PPI.

STAGES OF THE INTERVIEW

There are 3 stages in the interview: initiation, or statement of the purpose of the interview; development or exploration; and closure.

1. The initiation of the interview takes place as you, the interviewer, explain who you are, why you are here, and the purpose of the interview.

2. The body of the interview is the development or exploration stage. In it, the interviewer leads an exploration on the part of the patient, perhaps beginning with the open-ended question, "What brought you here today?" A good interviewer will guide the patient down a meaningful path, assisting the patient to explore his or her problem but not allowing the patient to go too far afield from the problem. Active listening helps the patient to clarify and zero in on the unique aspects of his or her situation. The interviewer listens carefully and sorts the information, jotting down significant revelations as he or she prepares for the clinical examination. The body of the interview unfolds in a unique story that the patient is invited and encouraged to tell. The helpful interviewer confirms to the patient that he or she is being carefully and humanely listened to by a skilled and caring health care professional. When moving from one topic to another, it is helpful to use a transition statement. An example would be, "I think I understand the nature of your headaches; is it okay with you to shift now to the pain in your lower back?"

3. The closing of the interview takes place at a time that has been predetermined by the interviewer. If it becomes obvious that the interview is not complete, the interviewer does not just let the session drop but says, for example, "We're beginning to run out of time for this session and I realize you haven't yet finished. What still needs to be covered?" Then a second session is scheduled, or the interviewer may begin the physical examination and continue discussing the problem with the patient during the exam. I offer a note of caution here, however. To begin the physical examination before allowing the patient to tell as complete a personal story as time allows is a mistake. As an interviewer, you cannot expect to establish a relationship and obtain meaningful information while engaging in palpation and physical evaluation methods. Your brain will attend to what you see and feel before it will attend to what it hears.

BODY OF THE INTERVIEW—INFORMATION GATHERED

The key questions that form the structure of the body of the interview and that set the boundaries for a meaningful story from the patient include the following:

- What is the patient's reason for seeking health care? Why did he or she come today?

- What is the patient's perception of the problem? What is it? Why did it begin? What are the consequences of the problem?

- What impact, if any, does the problem have on the patient's life? How does he or she feel about it? Does it affect work, relationships, and quality of everyday life?

- What are the characteristics of the problem? When did it begin? Precipitating factors? Where is it located? What is its quality and severity? What alleviates the problem? What makes it worse? What factors are associated with it?

- What does the patient expect from this visit? What does he or she hope that you will do?

NONVERBAL COMMUNICATION

The nonverbal communication by the interviewer can facilitate or hinder the quality of the interview. Revisiting Chapter 11 on neurolinguistic psychology and Chapter 12 on cultural sensitivity and reviewing nonverbal communication in more depth will help you develop your use of this important communication skill.

Key nonverbal elements of a helping interview include wise use of space and the environment (posture toward each other and at the same eye level, eliminating physical and perceived barriers); time (uninterrupted level of involvement; sufficient and adequate overall time, allowing for needed breaks); appropriate posture (leaning in, avoiding rigid posture or slouch or defiant gestures, keeping both feet on the ground, open arms); voice inflection (appropriate speed and volume, warmth, and genuine curiosity conveyed vs flatness or excessive use of "you know" or "like"); elimination of distracting body movements (twitching, shaking foot, tapping pencil); avoiding closed postures (no crossed legs, ankles, arms); and maintaining good eye contact (not constantly looking down at your paper or clipboard) so that you can utilize good pacing and timing, along with monitoring the patient's nonverbal communication and being fully present with the patient in the moment (so you can readily and responsively match, pace, and lead); and eliminating any and all distractions (social media, audible sounds from your devices, documentation barriers [ie, looking at a computer screen instead of the patient; interruptions by support staff, etc]).

THE INTERVIEW—A UNIQUE COMMUNICATION FORM

The interview represents a different form of communicating than we've learned growing up in our families and with our friends. The interview is the very first opportunity to convey a professional healing attitude, and it must be learned and practiced in order to develop skill. Behind every word needs to be an attitude of willingness and awareness that will result in congruence.

The words and the inner attitude must be in harmony in order for the interview to be therapeutic. The interviewer must feel confident, peaceful, at one with self, and genuinely willing to establish a healing relationship. You will need to practice many times before you feel fully comfortable, even with the process. Each time, you shall gain in skill level and become more comfortable in establishing the healing relationship, which is essential to the work of the health care professional in PPI.

MORE ON THE INTERVIEW ATTITUDE—WHAT WE ARE

Alfred Benjamin[4] said:

When interviewing, we are left with what we are. We have no books then, no classroom lessons, and no supporting person at our elbow. We are alone with the individual who has come to seek our help. How can we assist him (or her)? The same basic issues will confront us afresh whenever we face an interviewee for the first time. In summary they are:

1. *Shall we allow ourselves to emerge as genuine human beings, or shall we hide behind our role, position, and authority?*

2. *Shall we really try to listen with all our senses to the interviewee?*

3. *Shall we try to understand with him empathetically and acceptingly?*

4. *Shall we interpret her behavior to her in terms of her frame of reference, our own, or society's?*

5. *Shall we evaluate his thoughts, feelings, and actions and if so, in terms of whose values: his, society's, or ours?*

6. *Shall we support, encourage, urge her on, so that by leaning on us, hopefully she may be able to rely on her own strength one day?*

7. *Shall we question and probe, push and prod, causing him to feel that we are in command and that once all our queries have been answered, we shall provide the solutions he is seeking?*

8. *Shall we guide her in the direction we feel certain is the best for her?*

9. *Shall we reject his … thoughts and feelings, and insist that he become like us, or at least conform to our perception of what he should become?*

These are the central attitudinal questions that underlie every helping interview, and the response to each reveals the values that form our attitudes. When you read the above questions carefully, you will see that Benjamin[4] phrased a few to encourage a negative response, as if to have us examine our attitudes very carefully in order to be clear about our helping intentions. The humanistic values (and their subsequent actions) we discussed in previous chapters lead to developing a healing attitude. Once that attitude is established, skillful and artful questions will become second nature, and the interview will become one of the most important tools in the health care professional's repertoire of healing behaviors. Automatically, you will assume an active listening stance and convey a warm and genuine interest in your patient. Once this practiced routine becomes second nature, less stress will be attached to it, and you will experience great pleasure listening to most of your patients tell their stories.

THE NONHELPFUL INTERVIEW

What would a nonhelpful interview look and sound like? Sometimes it is useful for us to explore a concept by describing its opposite. One interpretation of the opposite of a healing interview might go like this:

> The clinician enters the treatment area where the patient has been waiting for quite a while. Without looking up from the patient record or acknowledging the patient in any way, the clinician begins to read the chart and mumbles, "Mr. Zuck?"
> The patient replies, "Yes," and the clinician continues to read.
> Clinician: "So, what's wrong with you?"
> Patient: "I'm not sure. I hurt my back. I can't work."
> Clinician: (No response but thinks to herself, *Oh no, another back. This is the third malingerer I have seen today.*)
> Clinician: "Well, take off your shirt and climb up on the table."
> She leaves the area, returns 10 minutes later, and, without speaking, begins the physical examination.

This, as you can see, is not really an interview at all. No rapport has been established, no active listening was done, and no meaningful information was gathered. The health care professional valued only the information she would get from her physical examination. The patient was reduced to a thing—another low back in a parade of low backs.

How would you feel if you were the patient? Would you, as many patients do, make excuses for the poor, overworked therapist whom you are grateful has made the time to see you? Or have you decided already that here is a person without manners who will treat you only as a thing, another event in a long and uninteresting day? Would you throw up your hands in frustration and bury your disappointment one more time, further convinced that no one really cares about your pain and that you must endure this alone without the understanding help of another person?

Whatever treatment gets accomplished in the previous example, it will be of far less quality than it could be had the clinician used helping interview skills.

RUMINATIONS AND CONCLUSION

If you have ever been fortunate enough to have observed a master clinician at work, you have seen a person who truly values the interview and devotes the kind of attention to it described in this chapter. The greatest obstacles to consistent use of the helping interview are overwork and burnout (see Chapter 5). The more we feel overextended in our day, and the more we feel that we are repeatedly facing irresolvable problems, the more difficult it will be to come outside of ourselves with a therapeutic presence for the interview. Therefore, the very foundation of the helping interview is a commitment to the discipline required to keep a balance in our lives so that we are rested and have good energy to give to our work. Also, we are required to keep a rein on the extent to which we commit ourselves to the work that must be done, avoiding giving up the right to keep a reasonable pace.

People who feel consistently overworked are avoiding the responsibility they have to keep control of the workload and to fight for that right. Each patient we see ideally deserves 100% of our professional ability. It is our responsibility to make sure that we have as much of ourselves to give as we can. Chapter 5 expanded on burnout and helped you learn to balance your life so that this ideal is more reachable.

The exercises for this chapter are critical to effective learning. Conducting a useful interview requires maturation, experience, and practice. Practice in peer and self-assessment shall assist you in developing as a mature health care professional. As discussed in Chapter 9, Musolino[5] described self-assessment skills as not only essential for health care professionals, but crucial to becoming a reflective practitioner[6,7] and moving along the professional development continuum from novice to expert practice.[8] Musolino's[5] study findings paralleled Schön's[6,7] concept of reflective practice and supported Bandura's[9-12] social learning theory in the resulting developed, conceptual model of self-assessment. Recall that feedback is necessary to convert reflective practitice didactic skills into actual clinical abilities and may require a transformative process for novice clinicians.[5,12] Musolino[5] emphasized the influence of critical thought and reflective action through the process of self-assessment and need for guided feedback to effect a change toward mindful practice.[13] Constructive feedback is not only a gift, but an art of sharing crucial insights to assist another to be an excellent health care professional in PPI. Doing peer and self-assessment and truly critically reflecting and being mindful shall enhance not only your interview skills, but also your communication skills as a developing reflective practitioner and health care professional. It is challenging and uncomfortable at first, but thriving on feedback shall assure that you reach your full potentials, along with your abilities to truly help your patients and clients. Do not forget that your patients are also great resources for feedback too.

One of the most efficient ways to correct mistakes and improve style is to review videos of yourself interviewing in a role-play and, if possible, with a patient, then to receive specific feedback as you watch the video. In this chapter's exercises, you shall find that the reviewer assessment forms are exceptional guidance documents for your practice sessions with peer and self-assessment to facilitate your progress toward reflective practice. Maturation and experience lead to quiet self-confidence and relaxation wherein the "third ear" is automatically engaged. Practicing interviewing will help you value and develop the artful balance of scientific discovery with compassionate intuition—the true marriage of the art and science of reflective practice health care in order to help others reach the full potential of their movement system.

Remember to be honest, objective, and constructively critically in your peer and self-assessment feedback. Feedback is a true gift, and your future patients are counting on your abilities to be a true partner in the care of their health. The only way to achieve an effective patient–health care professional partnership is through the initial establishment of good rapport.

Seif and Brown[14] described a similar learning activity using videotaping. They described physical therapy students who participated in 2 video-recorded sessions of simulated interviewing and examinations and completed peer and self-assessment during a 3-part musculoskeletal series prior to their first clinical education experience. The peer and self-assessment debriefing sessions provided feedback on areas for improvement and continued growth in areas of strength, with detailed specific information for continued progression in interviewing skills. The students in this study described the learning activity of peer and self-assessment, utilizing video recordings for assisting in the development of clinical and communication skills for patient care. Additional helpful health care professional resources for screening,[15] measurements,[16] and interviewing skills for self-assessment[17] are available at the end of the chapter.

Don't forget to journal about this experience. What did you learn about yourself as an interviewer? What feelings did you have as you received feedback and/or watched yourself on video? Does videotaping help you identify with patients even more than simply role-playing? Again, have fun as you learn and grow and mature into the role of the healing health care professional.

REFERENCES

1. Perlman HH. *Relationship: The Heart of Helping People*. Chicago, IL: University of Chicago Press; 1979.
2. Enelow AJ, Forde DL, Brummel-Smith K. *Interviewing and Patient Care*. 4th ed. New York, NY: Oxford University Press; 1996.
3. Friedman LS. Adolescents. In: Feldman MD, Christensen JF, eds. *Behavioral Medicine in Primary Care*. 2nd ed. New York, NY: Lange Medical Books/McGraw Hill; 2003:86-93.
4. Benjamin A. *The Helping Interview*. 3rd ed. Boston, MA: Houghton Mifflin; 1981.
5. Musolino GM. Fostering reflective practice: self-assessment abilities of physical therapy students and entry-level graduates. *J Allied Health*. 2006;35(1):30-42.
6. Schön DA. *Educating the Reflective Practitioner: Toward a New Design for Teaching and Learning in the Professions*. San Francisco, CA: Jossey-Bass; 1990.
7. Schön DA. The theory of inquiry: Dewey's legacy to education. *Curriculum Inquiry*. 1992;22:119-140.
8. Jensen G, Denton B. Teaching physical therapy students to reflect: a suggestion for clinical education. *J Phys Ther Educ*. 1991;5:33-38.
9. Bandura A. *Self-Efficacy: The Exercise of Control*. New York, NY: W.H. Freeman; 1997.
10. Bandura A. Self-efficacy: toward a unifying theory of behavioral change. *Psychol Rev*. 1997;84(2):191-215.
11. Bandura A. *Social Learning Theory*. Englewood Cliffs, NJ: Prentice-Hall; 1977.
12. Bandura A. The self-system in reciprocal determinism. *Am Psychologist*. 1978;33:344-358.
13. Epstein RM. Mindful practice. *JAMA*. 1999;282(9):833-839.
14. Seif GA, Brown D. Video-recorded simulated patient interactions: can they help develop clinical and communication skills in today's learning environment? *J Allied Health*. 2013;42(2):e37-e44.
15. The Psych Congress Network. http://www.psychcongress.com/saundras-corner. Accessed April 27, 2015.
16. Carlson JF, Geisinger KF, Johnson JL. *The Nineteenth Mental Measurements Yearbook*. Lincoln, NE: Department of Educational Psychology, University of Nebraska-Lincoln; 2014.
17. Boissonnault J, Boissonnault WG, Hetzel SJ. Development of a physical therapy patient-interview student assessment tool: a pilot study. *J Phys Ther Educ*. 2013;27(1):35-47.

ADDITIONAL RESOURCES FOR SCREENING AND MEASUREMENTS

Psych Congress Network

As you may have discovered already in your helping interview practice sessions, even the apparently healthy may present with the need for screening for other issues and concerns. There are many standardized screening tools to help you screen for psychological concerns if your health care professional PPI and helping interview lead you to believe that further workup and referral may be appropriate for your patients and clients (eg, the Beck Depression Inventory-II, which is a 21-item self-report, multiple-choice inventory with a resulting scaled score of severity, with 81% sensitivity and 92% specificity).[15] The Psych Congress Network houses much information about many of the health care professional practice tools for scales and screeners for diagnoses, such as attention deficit hyperactive disorder, alcohol abuse, anxiety disorders, Asperger's, bipolar disorder, cognitive impairment, depression, psychosis, posttraumatic stress disorder, sexual dysfunction, and suicide, as well as Structured Diagnostic Interview Instruments for neuropsychiatric function, Drug Use Questionnaire, and Well-Being Index. The Psych Congress Network serves as a resource to get you started and also includes trending topical information. Topics vary and include exploration of topics such as caregiver burden, blogs for health care professional support, and health care professional expert interviews. The site covers additional psychological aspects of trending areas, such as the effects of pharmacotherapeutics, current efforts related to medical marijuana, the changing legal landscape related to curbing cannabis use during the evolution toward legalization, and related approaches for health care professional of motivational interviewing (http://www.psychcongress.com/saundras-corner).

The Psych Congress Network site also includes mental health and wellness apps related to meditation, nutrition, exercise, mental health, cognitive behavioral therapy, and sleep applications. As a health care professional in training, you may also find it helpful to explore and try the applications as you go through the stressful times and the best of times (http://www.psychcongress.com/saundras-corner/apps)!

The Mental Measurements Yearbook

Founded in 1938 and published by the Buros Center for Testing, named for late author Oscar Krisen Buros, *The Mental Measurements Yearbook*[16] is the classic biannual text that includes timely, consumer-oriented test reviews; provides evaluation information; and aids health care professionals in selecting, promoting, and encouraging informed test selections. *The Mental Measurements Yearbook* includes descriptive information and professional reviews and is updated every 2 years. The tests cover psychology and education mental measurements. It is the classic go-to text to determine best tests for target populations, scoring, publication resources, and access information (http://buros.org/mental-measurements-yearbook).

ECHOWS Tool

The ECHOWS Tool[17] (E: Establishing rapport; C: Chief complaint; H: Health history; O: Obtain psychosocial perspective; W: Wrap-up; and S: Summary of performance) is an instrument for assessment of physical therapist students' patient interviewing skills with standardized patients. The ECHOWS instrument maintains excellent intrarater reliability and moderate interrater reliability. A training guide for users is provided with the ECHOWS instrument. The ECHOWS is a helpful assessment to use for additional practice and allows for student, peer, and faculty/clinical instructor feedback for interviewing skills, with either standardized or real patients. The ECHOWS may also be used as an assessment tool for debriefing purposes, with videotaped interviews and role-play practice with standardized or real patients, as in Exercise 2 at the end of this chapter.

EXERCISES

EXERCISE 1: RESPONDING TO SITUATIONS

The following are situations in which you might likely find yourself as you interact with patients in the clinical setting. These situations are posed to help you explore in advance what you might feel in the situation, what underlying concerns may be in the situation, and some specific things you might say or do in a situation such as this.

1. You are scheduled to interview Dr. Reynolds and report your findings to your clinical supervisor. Dr. Reynolds has been waiting for you for more than an hour, pacing up and down in the waiting area. When you go out to introduce yourself to her, she turns to you angrily and says, "You clinicians don't give a damn about other people's time. Do you realize how long I've been waiting out here?" How might you feel at this moment?

    What might the patient's underlying concerns include?

    What are some specific things you might say or do at this point to try to salvage the interview?

2. You walk into the patient's room, and he is watching television. You introduce yourself, and the patient never even takes his eyes off the TV. He acts as if you are not present in the room. How might you feel?

    What might the patient's situation be?

    What are some specific things you might say or do in this situation?

3. The person you are interviewing is a street person who has not bathed in a long time. She has severe body odor and an open sore on her leg that is infested with maggots. As she begins to speak to you, she asks for something to spit her tobacco into. What might you feel?

    What might be underlying the patient's behavior?

    What might you say and do to ensure a helping interview?

4. You begin an interview with Mr. Selker, who is 89 years old, with a good, open-ended question but soon after you begin he starts talking about his favorite football team. As you try to keep him on track about his problem, he consistently digresses to the topic of football. He is hard of hearing and seems to not understand what you are saying to him. How might you feel?

    What may be underlying this patient's behavior?

    What might you do to salvage the interview in the given amount of time allotted?

5. You are trying to conduct an interview with a patient, but each time you ask her a question, she looks to her husband and he answers it for her. What might you feel?

    What might be underlying this situation?

    What are some things you might say or do to get more information from the patient herself?

6. You are interviewing a teenager who has a sports injury. She has had type 1 diabetes mellitus since childhood and indicates that she is very tired of having to have insulin injections each day. She feels like an outsider with her friends. She loves playing sports, but it interferes with her insulin regimen, and she is feeling pretty hopeless that she will never be accepted as a normal person. She tells you she wants to die. What might you feel?

    What might be underlying this situation?

What might you say or do at this point to maintain a helping quality to the interview? (Practice your active listening skills of reflection and clarification. How serious is this wish to die, and has it been followed up by others?)

7.   You are interviewing a patient, and the patient suddenly leans forward, grabs your arm, and says, "You are so attractive. I'd like to see you, you know, have a date with you. How about it?" How might you feel?

What might be underlying the patient's behavior?

What might you say or do to get the interview back on track?

8.   You are interviewing an elderly patient who is sitting in a wheelchair. You believe that he is able to understand you, but his responses are quite slow and labored. Suddenly you notice a stream of urine running down his leg and onto the floor. He seems not to pay attention to this. What might you feel?

What decision must you make at this point of the interview?

What might you say or do to ensure that the interview remains helpful in nature? (Practice self-transposal. What would you want someone to say to you? To do?)

9.   You are asked to interview a patient who only speaks Spanish. You cannot elicit meaningful information using rudimentary sign language. No one is close by who could translate for you. What might you feel?

What decision must you make at this point?

How can you solicit accurate information and informed consent? Be creative. (Sign language alone is not legally adequate.)

Can you ethically or legally proceed without informed consent?

EXERCISE 2: VIDEOTAPING AN INTERVIEW

This exercise is offered to help you develop skill in conducting the helping interview and in critiquing your skills and the skills of your classmates. It consists of a role-play of an interview that, ideally, should be videotaped. Divide the class into several small groups, with each small group serving as an observation and feedback unit.

The exercise begins with each class member receiving a description of the patient he or she is to portray. This description should include all pertinent personal and illness (symptom) information so that the actor/actress can carry out the role completely. Completion of the Patient Information Form (pp. 236-237) is important to this process. Students are to be invited to submit patient descriptions from their experiences or simply make up a description of a patient's situation. Each student should complete a Patient Information Form.

Class members number off, but first divide the class in half. If there are 50 students, number off 1 through 25, then start over and number 1 through 25 again. The 2 number 1s will interview each other. Each will role-play his or her own patient described on the Patient Information Form. Some rearranging may take place (eg, a female student may prefer to interview another woman, or a man, whichever she feels she needs most practice with), but it is unwise to do much shifting around once the roles with numbers have been drawn.

When videotaping is done in small groups, an instructor should be with each group. The group should meet for as many sessions as it takes for each person to interview for 5 to 8 minutes. At that time the interview may not be over, but the instructor will call for an end.

During the interview, many thoughts and feelings are taking place. During the video playback, the interviewer has control of the pause button and should stop the tape at any point he or she wishes to discuss the action and to review the various options that are available at that moment.

The patient is invited to ask for the film to be stopped as well, but the interviewer is in charge of the playback. Once the tape is stopped, the interviewer and the patient are invited to discuss thoughts and feelings, and classmates may feel free to question, emphasizing a noncritical, curious attitude.

During the interview, observers are asked to complete the Reviewer Assessment Form (pp. 238-239). After the interview, the patient is asked to complete the Patient Assessment Form (p. 240).

During the discussion of the interview, reviewers may add comments on their assessment form. At the end of the entire process, the interviewer completes the Interviewer's Self-Critique Form (pp. 241-242).

The total time for each interview session should be 20 to 30 minutes.

An Alternate Plan

Time and resource constraints may require that the patient and clinician meet outside class, arrange to have their interview videotaped, and then bring the video to class for discussion and feedback. Classmates (reviewers) should have a summary description of the patient before viewing the video, but again, the class completes the Reviewer Assessment Form (pp. 238-239) as they are watching the video for the first time.

The most important learning for this exercise grows out of the class discussion, not out of the video itself. Feedback is best received when it is specific and given with kindness. Insights that contribute to learning are most effective when they are stimulated in a supportive and nonpunitive atmosphere.

You are reminded to journal about the experience. What was it like to play the role of an interviewer in front of a camera and your classmates? What did you learn about yourself? What behaviors do you intend to develop?

Patient Information Form

Please answer the following questions about the situation you will be representing in your role as a patient. This exercise will be most useful if you answer each item as accurately, completely, and authentically as a patient would who actually has the problem.

1. What is your reason for seeking care?

2. Why are you coming in to see the clinician now?

3. What other complaints or concerns have you had?

4. What do you think or fear the problem might be?

5. What do you think the consequences of the problem might be?

6. What are your past experiences with this problem?

7. How have your activities of daily living been modified as a result of this problem?

8. What other impact has this problem had on your life?

9. What has been the chronology of events in the development of this problem?

10. What is (are) the location(s) of the symptom(s)?

11. What is (are) quality(ies) of the symptom(s)?

12. What is (are) the quantity(ies) of the symptom(s) (eg, frequency, duration)?

13. What factors have you noted aggravate or alleviate the problem?

14. In what setting does the problem seem to occur (ie, what have you noted seems to precipitate the problem)?

15. What other manifestations or symptoms have you noted that seem to be associated with the problem?

16. What are your expectations of this visit to the therapist?

17. Describe your personal situation and characteristics.

18. What is the state of your underlying health?

19. What has been your past personal and medical history?

(Adapted from Course in Health and Human Values, University of Miami School of Medicine, 1982-1985.)

Reviewer Assessment Form

Circle the appropriate letters. Y=yes, N=no, NA=not applicable.
(Note: Where indicated, use space under items to describe and give specific examples of what the interviewer did.)

Your Name: _____

Interviewer's Name: _____

BEGINNING OF THE INTERVIEW

Did he or she:

1. Greet the patient in a friendly, attentive, respectful manner?....................................Y   N   NA

2. Attend to introductions of him- or herself and the patient,
    using the patient's name and his or her own name?..Y   N   NA

3. Define the purpose of the interview? ....Y   N   NA

4. Help the patient get physically comfortable? ....Y   N   NA

EXPLORING THE PATIENT'S CONCERNS: GATHERING INFORMATION

Did he or she:

5. Use questions appropriately?

    a. Use a general open-ended approach to help establish the reason(s) for the patient's visit?.........Y   N   NA

    b. Use a topic-oriented approach to explore new topics, using specific questions only as needed?......Y   N   NA
        Give example:

    c. Avoid premature closed questions that can be answered "yes" or "no"? ....Y   N   NA

    d. Ask one question at a time? ....Y   N   NA

    e. Refrain from using leading questions?..Y   N   NA
        If used, give example:

6. Nonverbally communicate attentiveness and openness?

    a. With a relaxed, open posture? ....Y   N   NA

    b. With facilitating gestures, like head nodding? ....Y   N   NA

    c. With natural, varied eye contact? ....Y   N   NA
        Describe:

7. Verbally communicate attentiveness and openness?

    a. Using encouraging phrases, like "Please, go on"?....................................Y   N   NA

    b. Repeating key words or feelings?..Y   N   NA

    c. Paraphrasing, reflecting back the essence of what the patient is saying and/or feeling?..........Y   N   NA
        Describe:

8. Remain silent where appropriate?

    a. Give patient an adequate opportunity to ask questions?.....................................Y   N   NA

    b. Not interrupt patient? ....Y   N   NA
        Describe:

9. Respond to patient in a warm and sympathetic manner?.....................................Y   N   NA
    Describe:

10. Organize interview in orderly fashion?

    a. Proceed from the general to the specific?...Y   N   NA

    b. Proceed from the less personal to the more personal?....................................Y   N   NA

    c. In history taking, proceed from present to past history? ....Y   N   NA

    d. When changing topics, make transitional statements? ....Y   N   NA
        Describe:

11. Speak clearly, using appropriate language without jargon?.................................Y   N   NA

Closing the Interview (Complete Only if Interviewer Got This Far)

Did he or she:

12. Summarize what was said? ....Y   N   NA

13. Check whether there were any further concerns or questions? ....Y   N   NA

14. Let patient know what will happen next?...Y   N   NA

15. Other strategies interviewer used that facilitated the interview:

16. Other strategies interviewer used that blocked the interview:

(Adapted from Course in Health and Human Values, University of Miami School of Medicine, 1982-1985.)

Patient Assessment Form

Name of Patient: _____

Name of Interviewer: _____

In response to the following, please be as specific as possible.

1. Behavior that facilitated my ability to communicate (eg, your use of silence, which gave me a chance to collect my thoughts).

2. Behaviors that blocked my ability to communicate (eg, your use of leading questions, like "You don't have a sore throat, do you?").

3. Information and feelings, if any, that I was unable to share with you.

4. What I wished you had done or asked me.

(Adapted from Course in Health and Human Values, University of Miami School of Medicine, 1982-1985.)

Interviewer's Self-Critique Form

Circle the appropriate letters. Y=yes, N=no, NA=not applicable.
Note: Where indicated, use space under items to describe and give specific examples of what you did.

Name: _____   Date: _____

BEGINNING OF THE INTERVIEW

Did I:

1. Greet the patient in a friendly, attentive, respectful manner?.................................Y   N   NA

2. Attend to introductions of myself and the patient, using the patient's name and my own name? .....Y   N   NA

3. Define the purpose of the interview? ....Y   N   NA

4. Identify and reflect on my initial impressions of the patient? ....Y   N   NA

EXPLORING THE PATIENT'S CONCERNS: GATHERING INFORMATION

Did I:

5. Use questions appropriately?

    a. Use a general open-ended approach to help establish the reason(s) for the patient's visit?.........Y   N   NA

    b. Use a topic-oriented approach to explore new topics, using specific questions only as needed?......Y   N   NA

    c. Avoid premature closed questions that can be answered "yes" or "no"? ....Y   N   NA

    d. Ask one question at a time? ....Y   N   NA

    e. Refrain from using leading questions?..Y   N   NA
        If used, give example of leading questions to avoid in future:

6. Nonverbally communicate attentiveness and openness?

    a. With a relaxed, open posture? ....Y   N   NA

    b. With facilitating gestures, like nodding my head?..Y   N   NA

    c. With natural, varied eye contact? ....Y   N   NA
        Describe how use of nonverbals felt during interview:

7. Verbally communicate attentiveness and openness? ....Y   N   NA

    a. Using encouraging phrases, like "Please, go on"?...Y   N   NA

    b. Repeating key words or feelings?..Y   N   NA

    c. Paraphrasing, reflecting back the essence of what the patient is saying and/or feeling? ....Y   N   NA
        Describe:

8. Remain silent where appropriate?

    a. Give patient an adequate opportunity to respond to questions? . . . . .Y   N   NA

    b. Not interrupt patient? . . . . .Y   N   NA

       Describe positives and negatives of verbal communication:

9. Reflect on my own feelings and attitudes toward the patient? . . . . .Y   N   NA

    Describe:

10. Organize interview in an orderly fashion?

    a. Proceed from the general to the specific?. . . . . .Y   N   NA

    b. Proceed from the less personal to the more personal?. . . . . .Y   N   NA

    c. In history taking, proceed from present to past history? . . . . .Y   N   NA

    d. When changing topics, make transitional statements? . . . . .Y   N   NA

       Describe:

11. Speak clearly, using appropriate language without jargon?. . . . . .Y   N   NA

CLOSING THE INTERVIEW (COMPLETE ONLY IF YOU GOT THIS FAR)

Did I:

12. Summarize what was said? . . . . .Y   N   NA

13. Check whether there were any further concerns or questions? . . . . .Y   N   NA

14. Let patient know what will happen next?. . . . . .Y   N   NA

15. Other strategies I used that facilitated the interview:

16. Other strategies that blocked the interview:

(Adapted from Course in Health and Human Values, University of Miami School of Medicine, 1982-1985.)

The exercises at the end of this chapter are also available online.
Please refer to the sticker in the front of the book and enter the access code provided.

14

SPIRITUALITY IN PATIENT CARE

Darina Sargeant, PT, PhD

"The best teachers are those who show you where to look, but don't tell you what to see." –Alexandra K. Trenfor

OBJECTIVES

- To explore the role of the spiritual domain in providing spiritual care for patients/clients.
- To review the components of the biomedical and biopsychosocial models of health care and contrast their implications to holistic care and the relationship to the human movement system.
- To define the constructs associated with the spiritual domain: spirituality, spirit, religion, religiousness, and religiosity.
- To recognize the interaction between the spiritual domain and health and wellness.
- To describe various levels of spiritual distress in patients.
- To recognize challenges, barriers, and opportunities to address spiritual care in health care.
- To provide examples of spiritual assessment tools and illustrate the use of a screening tool.
- To assist students in exploring their personal level of comfort with the spiritual domain.

Spirituality is a tool that can assist the practitioner in providing holistic patient-centered care and enhanced patient outcomes. The literature supports the inclusion of spirituality and/or religion as a coping tool, a method to reduce pain and anxiety, a means to improve quality of life, and a source of hope. Health care professionals (HCPs) are often uncomfortable with the provision of spiritual care because health care professionals perceive it to be beyond their scope of practice, express concerns about productivity, and feel unprepared to recognize and address spiritual issues. Chapter 14 provides you with the opportunity to explore personal beliefs about the spiritual domain. The definition of spiritual care, including spirituality and religion, are presented. Spiritual distress is identified, and examples of spiritual distress are shared. Evidence for the inclusion of spiritual care is included, as are models of health, illness, and wellness. Barriers and challenges to the inclusion of spiritual care are discussed, and tools for spiritual screening are introduced. Spiritual care is not limited to palliative and/or hospice care, but also has a role in wellness and any situation in which the patient/client or family/caregiver needs spiritual support. Strategies to incorporate spiritual care are explored, along with examples of spiritual

Davis CM, Musolino GM. *Patient Practitioner Interaction: An Experiential Manual for Developing the Art of Health Care, Sixth Edition* (pp 243-262).
© 2016 SLACK Incorporated.

care. The student will have opportunities to practice the strategies to improve their comfort and skills with spiritual care though use of exercises at the end of the chapter.

Health care professionals work with patients/clients from diverse cultures who have spiritual needs ranging from maintaining health and wellness to facing life-altering circumstances. As culturally competent practitioners and moral agents, health care professionals are expected to interact with patients/clients using ethically caring responses. Because spirituality and religion are part of an individual's cultural identity, knowledge of the spiritual domain can be used by health care professionals to enhance culturally competent and ethically caring responses.[1,2] The spiritual needs of the patient are not always obvious, so the practitioner must be mindful and listen for them, as in the following example:

> Ray is a 45-year-old over-the-road truck driver who recently had a repair of a right rotator cuff tear. Ray's surgeon believes the surgery was successful and anticipates that Ray will be able to return to driving his truck without residual problems. Ray has expressed to his physical therapist, Amy, that he still has a lot of pain and expected to be moving better by now. He tells Amy, "As a young man, I led a pretty wild life, so maybe God is punishing me—maybe that's why I am not getting better." Amy thinks she should talk with Ray about his statement, but she is afraid that her employer or coworkers may think she is overstepping her boundaries as a physical therapist. She decides not to talk to Ray and to just drop it, even though she can see he is very upset and his focusing on this issue seems to be primarily on his mind. She actually believes that this preoccupation is interfering with motivation to do his home exercises, almost as if he feels that he deserves to be punished.

Spiritual Versus Religious

In this chapter, the term *spiritual domain* is used to mean any concepts associated with the patient's religious and spiritual needs. The spiritual domain influences the patient's/client's perception of the impact of illness and assists the individual in coping with the illness and promoting psychological well-being.[2-4] Knowledge of illness and health models, the spiritual domain, spiritual distress, coping strategies, and aspects of health and wellness will assist the health care professional in assessing the patient's/client's spiritual needs. The spiritual domain cannot be limited to illness alone because it is a component of wellness and is a growing focus area for health care professionals interested in the overall health of the general population and themselves.

Jensen and Mostrom[5] indicated that the level of comfort a physical therapist has in addressing the patient's spiritual/religious needs is related to the health care professional's personal comfort with the spiritual domain. The purpose of this chapter is to introduce student health care professionals to key concepts about the spiritual domain, allowing students to explore personal beliefs about the spiritual domain and apply that knowledge to ensure a caring response with all patients/clients and their families.

Models of Illness and Health

Historically, health care professionals have practiced in an environment guided by the biomedical model of illness in which the focus of treatment is primarily on illness as a biological process. This model is reductionist or single factor in nature and focuses on a biochemical explanation of illness, such as a disease process, presence of microorganisms, or accidents and their resulting biochemical and physiological changes. This is not a holistic model of care. Little attention is given to psychological or social factors present in the individual's life. According to Wade and Halligan,[6] the patient is viewed as victim and, as such, has limited to no responsibility in the cause or outcomes. The biomedical model of illness reflects the separation of mind and body, with a focus on illness, rather than health.

Most health care professionals are moving away from this unifactorial view of illness and disease. For example, in 2008, the American Physical Therapy Association (APTA) adopted the World Health Organization's (WHO) International Classification of Functioning, Disability and Health (ICF) that is grounded in the biopsychosocial model of health,[7] which considers physical, emotional, and environmental factors present in the individual's life. In the profession of physical therapy, Sahrmann[8,9] focuses on the movement system in physical therapy and not only considers the physiological system that produces movement in the body at all levels (subcellular, cellular, and system), but also on interaction with the environment; modifiers in the nervous system, including psychosocial factors; and personal characteristics, thus building on the ICF model. The individual's accessibility to preventative care, routine health practices, social support, and exposure to various toxins and environmental pollutants can all impact the individual's health and wellness. Thus, the individual has the responsibility to make choices that lead to improved health. The patient/client becomes an active participant in the health care process. The biopsychosocial model of health is rooted in the unity of the mind, body, and spirit and, hence, is multifactorial in nature.

The biopsychosocial model recognizes that there are micro- and macro-level processes that influence health. The micro-level processes include cellular disorders and chemical imbalances. Macro-level processes consider social support, including cultural, family, religious, and spiritual support systems; psychological well-being, including the presence of depression; and environmental factors, such as pollution, accessibility of health care, and education. In sum, the WHO model includes all of the factors in the ICF and recognizes that health is dependent on attention to the biological, social, and psychological needs of each person. In addition, Puchalski[10] suggested that the patient-centered care model, along with the biopsychosocial model, supports the inclusion of spiritual care because these models consider not only the physical aspect of an illness, but also the emotional, social, and spiritual aspects of care. Patient values and preferences, including quality of life and religious/spiritual beliefs, are considered and inform the decision-making process in the patient-centered model of care.

Patient's/client's/family's beliefs about their health locus of control can also be a determinant in clinical outcomes. Patients/clients and their families may or may not believe that they are responsible for their health or that they can return to a healthy state even in the presence of a disability or illness. Contemporary health care professionals must be aware of each of these factors in screening patients/clients and in developing a plan of care that is individualized and achievable and addresses health and wellness, healing, pain mediation, coping strategies, quality of life, and end-of-life care.[11,12]

The assumptions associated with the models of health and illness can lead to very different patient-practitioner interactions. In the most simplistic terms, the biomedical model is hierarchical in nature, with the health care professional supplying answers to the health problems and providing a "cure." The patient is the passive recipient of care. Although the patient is not an equal partner in the decision-making process, the health care professional expects cooperation from the patient. The cooperative or fully engaged patient will follow the directions given by a health care professional without fail, whereas the uncooperative or less engaged patient does not (see Chapter 15) follow the health care professional's instructions.

In contrast, the biopsychosocial and patient-centered care models encourage health care professionals and the patient to work together to find solutions to problems in order to enhance the healing process. Understanding the complexity of pain and its impact on the movement system[8] necessitates attention to the contextual factors present in the patient's/client's life. Deep listening and attention to the patient's values and beliefs are critical in understanding how these contextual factors affect healing and the return to a functional and meaningful life. Patient and practitioner communication needs to be an exchange of ideas, with all participants valuing the shared information.[13] The relationship between the patient/client and the health care professional may serve as a motivator and source of support to the patient and is more egalitarian in nature. The health care professional's attitude toward the patient can become a barrier to health and healing if the relationship between the patient and therapist is not based on mutual trust and acceptance. Knowledge of and comfort with the spiritual domain can help prepare the health care professional as a positive influence in the healing process.[10]

RELIGION, RELIGIOUSNESS, RELIGIOSITY, SPIRIT, AND SPIRITUALITY

The literature pertaining to the spiritual domain is complex and multidimensional and focuses on the impact of religion, religiousness, religiosity, and spirituality related to patient outcomes with varying levels of consensus.[2,14-21] Definitions of religion and spirituality are different depending on the approach of the researcher or authors. In general, many authors consider *spirituality* an internal search for the transcendent or sacred based on a personal belief system, and religion is considered external to that process. One view of religion defines it as the rules, rites, and rituals that are an external or exoteric manifestation of beliefs and, as such, separate from spirituality.[22] However, according to Zinnbauer and Pargament,[23] spirituality is the search for the sacred and forms the substantive approach to religion. "The sacred is the common denominator of religious and spiritual life. It represents the most vital destination sought by the religious/spiritual person, and it is interwoven into the pathways many people take in life."[24]

Other views of religion consider spiritual or internal beliefs as essential and inseparable components of religion. Psychologists who center their work in the spiritual domain speak of religion as having a substantive and functional purpose in an individual's life. This description of religion is characterized by the search for meaning "related to the sacred" or religiousness.[23] *Religiosity* is a term used in the literature to describe the degree to which a person's life is influenced by religious beliefs and practices.

When spirituality is solely viewed as an extension of religion, it is labeled *religious spirituality*. When spirituality is perceived as independent of religion, it is labeled *secular spirituality*. Hill and Pargament[24] contended that the division of religion and spirituality implies that spirituality is good, whereas religion can be bad. Although some patients/clients may have a poor or negative experience with traditional religion, that experience tends to be the exception for the majority of people.[24] Individuals display varying levels of conviction in their religious beliefs, so it is important for health care professionals to listen for clues about the level of importance of religion, faith, and spirituality in the patient's/client's life. For many patients/clients, religion is a guiding force at all times, whereas for others it becomes more important during times of illness or injury.

Religion, Spirituality, and Health Care

Strict religious beliefs can sometimes be at odds with medical practice, such as when a religion forbids the use of blood or blood products or the use of vaccines for prevention of illness. For many people, however, religion, faith, and/or spirituality offer tremendous help in coping with pain, uncertainty, spiritual suffering, and change that they may be experiencing.[25-29]

Some individuals may also use religion in a maladaptive manner; just as in the case of Ray, they may believe that the pain or illness they are experiencing is a punishment for a past transgression and decide against treatment that could restore their health.[30] It is important to gather information about a patient's spiritual needs during initial assessment in order to provide holistic care. But all health care professionals must exercise caution not to proselytize or force their own religious beliefs on others, judge individuals with different belief systems as inferior or unworthy of assistance, or in any way discriminate based upon the patient's or their own religious beliefs.[2,15,31] Also, one must not assume that because a person ascribes to a certain religion that they practice every tenet of that faith or belief in daily life. Practitioners should explore how faith and religion, beliefs, and practices are part of those individuals' spiritual practices or not. A sample of some common health beliefs of some regions and peoples of the world is explored in the Providers' Guide to Quality and Culture (http://erc.msh.org/mainpage.cfm?file=5.3.0a.htm&module=provider&language=English). Practitioners should become familiar with these practices but make no assumptions for individual patients and consider each patient's/client's individual spiritual history.

For individuals who harbor negative feelings toward traditional religions, spirituality viewed separately from religion can be a reasonable alternative coping strategy. They can ignore the negative thoughts associated with religion and focus instead on hope and finding meaning in the situation. Leaders in the area of patient-centered spiritual care include physicians Koenig[16] and Puchalski,[10] who believe that health care professionals cannot ignore a patient's/client's spiritual or religious beliefs because both assist the patient to cope and find meaning for what he or she will experience.

Spirituality

Although spirituality has numerous definitions in the literature, the consistent components include the search for meaning and purpose in life; connection with others, nature, or a higher being; and transcendence or movement beyond oneself.[2,24,32] Spirituality is a characteristic of all cultures.[2] In Western culture, spiritual development is grounded in the theories of Jung, Erickson, Frankl, Kohler, and Fowler and is influenced by Eastern cultural beliefs and practices.[33] Scandurra's[34] definition—"[s]pirituality is a fundamental, everyday-life process involving and connecting to self, others, nature, and to a larger meaning or purpose"—is useful for persons who may not have a belief in a supreme being. For the purposes of this chapter, we will refer to spirituality as an internal set of beliefs and needs that function to help discover the sacred and meaning in life, and religion will refer to one external way that people act on their need for spirituality in their lives.

As altruistic health care clinicians, we want to do everything possible to help our patients get back into functional life again, to heal and thrive. That is our primary purpose, no matter what discipline we practice. Illness and injury interrupt our lives, and once the original insult has been assimilated or chronic disease becomes a reality of their lives, patients often start asking the larger questions about meaning and purpose of these events in their own lived experiences.

In addition, spirituality is considered a component of wellness that can contribute to health and well-being. Hettler[35] defined wellness as "an active process through which people become aware of, and make choices toward a more successful existence." Hettler[35] developed a hexagon model of wellness in which he identified 6 dimensions of wellness: social, occupational, spiritual, physical, intellectual, and emotional. Spirituality as a component of wellness is associated with balance in life, as well as quality of life. As noted by Rush Thompson in *Prevention Practice: A Physical Therapist's Guide to Health, Fitness, and Wellness*,[36] other wellness models, such as Ardell's Model in Three Domains or Robins' Seven Dimensions of Wellness, offer similar categorizations and either implicitly or explicitly include spirituality as a dimension.[36] Ardell's model explores wellness in 3 domains: physical, mental, and meaning and purpose.[36] Although not mentioned explicitly in Ardell's wellness model as a domain, spirituality is implicitly contained in the meaning and purpose domain as supported by Scandurra's definition of spirituality.[34] Spiritual well-being is one of the Seven Dimensions of Wellness.[36]

As individuals, health care professionals give so much of themselves to others, and in the care of others, we need a place to replenish ourselves. Assuming that spirituality is a connection with others or with a greater being and nature and/or transcendence beyond self, health care professionals can utilize spirituality to help their patients find meaning in their lives and to find balance in their own personal and professional lives. In addition, health care professionals have a professional responsibility to address the health and wellness of society and of individuals in special populations.[37] The House of Delegates of the APTA[38] has encouraged knowledge of all components of wellness as essential for physical therapists because, as professionals, health care professionals must play a positive role in the promotion of healthy lifestyles for persons with and without existing disabilities and must advocate and create programs for wellness, injury prevention, and improved quality of life.[39] The APTA Vision (discussed in Chapter 10) for the profession embraces the impact on society (http://www.apta.org/Vision/): "Transforming society by optimizing movement to improve the human experience."

What is the vision of your chosen profession and the tenets or guiding principles to uphold or achieve the vision? Explore how you have seen health care professionals impact society or how you plan to within your chosen profession. Consider the impact on the human spirit in your explorations.

RESEARCH EVIDENCE SUPPORTING SPIRITUAL CARE— POSITIVE HEALTH IMPACTS

The incorporation of spirituality into holistic patient care is reported to contribute to health, wellness, pain control, delayed morbidity, reduction of depressive symptoms, and healing. Koenig[2,16] cited numerous studies that support the role of spirituality and religion in the promotion and maintenance of health. Udermann[40] conducted a review of the literature on the role of spirituality on health and healing and reported a positive association between spirituality and health.

The field of psychoneuroimmunology considers the complex interconnection of the mind, body, and spirit through the study of the limbic system and its influence on the autonomic nervous system. Chronic stress is linked to the development of autoimmune diseases, chronic illness, and pain.[41] Seybold,[42] in a review of the literature relating health to religiosity and spirituality, reported the following health benefits associated with spirituality and religious practices:

- Increased longevity and decreased morbidity as result of healthy habits (no smoking, moderate diet, and alcohol intake)
- Social support
- Increased self-esteem
- Increased self-efficacy
- Increased levels of serotonin during meditation
- Decreased pain
- Decreased cortisol levels
- Increased blood flow to the frontal lobes with decreased blood flow to the parietal lobes during prayer and meditation
- Reduced sympathetic nervous system activity and increased parasympathetic nervous system activation

Increased activation of the parasympathetic nervous system through religious or spiritual engagement promotes relaxation, improved sleep, decreased heart and respiratory rates, and decreased blood pressure and can result in improved autoimmune function, less depression, and an improved sense of well-being and general health.[43-45] The literature supports the use of the spiritual in assisting patients/clients and families in coping with life-altering events and pain.[14,16,46] Mactavish and Iwasaki[47] reported that individuals with disabilities utilize the spiritual domain for stress coping in different ways—through organized religion, culturally defined activities, prayer, meditation, exercise, or time away from others spent in connecting with the transcendent. Idler and Kasl[48] found that elderly persons who attended church services regularly demonstrated less functional decline or disability over time. A recent study with 132 men and women with stage B heart failure (asymptomatic, but at high risk for the development of symptomatic heart failure due to structural changes in the heart) focused on a potential association between depression and spiritual well-being in patients with asymptomatic heart failure as a means of slowing disease progression, improving quality of life, and reducing death. The authors in this study determined that higher levels of spiritual well-being and greater sense of life meaning and peace were positively associated with fewer depressive symptoms.[49] The authors suggested that spiritual care interventions could be a potential treatment consideration for patients with asymptomatic heart failure. These spiritual interventions can include such activities as journaling, having a connection to nature, meditation, prayer, yoga, utilizing a spiritual coach, art, music, and guided imagery.

There is not a large amount of research in the area of physical therapy, but the research that does exist supports the value of the spiritual domain in physical therapy patient care in building trust, coping with pain and improved outcomes, discovering a sense of purpose, interacting with compassion, and promoting relaxation during physical therapy procedures.[50-53] Pressman et al[53] used an index of religiousness and ambulatory status at discharge to demonstrate a correlation between distances walked and level of religiousness. Elderly woman with higher levels of religious practice exhibited better ambulation status and a lower level of depression following hip fractures.[53] The researchers concluded that the lower level of depression present in elderly women with strong religious practices contributed to improved physical therapy outcomes. Mackey and Sparling[54] reported in their qualitative study that older women with terminal cancer found strength, acceptance, and improved quality of life through their spiritual beliefs. They identified that this acceptance and improved quality of life were accomplished by the physical therapist listening carefully to reminiscences and stories about the important meanings in their lives. Similar skills are utilized in nursing. Johnston-Taylor[55] addressed dimensions of listening that health care professionals can use in being holistically present for the patient in her book *What Do I Say? Talking With Patients About Spirituality*.

Johnston-Taylor's[55] dimensions of listening include the following:

- Intellectual—The health care professional is able to reiterate the intellectual or factual content of what the patient has said in a way that the patient recognizes.

- Emotional—The health care professional can identify and reflect back to the patient the deepest feelings or significance of what he or she has said.

- Physical—The health care professional maintains an awareness of the nonverbal and postural messages sent from the patient's body (eg, voice quality, posture, facial expressions, the look in his or her eyes) as well as the health care professional's own body's physical responses to the incoming messages (eg, neck tension, flushed face, knot in the stomach). These messages then inform the health care professional's responses. For example, a nurse feels exhausted and slumps her shoulders while listening to a patient talk about several losses. Such information can inform the nurse that the losses are tiring to the patient, as well as for herself.

- Spiritual—The listener has an awareness of the Holy in the relationship, a sense of divine presence, and consequently an openness to whatever transpires in the conversation.

Quality of life is individually determined and has different meanings for different persons. Stuifbergen et al[39] indicated that quality of life is a complex construct dependent on 3 sets of factors: context, antecedent variables, and health-promoting behaviors. It is highly subjective and depends on context, such as the perceived severity of the condition. Antecedent variables include barriers, resources, self-efficacy, and acceptance. Barriers may include those imposed by society or those perceived by the person. Resources may include financial, emotional, and cultural resources, to name a few. Religious and spiritual support has been shown to be a positive influence in an individual's quality of life. Belief in self and the ability to overcome a circumstance can influence an individual's health and quality of life.[56] Acceptance of what has occurred or will occur allows the individual to focus on the possibilities rather than the limitations. As noted earlier, the presence of health-promoting behaviors demonstrates the individual's belief in the ability to influence outcomes.

Despite so many positive outcomes reported in the literature, several researchers believe that many of the study methodologies are flawed.[57] Therefore, health care professionals must approach the literature critically while considering the expressed needs of the patient/client/family when making decisions about the inclusion of spiritual care. One cannot ignore the potential ramifications of the growing body of literature, and practitioners are encouraged to be ever-mindful of the spiritual influence in their patients'/clients' lived experiences within the health care arenas.

The spiritual domain can be an excellent source of strength for coping with loss, potential loss, pain, and the dying process. It can also contribute to an improved quality of life and improved ability to cope with depressive symptoms, such as loss of hope and withdrawal from social interaction.[2,16,53,58-61] In a study reported by Murphy et al,[62] patients with amyotrophic lateral sclerosis "who were more religious or spiritual had more hope" and used prayer and attendance at church to help them cope with the changes the patients experienced. In a study by Anderson et al,[63] 74% of individuals who sustained spinal cord injuries as children or adolescents reported that their spiritual beliefs helped them to cope with the injury. Kaufman et al[64] reported a slower progression of Alzheimer's disease in people with higher levels of spirituality and private religious activities. In a study conducted with 293 Indonesian individuals with congestive heart disease, the researchers concluded that higher levels of spirituality were associated with less depressive symptoms, less anxiety, and less anger.[65] Now, let's reflect on the action of a caregiver by considering the following example of spirituality and religious faith in action:

Louise is a professional woman, age 58 and married with 3 children, who was diagnosed with pancreatic cancer. Louise receives chemotherapy on a weekly basis depending on her blood counts. One evening, Louise experienced extreme nausea and vomiting that was accompanied by severe pain. She was unable to take oral pain medications due to nausea. As she lay on the bathroom floor, she said out loud, "God, you promised me that you would not give me more pain than I could handle. I cannot handle this. You have to take it away." Louise considered going to the emergency department for a pain shot but believed that she would not be a priority there and was afraid that she may be even more uncomfortable lying on a stretcher. Her husband lifted her from the floor and took her to her bed. As she lay down, she continued to pray to God to uphold His promise. Louise reported that she fell asleep and was pain free when she awoke. She remained pain free throughout the night. Louise reported that her pain returned in the morning but not at the level she had experienced the preceding evening. Louise believed that God kept His promise. She said that she knew that pain was a reality in her life, but she said she could cope with it knowing that God had not deserted her.

In this example, Louise used her spiritual and religious beliefs to provide hope that she would not be abandoned and that her pain could be controlled. Her belief in a power beyond herself provided her with hope, which allowed her to relax and sleep. Recent science has confirmed that negative symptoms can be mitigated by a change in belief emphasizing hope and optimism.[66]

What would be your level of comfort if Louise shared her story with you the next day? As a health care professional working with special populations, in this case a person who has cancer, you must not only be aware of the specific physical and cognitive needs of the patient, but you must also be aware of the patient's spiritual needs. As a future health care professional, you must ask yourself, "Would I be able to listen and respond to what Louise has shared?" Or would you quickly move past it by changing the focus of the conversation?

Discomfort with a patient's/client's/family's spiritual needs may be a reality, but ignoring a patient's religious or spiritual needs is not acceptable. By ignoring their statements, you may cause the patient/client embarrassment and undermine the trust relationship you established. Baetz and Bowen[26] shared important perspectives:

> *Asking patients about their religious or spiritual beliefs may allow for exploration of potential positive or negative forms of coping or beliefs that would otherwise go unnoticed. Sensitive inquiry and referral to appropriate sources to deal with spiritual struggles are encouraged as part of patient-centered care.*

Redirection of the conversation away from personal disclosures, such as religious, faith, or spiritual beliefs, undermines the patient-therapist relationship and ultimately diminishes the likelihood that the health care professional's interventions will be successful. The patient will likely feel embarrassed and be less likely to share other personal information that could inform the health care professional's clinical decisions. Mackey and Sparling[54] believed that physical therapists can help patients who are receiving hospice care to improve the quality of life by listening to the patient's thoughts about the meaning of life through reminiscence. This is an excellent illustration of using spiritual care and listening to help a patient cope with impending death (see Chapter 18). On occasion, differences in religious beliefs between patients and caregivers can lead to misunderstanding. Consider the following example:

Kathy Winslow is a nurse in a skilled nursing facility who is working with Mrs. Randall, a 78-year-old patient with a diagnosis of congestive heart failure and Parkinson's disease. Mrs. Randall asked Kathy if she would have a priest come to see her for anointing of the sick. Kathy is concerned that Mrs. Randall is depressed and is giving up rather than fighting to get better. Kathy tells Mrs. Randall that she will contact the priest for her. Kathy feels very troubled and considers calling the doctor to report Mrs. Randall's depression.

In this situation, the nurse is not comfortable with a religious ritual requested by the patient. Kathy does not realize that Mrs. Randall finds solace in receiving grace afforded through the anointing of the sick sacrament. On the surface, she is being supportive of Mrs. Randall's wishes by agreeing to contact the priest. However, her concern about the patient being depressed may be unfounded and may lead to unnecessary medical and pharmaceutical interventions and result in Kathy being less emotionally available to Mrs. Randall. If Kathy speaks with the chaplain/priest and shares her concerns, the chaplain/priest can explain the purpose of this particular ritual as not preparing the patient for death, but rather as providing spiritual strength for healing. Open dialogue about spirituality and religion is paramount in providing patient-centered care.

OVERCOMING DISCOMFORT

How can you address the person's spiritual needs if you are not comfortable with the spiritual domain? Becoming familiar with signs of spiritual distress can be helpful in identifying an individual who is at risk and could benefit from spiritual care. At the very least, you must acknowledge the sacredness of the person's statement by reflecting back to the person the importance of the statement (see Chapter 7). In the example of Louise, you might say, "Your faith in God seemed to help you relax enough to get the rest you needed last night" or "I have worked with other people who had similar experiences." The patient then knows that you have heard what was said and recognizes that you did not negatively judge his or her admission. Depending on your level of comfort, you might disclose more in your response with a statement such as, "Focusing on God has helped me deal with pain in my life, also." Then you must assess the patient's reactions to determine whether there is any level of discomfort present for the patient, and you would need to modify your actions accordingly. Once again, it is never appropriate to detail your own religious beliefs in the hopes of convincing patients to believe as you believe (proselytizing). Your role as a clinician is to support and assist through active listening and empathy. Even if patients ask you to go into detail about your beliefs, the patients are most often seeking support of their own beliefs. Simply redirecting the conversation to them and the patient's concerns will be most helpful. For example, say, "I'm more interested in what you believe and how that is helping you cope, or not, at this time."

SPIRITUAL DISTRESS

O'Brien[67] indicated that patients in religious- and nonreligious-based institutions experience varying levels of spiritual distress: spiritual pain, spiritual alienation, spiritual anxiety, spiritual guilt, spiritual anger, spiritual loss, and spiritual despair. Likewise, the concept of spiritual care has implications for health care professionals in any setting—inpatient, outpatient, home care, and school systems. Health care professionals who work closely with patients are often the first to notice the signs of spiritual distress. The most basic level involves spiritual pain, in which patients may experience a loss of support from their normal spiritual or religious sources. The patient may be physically unable to attend services if he or she is homebound or lacking transportation resources; may be unable to watch religious programs on the television; may be hesitant to read the Bible late into the night out of concern for disturbing a roommate, if hospitalized; or may feel unable to pray or find a sense of peace because of feeling overwhelmed with the situation. Spiritual alienation is precipitated by material concerns, such as financial resources, pain, and an inability to take care of family obligations or fear of the unknown that takes the person's attention.

Patients often express their concerns to health care professionals by indicating that they need to return home to take care of a loved one or that they do not know how they will pay for all the care they are receiving. Spiritual anxiety is the fear that the persons or group who normally provide spiritual support will judge the person as no longer worthy of such support. Spiritual guilt is associated with feelings of sinfulness, such as the person who believes that somehow having more faith would have protected him or her from this situation or the belief that he or she is being punished for leading a bad life. Patients sometimes say this in jest, but further probing by the health care professional may reveal that these are very real concerns for the person. Spiritual anger may be manifested by blaming others or God for what has happened. Spiritual loss is the feeling that the patient no longer has the support of others or God, and there is a loss of meaning in life. The most severe manifestation of spiritual distress is spiritual despair. Once hope is lost, the person believes that he or she has no future and often gives up. Any level of spiritual distress could affect the health care outcomes because the patient's/client's ability/desire to focus on tasks will likely diminish. The health care professional is responsible for noticing spiritual distress and communicating that observation to the appropriate persons. This may involve a referral to pastoral care; contact with nursing, physicians, psychology, or social service; contact with family members with the patient's permission; or a gentle encouragement to the patient to contact his or her clergy/rabbi, pastor/priest, or other spiritual leader.

SPIRITUAL DOMAIN IN PATIENT CARE

Not all health care professionals are involved in end-of-life care or in care of patients with permanently life-altering events. However, every health care professional has or will have patients who are afraid of the potential outcome of their injuries or illnesses, who have short-term life-altering events with which they have to cope, or who have acute or chronic pain. It is irrelevant whether the injury/illness is transient or permanent because the normal routine of the patient is altered and coping strategies will need to be adapted to meet his or her changing emotional, physical, and spiritual needs.

Health care professionals must recognize when to incorporate spirituality into patient care as well as when a patient's spiritual needs are beyond their scope of practice. Clinicians should pay attention to cues that patients may give, such as religious symbols in their room, statements about God, search for meaning or purpose in what they are experiencing, feelings of despair or loss of support, and the methods they use to cope with the situation.[68] As stated previously, at the very least, health care professionals have a responsibility to provide holistic, patient-centered care, which includes responding to the patient's physical, intellectual, emotional, and spiritual needs. Hospitalized or homebound persons often lose their spiritual and social support systems because they cannot physically attend religious services or have more limited contact with persons who normally provide them with spiritual support.[41] At a time when individuals require additional emotional and spiritual support, there is generally less support available. The Joint Commission recognized this need and created the regulation RI-1, which requires health care professionals to consider the spiritual and religious needs of patients.[69] The regulation may be technically addressed by asking patients about their religious affiliation, but that question alone does not truly assess the spiritual and religious needs of the patients/clients. It cannot be stated often enough that health care professionals must be vigilant to avoid judgment about a person's beliefs or nonbeliefs. Health care professionals should not make patients feel uncomfortable with explicit and/or unsolicited conversation about personal religious or spiritual beliefs. Although the health care professional may feel comfortable offering to pray for the patient, this should only be done after the health care professional has clearly established that the patient values prayer. For some patients, the offer for prayer would be viewed as proselytization, and the patient-practitioner relationship could be negatively impacted.

What should the practitioner do if the patient discloses that he or she feels that he or she deserves this illness? When a patient discloses this level of spiritual distress, it is imperative that the health care professional recognizes that the level of spiritual care needed by the patient is beyond his or her skills. Referral to persons trained in spiritual care is required. The health care professional can remain aware and supportive of the patient's spiritual care but cannot be the sole source of spiritual care when the individual's needs are more complex.

HELPFUL TOOLS TO ASSIST

How can the health care professional address the patient's spiritual needs given limited time with patients and limited knowledge of world religions? Knowledge of all the religions that exist is not an expectation health care professionals should have for themselves because that would be unrealistic. The nuances are too complex and too subject to personal interpretation to allow accurate understanding across multiple religions. Instead, it is appropriate to ask the patient questions about how the clinician can support his or her spiritual or religious beliefs and needs. The patient should be able to identify rules and rituals that may alter how you interact with the individual and family. A spiritual history, which is a screen for spiritual needs, can be quickly conducted by the health care professional. Short questionnaires exist that allow the clinician to quickly determine how to support the patient and can be readily incorporated into the initial subjective examination or at a later time as needed. Tools such as FICA,[19] SPIRITual History,[22] B-E-L-I-E-F,[70] and HOPE[71] provide the health care professional with the information in 5 minutes or less. Each of these questionnaires has common elements related to inquiry about the beliefs or faith life of the patient, how the beliefs support the patient in daily life and during times of stress, and how the health care professional can support his or her beliefs during care. Health care professionals should familiarize themselves with these tools to determine which tool works best for a given patient or situation. Although the health care professional may be the person who initially identifies spiritual distress, referral to the chaplain or spiritual advisor is necessary because the spiritual staff have the training to perform a more formal spiritual assessment and formulate a spiritual plan of care.[2,72,73] The most basic method a health care professional can use to determine whether a patient would like spiritual assistance is by asking the person for permission to contact pastoral care personnel or a chaplain and requesting a visit if the patient displays signs of spiritual distress. A team approach to spiritual care is essential and demands ongoing communication with the patient/client, family members, spiritual leaders, and health care professionals.

Mr. Cunningham experienced a myocardial infarction 3 days ago, which has left him reeling with confusion and fear. He is currently awaiting discharge from a stepdown unit following the insertion of a stent, and his physician has ordered physical therapy for weakness and fatigue. He is scheduled to begin cardiac rehab in 2 weeks. When his physical therapist, Erin, came to his bedside to evaluate and examine him, she recognized immediately that his anxiety and fear seemed to dominate his responses to her questions. More than once, he mentioned that he did not understand how God could allow this to happen after all he had done to take care of himself, and he felt afraid to get back into life again for fear of what God would do next. He asked Erin, "Why do you think this happened to me?"

(continued)

Erin decided to do a quick FICA[19,72-74] spiritual history and screening in order to plan how to arrange for Mr. Cunningham's support. She told him she recognized that he seemed to be struggling with spiritual questions, and although this was not her area of professional expertise, she asked his permission to gather a little more specific information to better know how to help him. Here is how she proceeded with the FICA[19,73]:

- **F (Faith):** "Mr. Cunningham, do you consider yourself a religious or spiritual person?" He responded, "Yes, I've gone to the Lutheran church regularly since I was a child."

- **I (Importance and influence):** "How important is your religion to you?" He responded, "It really serves as a cornerstone of my life. My faith in God and my ability to worship regularly keeps me going."

- **C (Community):** "Besides attending church regularly, do you feel like you are a member of a spiritual community?" He said, "Yes, I look forward to meeting my pastor and my friends after church for coffee hour, and I am a Deacon in the church, so I help serve the congregation."

- **A (Address or application):** "It seems as if these questions are foremost on your mind, and your rehab will benefit greatly once you get a chance to talk about this with your pastor or spiritual community members. What can I do to help you get your religious and spiritual questions answered?" Mr. Cunningham hesitated and then said, "Well, I have been fussing about calling my pastor. He is so busy. And I just can't shake this feeling that somehow I am at fault for all of this and I feel so guilty."

Erin then offered to have a chaplain talk with him. She also offered him the option to have his social worker help contact his pastor. Both solutions reinforce the idea that once these issues around faith and meaning were talked out, he very likely would feel more at ease and more free to engage fully in his rehab program.

Sometimes a full screening evaluation is not even necessary. If the health care professional practices in a hospital, assisted living, skilled nursing facility, or other inpatient facility, spiritual care can be accomplished in several ways: by listening attentively to the patient, using reflective communication skills (ie, reflection of content, feeling, and meaning), offering a warm blanket when the patient is cold, remarking on pictures of family and friends at the patient's bedside or in the home, or offering to keep the person in his or her prayers if the patient has made it clear that prayer is important to him or her. If the health care professional is seeing the patient in an outpatient setting or home care, the clinician could ask the patient whether he or she has someone with whom to discuss spiritual or religious questions or who can provide spiritual support. The health care professional should feel comfortable enough to ask probing questions if the patient discloses spiritual concerns during the subjective interview or during normal conversations. In addition, clinicians can be respectful of the spiritual care of the patient if they happen upon a shared spiritual interaction by stepping outside or silently standing by during a spiritual interaction between the patient and pastoral care personnel. The presence of the health care professional is comforting to the patient and indicates that the therapist recognizes the value of prayer for the patient.

Sometimes a patient may ask the health care professional to pray with him or her during the course of care. This can be an uncomfortable situation for many health care professionals. It may be more comfortable to ask the patient to lead the prayer because the patient knows what petitions to include in the prayer. For the health care professional who is comfortable leading prayer, it is generally less likely to offend the patient if the clinician invokes guidance throughout the treatment session, as well as patient relaxation, as part of the prayer.

CHALLENGES SUPPORTING PATIENTS' SPIRITUAL NEEDS

What should the health care professional do if the patient is offended by questions within the spiritual domain? Just as many health care professionals are not comfortable with the spiritual domain, there will patients/clients who prefer not to talk about personal beliefs. In approaching a delicate subject such as spirituality or religion, it is helpful to preface the interaction with a statement such as "Sometimes patients want their health care professional to be aware of religious or spiritual beliefs, so I need to ask you some questions about that. Is that okay with you?" If the patient says no, then naturally you would not proceed further. If the patient says yes, you can ask him or her to tell you what is important for you to know. Another approach would be to say, "I need to ask you some questions about how I might support your religious or spiritual beliefs while you are my patient." You would then proceed with one of the tools noted earlier (FICA,[19,72-74] SPIRITual History,[22] B-E-L-I-E-F,[70] and HOPE[71]).

What should the health care professional do if the patient loses focus on therapy and focuses instead on converting the health care professional to his or her religious beliefs? There is a danger in asking about religious and spiritual beliefs because the individual may view the question as an opportunity to convert you to his or her religious beliefs. The health care professional can handle this situation by thanking the patient for sharing information about his or her religious beliefs and then redirect the conversation to the task at hand.

In summary, health care professionals must stand with patients/clients in their spiritual pain. How can health care professionals accomplish this when health care professionals do not have training as spiritual leaders? When the health care professional remains in touch with his or her humanity and acknowledges personal mortality, it is easier to be present with the patient. Quite simply, a gentle touch, a nod, or some other affirmation that the patient is not alone can be shared by the health care professional, thereby establishing the human connection during a time of potential alienation and fear.

There are times when the patient's spiritual needs are more intense and require more advanced skills than reminiscencing, listening, or standing silently as prayer occurs. During the patient's/client's times of escalated spiritual needs, the health care professional should make a referral to professionals trained in spiritual care, such as chaplains and/or pastoral care personnel.

BARRIERS TO INCORPORATING SPIRITUAL CARE

As noted earlier, barriers to incorporating spiritual care are ever-present. Barriers may include concerns regarding scope of practice, preference for the biomedical model, productivity requirements, and personal discomfort with the spiritual domain. For many health care professionals, one barrier to providing spiritual care to the patient is the concern that spiritual care is beyond one's scope of practice and should not be part of the health care professional's plan of care. As noted earlier, in order to give holistic care, the patient's spiritual domain and care must be considered because physical symptoms and signs are affected by the mind and spirit.

A second possible barrier to incorporating spiritual care for some health care professionals is that they may be more comfortable with the reductionistic point of view afforded by the biomedical model, preferring not to delve into the societal, spiritual, and personal factors that influence health and return to a meaningful life. Because many professional associations have adopted the WHO model of the ICF and the patient-centered care model, it is less likely today that health care professionals will consider the biomedical model superior to the biopsychosocial model.

A third possible barrier is productivity, which is a very real concern for health care professionals. Listening to patients and addressing their spiritual needs appear to use more time, but when a patient believes that the clinician has his or her best interest in mind, the level of trust increases, and the patient is more likely to respond in a positive manner to the interventions suggested by the health care professional, therefore resulting in less time needed overall. Ultimately, this often results in fewer refused treatments, better control of pain, and increased functional ability when the patient-practitioner relationship is based on mutual trust and an ethically caring response that is attentive to the patient's values, beliefs, and practices.

Finally, the health care professional's level of comfort with the spiritual domain can be a barrier to implementing spiritual care. In a study conducted with 108 pediatricians, the researchers noted that physicians who were less comfortable in addressing spirituality/religion were less likely to value referral to pastoral care personnel/chaplains than those physicians who recognized the value of the chaplain in the pediatric and oncology settings.[75] Increasing your knowledge about the spiritual domain and pastoral care professionals/chaplains will be helpful, and exploration of your level of comfort with the spiritual domain is necessary. At the end of this chapter, you will find exercises to assist you in reviewing and/or developing your comfort zone with the spiritual domain.

CONCLUSION

Health care professionals are able to enhance the quality of patient-practitioner interactions by increasing their level of comfort with the spiritual domain. Knowledge of the evidence that supports and refutes the inclusion of spiritual care as part of holistic patient care remains essential in order for the clinician to determine the value of including spiritual care as part of the plan of care. Exploration of the spiritual domain informs health care professionals on the most effective and efficient methods to include spiritual support to patients as an important aspect of holistic, patient-centered care.

REFERENCES

1. Elkins M, Cavendish R. Developing a plan for pediatric spiritual care. *Holist Nurs Pract.* 2004;18(4):179-186.
2. Koenig H. *Medicine, Religion, and Health: Where Science and Spirituality Meet.* West Conshohocken, PA: Templeton Foundation Press; 2008:54-112.
3. Krok D. The role of meaning in life within the relations of religious coping and psychological well-being. *J Relig Health.* 2015;54(6):2292-2308.
4. Drutchas A, Anandarajah G. Spirituality and coping with chronic disease in pediatrics. *R I Med J (2013).* 2014;97(3):26-30.
5. Jensen GM, Mostrom E. *The Handbook of Teaching and Learning for Physical Therapists.* 3rd ed. St. Louis, MO: Elsevier, Butterworth-Heinemann; 2013.
6. Wade DT, Halligan PW. Do biomedical models of illness make for good healthcare systems? *BMJ.* 2004;329(7479):1398-1401.
7. Borrell-Carrió F, Suchman AL, Epstein RM. The biopsychosocial model 25 years later: principles, practice, and scientific. *Ann Fam Med.* 2004;2(6):576-582.
8. Sahrmann SA. The human movement system: our professional identity. *Phys Ther.* 2014;94(7):1034-1042.
9. Sahrmann S, Bloom N. Update of concepts underlying movement system syndromes. In: Sahrmann S. *Movement System Impairment Syndromes of the Extremities, Cervical and Thoracic Spines.* St. Louis, MO: Elsevier; 2011:1-34.
10. Puchalski C. Restorative medicine. In: Cobb M, Puchalski C, Rumbold B, eds. *Oxford Textbook of Spirituality in Healthcare.* New York, NY: Oxford University Press; 2012:197-210.
11. Hematti S, Baradaran-Ghahforokhi M, Khajooei-Fard R, Mohammadi-Bertiani Z. Spiritual well-being for increasing life expectancy in palliative radiotherapy patients: a questionnaire-based study. *J Relig Health.* 2014;54(5):1563-1572.
12. Siddall PJ, Lovell M, MacLeod R. Spirituality: what is its role in pain medicine? *Pain Med.* 2015;16(1):51-60.
13. May S. Patient satisfaction with management of back pain: part 2: qualitative study into patients' satisfaction with physiotherapy. *Physiotherapy.* 2000;87:10-20.
14. Astrow AB, Puchalski CM, Sulmasy DP. Religion, spirituality, and health care: social, ethical, and practical considerations. *Am J Med.* 2001;110(4):283-287.
15. Highfield MF, Cason C. Spiritual needs of patients: are they recognized? *Cancer Nurs.* 1983;6(3):187-192.
16. Koenig HG. *Spirituality in Patient Care: Why, How, When, and What.* 3rd ed. West Conshohocken, PA: Templeton Foundation Press; 2013.
17. Koenig HG, Larson DB, Larson SS. Religion and coping with serious medical illness. *Ann Pharmacother.* 2001;35(3):352-359.
18. Peterman AH, Fitchett G, Brady MJ, Hernandez L, Cella D. Measuring spiritual well-being in people with cancer: the functional assessment of chronic illness therapy—Spiritual Well-Being Scale (FACIT-Sp). *Ann Behav Med.* 2002;24(1):49-58.
19. Post SS, Puchalski CM, Larson DB. Physician and patient spirituality: professional boundaries, competency, and ethics. *Ann Intern Med.* 2000;132(7):578-583.
20. Zinnbauer B, Pargament K. Capturing the meanings of religiousness and spirituality: one way down from a definitional Tower of Babel. *Res Soc Sci Stud Relig.* 2002;13:22-54.
21. Zinnbauer B, Pargament K, Scott A. The emerging meanings of religiousness and spirituality: problems and prospects. *J Pers.* 1999;67:889-919.
22. Maugans T. The SPIRITual history. *Arch Fam Med.* 1996;5:11-16.
23. Zinnbauer B, Pargament K. Religiousness and spirituality. In: Paloutzian RF, Park CL, eds. *Handbook of the Psychology of Religion and Spirituality.* New York, NY: Guilford Press; 2005:21-42.
24. Hill PC, Pargament KI. Advances in the conceptualization and measurement of religion and spirituality. Implications for physical and mental health research. *Am Psychol.* 2003;58(1):64-74.
25. Delgado-Guay MO. Spirituality and religiosity in supportive and palliative care. *Curr Opin Support Palliat Care.* 2014;8(3):308-313.
26. Baetz M, Bowen R. Chronic pain and fatigue: associations with religion and spirituality. *Pain Res Manage.* 2008;13(5):383-388.
27. Wachholtz AB, Pargament KI. Migraine and meditation: does spirituality matter? *J Behav Med.* 2008;31(4):351-366.
28. Wachholtz AB, Pearce MJ. Does spirituality as a coping mechanism help or hinder coping with chronic pain? *Curr Pain Headache Rep.* 2009;13(2):127-132.
29. Wachholtz AB, Pearce MJ, Koenig H. Exploring the relationship between spirituality, coping, and pain. *J Behav Med.* 2007;30(4):311-318.
30. Groopman J. *The Anatomy of Hope: How People Prevail in the Face of Illness.* New York, NY: Random House; 2005.
31. Miller WR, Thoresen CE. Spirituality, religion, and health. An emerging research field. *Am Psychol.* 2003;58(1):24-35.
32. Narayanasamy A. Learning spiritual dimension of care from a historical perspective. *Nurse Educ Today.* 1999;19(5):386-395.
33. Sargeant D. Teaching spirituality in the physical therapy classroom and clinic. *J Phys Ther Educ.* 2009;23(1):29-35.
34. Scandurra A. Everyday spirituality: a core unit in health education and lifetime wellness. *J Health Educ.* 1999;30:104-109.
35. Hettler B. Wellness: encouraging a lifetime pursuit of excellence. *Health Values.* 1984;8:13-17.
36. Rush Thompson C. *Prevention Practice and Health Promotion: A Physical Therapist's Guide to Health, Fitness, and Wellness.* 2nd ed. Thorofare, NJ: SLACK Incorporated; 2015.
37. Emmons R, Paluotzian R. The psychology of religion. *Annu Rev Psychol.* 2003;54:377-402.
38. American Physical Therapy Association. Physical fitness for specialized populations. www.apta.org/PFSP/. Accessed March 25, 2015.
39. Stuifbergen AK, Seraphine A, Roberts G. An explanatory model of health promotion and quality of life in chronic disabling conditions. *Nurs Res.* 2000;49(3):122-129.

40. Udermann BE. The effect of spirituality on health and healing: a critical review for athletic trainers. *J Athl Train*. 2000;35(2):194-197.

41. Drench ME, Noonan A, Sharby N, Ventura S. *Psychosocial Aspects of Healthcare*. 3rd ed. Upper Saddle River, NJ: Pearson Prentice Hall; 2012.

42. Seybold KS. Physiological mechanisms involved in religiosity/spirituality and health. *J Behav Med*. 2007;30(4):303-309.

43. Daaleman TP, Kaufman JS. Spirituality and depressive symptoms in primary care outpatients. *South Med J*. 2006;99(12):1340-1344.

44. Daaleman TP, Perera S, Studenski SA. Religion, spirituality, and health status in geriatric outpatients. *Ann Fam Med*. 2004;2(1):49-53.

45. Yohannes AM, Koenig HG, Baldwin RC, Connolly MJ. Health behavior, depression and religiosity in older patients admitted to intermediate care. *Int J Geriatr Psychiatry*. 2008;23(7):735-740.

46. Banks JW. The importance of incorporating faith and spirituality issues in the care of patients with chronic daily headache. *Curr Pain Headache Rep*. 2006;10(1):41-46.

47. Mactavish J, Iwasaki Y. Exploring perspectives of individuals with disabilities on stress-coping. *J Rehabil*. 2005;71:20-31.

48. Idler EL, Kasl SV. Religion among disabled and nondisabled persons II: attendance at religious services as a predictor of the course of disability. *J Gerontol B Psychol Sci Soc Sci*. 1997;52(6):S306-S316.

49. Mills PJ, Wilson K, Iqbal N, et al. Depressive symptoms and spiritual wellbeing in asymptomatic heart failure patients. *J Behav Med*. 2015;38(3):407-415.

50. Reynolds F. *Communication and Clinical Effectiveness in Rehabilitation*. Edinburgh, Scotland: Elsevier; 2005.

51. Kim J, Heinemann A, Bode R, Sliwa J, King R. Spirituality, quality of life, and functional recovery after medical rehabilitation. *Rehabil Psychol*. 2000;45:365-385.

52. McColl M, Bickenbach J, Johnston J, et al. Changes in spiritual beliefs after traumatic injury. *Arch Phys Med Rehabil*. 2000;81:817-823.

53. Pressman P, Lyons JS, Larson DB, Strain JJ. Religious belief, depression, and ambulation status in elderly women with broken hips. *Am J Psychiatry*. 1990;147(6):758-760.

54. Mackey KM, Sparling JW. Experiences of older women with cancer receiving hospice care: significance for physical therapy. *Phys Ther*. 2000;80(5):459-468.

55. Johnston-Taylor E. *What Do I Say? Talking With Patients About Spirituality*. Philadelphia, PA: Templeton Foundation Press; 2007.

56. Womble MN, Labbé EE, Cochran CR. Spirituality and personality: understanding their relationship to health resilience. *Psychological Rep*. 2013;112(3):706-715.

57. Powell L, Shahabi L, Thoresen CE. Religion and spirituality. Linkages to physical health. *Am Psychol*. 2003;58(1):36-52.

58. Ecklund EH, Cadge W, Gage EA, Catlin EA. The religious and spiritual beliefs and practices of academic pediatric oncologists in the United States. *J Pediatr Hematol Oncol*. 2007;29(11):736-742.

59. Fanos JH, Gelinas DF, Foster RS, Postone N, Miller RG. Hope in palliative care: from narcissism to self-transcendence in amyotrophic lateral sclerosis. *J Palliat Med*. 2008;11(3):470-475.

60. Lin HR, Bauer-Wu SM. Psycho-spiritual well-being in patients with advanced cancer: an integrative review of the literature. *J Adv Nurs*. 2003;44(1):69-80.

61. Robinson MR, Thiel MM, Backus MM, Meyer EC. Matters of spirituality at the end of life in the pediatric intensive care unit. *Pediatrics*. 2006;118(3):e719-e729.

62. Murphy PL, Albert SM, Weber CM, Del Bene ML, Rowland LP. Impact of spirituality and religiousness on outcomes in patients with ALS. *Neurology*. 2000;55(10):1581-1584.

63. Anderson CJ, Vogel LC, Chlan KM, Betz RR. Coping with spinal cord injury: strategies used by adults who sustained their injuries as children or adolescents. *J Spinal Cord Med*. 2008;31(3):290-296.

64. Kaufman Y, Anaki D, Binns M, Freedman M. Cognitive decline in Alzheimer disease: impact of spirituality, religiosity and QOL. *Neurology*. 2007;68(18):1509-1514.

65. Ginting H, Näring, G, Kwakkenbos L, Becker ES. Spirituality and negative emotions in individuals with coronary heart disease. *J Cardiovas Nurs*. 2015;30(6):537-545.

66. Lipton B. *Biology of Belief*. Carlsbad, CA: Hay House; 2011.

67. O'Brien M. The need for spiritual integrity. In: Yura H, Walsh MB, eds. *Human Needs and the Nursing Process*. Norwalk, CT: Appleton-Century-Crofts; 1982:85-115.

68. Stanworth R. Spirituality, language and depth of reality. *Int J Palliat Nurs*. 1997;3:19-22.

69. *The Joint Commission: Advancing Effective Communication, Cultural Competence, and Patient- and Family-Centered Care: A Roadmap for Hospitals*. Oakbrook Terrace, IL: The Joint Commission, 2010.

70. Clark P, Drain M, Malone M. Addressing patients' emotional and spiritual needs. *Jt Comm J Qual Saf*. 2003;29:659-670.

71. McEvoy M. An added dimension to the pediatric health maintenance visit: the spiritual history. *J Pediatr Health Care*. 2000;14:216-220.

72. Anandarajah G, Hight E. Spirituality and medical practice: using the HOPE questions as a practical tool for spiritual assessment. *Am Fam Physician*. 2001;63(1):81-89.

73. Puchalski C, Ferrell B. *Making Health Care Whole: Integrating Spirituality into Patient Care*. West Conshohocken, PA: Templeton Foundation Press; 2010.

74. George Washington Institute for Spirituality and Health. FICA Spiritual Assessment Tool. https://smhs.gwu.edu/gwish/clinical/fica. Accessed May 5, 2015.

75. King SD, Dimmers MA, Langer S, Murphy PE. Doctors' attentiveness to the spirituality/religion of their patients in the pediatric and oncology settings in the Northwest USA. *J Health Care Chaplain*. 2013;19(4):140-164.

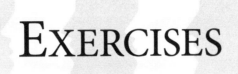

EXERCISES

EXERCISE 1: ASSESSING PERSONAL LEVELS OF COMFORT WITH SPIRITUALITY

1. What does the word *religion* mean to you?

2. What does the word *spirituality* mean to you?

3. Create a time line of meaningful spiritual or religious events in your life.

_____

4. How comfortable do feel you are with the idea of giving spiritual care as a health care professional? Please explain.

5. If there are aspects of giving spiritual care that make you uncomfortable, what are your plans to increase your level of comfort?

EXERCISE 2: INTERVIEW A FAMILY MEMBER OR FRIEND

1. If you have a spiritual or religious belief system, how do you use them to support you during times of illness?

2. How would you feel if your doctor or other health care professional asked about your religious or spiritual needs?

3. When do you think is the best time for the doctor or other health care professional to ask about your spiritual or religious needs?

4. How should your doctor or other health care professional support religious or spiritual beliefs?

EXERCISE 3: PRACTICE YOUR SKILLS

Case Study 1

Selma Brown is a 50-year-old female with a 20-year history of multiple sclerosis. During the interview, she shared with the health care professional that after her initial diagnosis she remained as active as possible. She exercised and walked regularly and was careful not to over fatigue herself. Prior to her diagnosis of multiple sclerosis, Ms. Brown was an avid bicyclist and hiker and worked as a flight attendant. She was able to work for almost 15 years after her diagnosis. As Ms. Brown shared the details of her life with you, she began to cry. About 6 years ago, Ms. Brown had a major exacerbation of her symptoms. While in the hospital, she tried to help herself as much as possible during bed baths and activities of daily living. One day a nurse asked her, "Why bother helping me so much? You're going to end up wheelchair dependent anyway." Ms. Brown said, "That was the day I gave up." Her husband divorced her 5 years ago because he could not "deal with her problem."

Ms. Brown lives alone in a one-story home. Ms. Brown shares with you that her house is totally accessible because, prior to her divorce, she had good insurance and had the house adapted for her use. She uses a motorized wheelchair and can transfer independently. She no longer has insurance and is seeing you as an outpatient at a county hospital.

When the physical therapist requested Ms. Brown's input on what she hopes to achieve by coming to physical therapy, Ms. Brown says she really wants to be able to stand again. She tells the therapist that she wants to be more independent and realizes that walking is out of the question. "I know I will never get back to where I was, but I really want to be as independent as possible. The people from my church offer me a lot of help, but I want to be able to reach plates in my cabinet without falling when the ladies are not around. I prefer to talk with them rather than having them doing everything for me. I just want to be me again. I can't go on this way!"

    1.   What information has she given you about her quality of life?

    2.   How will you address the despair Ms. Brown has shared with you?

    3.   What do you know about Ms. Brown's support system?

Case Study 2

Alma Bender is a frail, elderly female who is experiencing an overall decline in independent function. Her past history includes spinal stenosis, breast cancer, severe scoliosis, and an aortic aneurysm that needs to be repaired. Her 60-year-old daughter, who has bipolar disorder, lives with her. Mrs. Bender was admitted to the hospital 4 days ago secondary to a diagnosis of pneumonia. You received an order to evaluate and treat Mrs. Bender.

During your initial interview, Mrs. Bender indicated to you that she is very worried about her daughter because her daughter can't live alone. Mrs. Bender feels that she doesn't have much time left on this earth. She wakes up each morning with pain in her back and a feeling of impending doom about her health. She feels like she is failing her daughter. She is worried about what will happen to her daughter if she doesn't stay as independent as possible. She wants to be able to get home as soon as possible so that her daughter can come home from the nursing home in which she is currently living.

As her health care professional, you have listened carefully to Mrs. Bender and have reflected her content and feelings back to her. Mrs. Bender has expressed gratitude to you for being such a nice person and says, "Your mother must be very proud of you." Mrs. Bender then begins to cry. You feel awkward but ask her what is wrong. She shares with you, "I am afraid to die because my daughter needs me." As you work with Mrs. Bender on transfers, you hear her say under her breath, "Oh God, please help me. I need your help."

1. How can you communicate your awareness of Mrs. Bender's spiritual needs to her?

2. What is your level of comfort in discussing her spiritual health with Mrs. Bender?

3. What are the pros and cons of addressing Mrs. Bender's spiritual needs?

4. How has your ability to make a connection with Mrs. Bender assisted you in establishing a plan of care that is most likely to have a positive outcome?

Case Study 3

You are a health care professional working in a moderately large hospital with a rehab floor. Several of the patients you see participate in the endurance program developed for persons with cancer. Mr. Ryder was recently diagnosed with lung cancer. Surgery was performed, and Mr. Ryder has been referred to the endurance program. You will treat Mr. Ryder for the first time today. As part of your initial evaluation, you have decided to use the FICA[19,72-74] Spiritual History Tool. Go to the George Washington Institute for Spirituality and Health[74] website (https://smhs.gwu.edu/gwish/clinical/fica) to learn more about the FICA Spiritual Assessment Tool. Develop your FICA approach to gather Mr. Ryder's spiritual history. You may wish to refer back to the example earlier in the chapter utilizing the FICA questionnaire.

- F (Faith):

- I (Influence):

- C (Community):

- A (Address or Application):

1. Develop a transitional statement you will use to put Mr. Ryder at ease when asking about a sensitive issue such as spirituality/religion.

2. Mr. Ryder appears depressed with his diagnosis and unsure of the future. What are some tactics you could incorporate into your plan of care to address his needs?

3. Mr. Ryder is very concerned about his fatigue and his inability to get down on the floor because he wants to play with his grandchildren on the floor again. How would working on floor transfers support this man's spiritual needs?

EXERCISE 4: SPIRITUAL AUTOBIOGRAPHY

1. Clearly state your personal beliefs about spirituality, faith, and/or religion or state that after you reflected on your beliefs, you are not comfortable sharing this information.

2. Include examples of defining moments in personal spiritual, faith, or religious development, indicate that key moments have not been part of your experience, or indicate in #1 that you not comfortable sharing beliefs or examples.

EXERCISE 5: ANNOTATED BIBLIOGRAPHY

1. Provide a one-paragraph summary of the key points of an article (not the abstract) about spirituality or religion as related to the provision of spiritual care by health care professionals.

2. Craft a discussion question based on the article content that will stimulate discussion with your classmates.

15

HEALTH BEHAVIOR AND EFFECTIVE PATIENT EDUCATION

Kathleen A. Curtis, PT, PhD

"I did then what I knew how to do. Now that I know better, I do better." –Maya Angelou

OBJECTIVES

- To define health behavior and health literacy.
- To illustrate how the concept of responsibility makes its way into the messages we give patients by way of examining the 4 models of helping and coping reported by Brickman et al.[1]
- To examine various health behavior theories to better understand why patients sometimes act in ways that go against promoting their health.
- To examine the influence of language and culture on health-related communications.
- To review evidence supporting the use of technology and interactive approaches to promote health behavior change.
- To teach principles of effective patient education.
- To offer instructional planning guidelines when preparing patient and family education materials.
- To teach instructional tips when working with groups.

The health care professional (HCP) entered a note in the patient's medical record. An excerpt:

> The patient returns for follow-up today with essentially no change in his condition…Questionable compliance with the prescribed treatment program. Plan: review importance of continuing daily medication.

What happened? The patient forgot, didn't have time, didn't have the money, didn't want to? It was too much trouble, too complicated, didn't meet his needs, couldn't fit it in with his lifestyle? He didn't understand, doesn't speak English, has too many children, lost the instructions, or felt it was just not that important?

Davis CM, Musolino GM. *Patient Practitioner Interaction: An Experiential Manual for Developing the Art of Health Care, Sixth Edition* (pp 263-283).
© 2016 SLACK Incorporated.

Most health care professionals would find one of these reasons to explain the patient's noncompliance with the treatment program. The reasons may be valid, but the patient's inability or choice not to follow through with the provider's instructions may result in serious illness, disability, or death. If health care professionals really want to influence patient behavior, they must understand health behavior and health literacy.

WHAT IS HEALTH BEHAVIOR?

Health behavior is a series of actions we take to maintain, promote, or improve our well-being. This might include getting immunizations, making regular dental visits, having an annual mammogram or Pap smear, using condoms during sexual activity, doing activities designed to reduce anxiety or stress, being mindful of what you are eating and drinking, or starting a regular exercise program. What health behaviors do you practice regularly in the following categories?:

- Screening examinations
- Health promotion activities
- Treatment of chronic illnesses

WHAT IS HEALTH LITERACY?

Millions of adults have difficulty following self-care instructions due to limited health vocabulary and poor understanding of information and concepts. *Health literacy* is the patient's ability to read and understand all types of health-related materials. One of the first studies in health literacy work documented that 1 in 3 English-speaking patients, and 1 in 2 Spanish-speaking patients at public hospitals had marginal health literacy.[2] Estimates indicate that more than 90 million people in the United States experience difficulty understanding health-related information.[3] Individuals with low health literacy lack sufficient health background knowledge and often have difficulty reading and understanding labels, appointment slips, and instructions for taking medications.

The degree of health literacy makes a significant difference in health outcomes and is often overlooked. Individuals with lower levels of health literacy report worse overall health. When asked to self-report overall health, adults with higher degrees of health had higher average health literacy scores than did adults who self-reported worse overall health levels. Low health literacy is associated with poor health outcomes, including increased hospitalization rates, fewer preventive screenings, and higher rates of disease and mortality. In addition, Medicare and Medicaid enrollees and those without health insurance had lower levels of health literacy than did those who were insured by their employer or the military or purchased private insurance.[3] It takes additional time and costs more to provide quality care to patients with low health literacy. Persons with lower health literacy rates have longer hospital stays, require more care, and make more physician visits, which cumulatively accounts for more than $73 billion in increased health care expenditures.[4]

Compared with adults with higher levels of health literacy, more adults with lower levels of health literacy reported that they received information about health issues from radio and television, rather than from written sources, such as books, brochures, newspapers, or magazines.[3] In an era where cost containment has reduced the availability of follow-up services, low health literacy presents an ever-present danger to this population and raises the question of who is responsible for one's well-being: the patient or the provider?

WHO IS RESPONSIBLE...IN SICKNESS AND IN HEALTH?

If you are like most people, you are very likely to seek a physician's assistance when you have a painful problem. Imagine yourself visiting your physician for diagnosis and treatment of a minor but very irritating and painful skin infection. Your skin is cultured, and you are given a prescription medication to put on your skin every day and an oral medication to take by mouth for 10 days. After 4 or 5 days, the lesion clears up and you discontinue your oral medication. A resistant strain of the same organism then shows up in the same location 2 weeks later. Your physician tells you that you will now have to undergo a complicated, prolonged course of treatment that is riskier to you and those around you. In addition, you will not be allowed to work at your job in the hospital due to the possibility of spreading this infection to immune-compromised patients.

TABLE 15-1		
BRICKMAN'S MODELS OF HELPING AND COPING APPLIED TO PATIENT EDUCATION: PROVIDER PERCEPTIONS OF PATIENT RESPONSIBILITY		
	PATIENT RESPONSIBLE FOR CAUSING PROBLEM	**PATIENT NOT RESPONSIBLE FOR CAUSING PROBLEM**
PATIENT RESPONSIBLE FOR SOLUTION	*Moral Model* Patient admonished for causing problem. Patient education of high value but probably less likely to happen.	*Compensatory Model* Provider has sympathy for patient's problems. Patient education highly valued. Provider highly motivated to provide it.
PATIENT NOT RESPONSIBLE FOR SOLUTION	*Enlightenment Model* Patient education of less value. Patient likely to be admonished for causing problem. Provider will be responsible for solution, which minimizes need for patient education.	*Medical Model* Patient education of less value. Provider has sympathy for patient. Provider will be responsible for patient. Provider will be responsible for solution, which minimizes need for patient education.

Adapted from Brickman P, Rabinowitz VC, Karuza J Jr, Coates D, Cohn E, Kidder L. Models of helping and coping. *Am Psychol.* 1982;37(4):368-384.

Who Is Responsible Now?

If the patient doesn't do what he or she is told to do, is it the provider's fault? Most providers would say no! Do you believe the patient is responsible for the previous situation? How would you feel as the patient in this case?

Our beliefs about the patient's responsibility influence how willing we are to help our patients. Brickman et al's[1] 4 models of helping and coping provide a framework for understanding how the concept of responsibility ties into the messages we give to patients in many patient education situations. The 4 models vary in provider perceptions of the patient's responsibility for causing the problem and for taking action to solve the problem. Here are the rules[1]:

1. If providers believe that patients are not responsible for causing their problems, they are more willing to help (medical and compensatory models).

2. If providers believe that the patients are responsible for causing their problems, they are less willing to help (enlightenment and moral models). If patients see themselves as not responsible for their problem and providers see them as responsible for the problems, conflict may result. Patients may be angry and resentful of the providers' assigning blame to them.

3. If providers see patients as not responsible for the solutions to their problems (such as the treatment), they are likely to take most of the responsibility for patients and therefore do less patient education (medical and enlightenment models).

4. If providers see patients as responsible for the solutions to their problems, they are likely to involve the patient in solving the problem and then hold the patient responsible (compensatory and moral models).

Put yourself in the provider's shoes. What are your feelings about your patient's problems in this case? Who is responsible? If your provider holds you responsible for the solution, he or she may consider you unreliable and feel that his or her efforts have been wasted and are likely unappreciated, even though he or she may feel some sense of obligation to provide further treatment. Table 15-1 helps to explain the relationship of health care professionals' perceptions of responsibility to their willingness to help. As you can see, only one set of conditions (compensatory model) exists in which the provider is highly motivated to help and the patient is seen as responsible for participating in the solution to the problem.[4]

As you are reading, some of you have already begun worrying about your health. Consider your perceptions about your own illnesses or problems or commitment to your personal health. Then consider, would most patients see themselves as causing their obesity, their hypertension, their HIV infection? Do you think your health care professionals hold the same perceptions of your responsibility for these health problems? It would be interesting to find out because the answer to this question has everything to do with the way patients are treated and cared for by their health care professionals.

The behavior change exercise at the end of this chapter may help you gain insight into the challenges of changing your own personal health behaviors and what we are often imposing with our patients/clients as we facilitate their own health behavior changes. In designing effective patient education approaches, it is essential that we understand what influences health behavior. Researchers have published widely on this area for the past 50 years, and there are still many questions. However, there are several key schools of thought that can help health care professionals to feel more informed about how to proceed with their patients.

HEALTH BEHAVIOR THEORIES

Health Belief Model

Perhaps the most influential theory of health behavior is the *health belief model*.[5] This model explains why people fail to participate in programs or behaviors that prevent or detect disease.[5] For example, when the evidence is clear that smoking is harmful to one's health, why would a young person begin to smoke? Why would a health care professional, fully aware of the risks and diseases associated with smoking, continue to smoke?

The health belief model proposes that the likelihood of an individual doing something to protect against a health threat is related to his or her perceptions in 4 areas:

1. Susceptibility to the health threat? (eg, How likely is it that I will have this problem?)

2. Severity of the health threat? (eg, How serious is this problem?)

3. Benefits of the recommended behavior? (eg, What will I gain by doing this?)

4. Barriers or costs of the recommended behavior? (eg, What are the obstacles that stand in my way or the costs to me of taking this action?)

Essentially, what this model proposes is that a person's action has little to do with the types of messages received or the validity of the information communicated and received. Thus, a person could simultaneously hold the belief that smoking is a potentially harmful behavior and, because of conflicting beliefs such as "My grandfather smoked for 55 years and died when he was 80," or "I will gain weight if I attempt to quit," this person will not take the essential action to reduce the health threat he or she may cognitively recognize.

Locus of Control

Another widely accepted theoretical approach uses the concept of *locus of control*, which refers to our perceptions that the outcomes and rewards we experience are either under our control or out of our control.[6] Remember that we first discussed this theory in Chapter 8 on assertiveness.

Individuals with an internal locus of control generally believe that their personal actions and choices have a direct bearing on the outcomes they experience. In contrast, individuals with an external locus of control feel that events are caused by fate, powerful others, or other factors out of their control. This orientation has significance in information-seeking behavior because individuals with an internal locus of control are more likely to seek information about their health problems and choices. Some studies have reported that individuals with an internal locus of control experience more favorable health outcomes than matched subjects with an external locus of control.[7] However, an external locus of control may work very well for some individuals who prefer to follow the directions of an expert.

Health care professionals who are offering educational interventions for their patients or clients need to keep in mind that individuals may not only vary in beliefs regarding the problem and ease of solving the problem (health belief model), but they may also vary in the degree to which they believe that their choices and actions will influence the outcomes they experience. In a study at the Royal Free Hospital in London, physical therapists sent a letter designed to increase perceived control to 39 first-time patients with a variety of disabilities who were scheduled for outpatient physical therapy services.[8] The patients who received the letter reported significantly higher levels of perceived control and were more satisfied with information than the control group, who only received a letter about their appointment time.[8] The sample letter in Figure 15-1 illustrates an effective means to influence patient perceptions of locus of control.

Self-Efficacy

Another perspective in understanding health behavior comes from social learning theory (as discussed in Chapter 9).[9] Self-efficacy is an individual's sense that he or she can successfully carry out a particular health behavior needed to

Figure 15-1. Letter to patients at the Royal Free Hospital. (Adapted from Johnston M, Gilbert P, Partridge C, Coolins J. Changing perceived control in patients with physical disabilities: an intervention study with patients receiving rehabilitation. *Br J Clin Psychol.* 1992;31[pt 1]:89-94.)

Dear Sir/Madam:

This is to let you know that you are now being offered physiotherapy at the Royal Free Hospital to help you to overcome your particular health problem. By concentrating on your difficulties, you will be shown how you can control your symptoms and problems as quickly and as effectively as possible.

You may be offered advice and instructions about your symptoms or problems and given a home program. It will be up to you to follow these if you want to recover quickly.

Experience has shown that the more effort you can put in, the more quickly results will be achieved. The therapists are there to help you to resolve your problems.

You may find it helpful to enlist friends and relatives to help you to follow any home program you are given. May we wish you a speedy recovery.

Sincerely,
Royal Free Hospital

result in a desired outcome. Self-efficacy is influenced by one's own past experiences, observations of the experiences of influential others, and valued verbal and emotional support of others.[10] Self-efficacy and social learning theory have tremendous implications for patient education in that we can promote the use of peer counselors who can model the desired behavior in addition to providing emotional support.

Bandura[9,10] also discussed how the environment influences our choices. Providing and suggesting to patients a variety of environments in which to be successful may assist in compliance efforts. For example, a patient with a forward head position may benefit from simple chin tuck exercises; cue the patient to complete a few at every red stop light, rather than asking him or her to do multiple bouts all at once. By breaking down the exercise activity into simple cues and short periods of time, the patient may not be as overwhelmed. Incorporating the exercise into the patient's daily routine will assist in reminding him or her without being additive to his or her day. You may also cue the patient that every time he or she thinks about the time of day or answers a phone call or text, he or she should think about his or her posture and self-correct. Utilizing the environment and everyday occurrences that fit the patient's lifestyle may lead to greater degrees of compliance. A busy mother and wife with 3 young children who works full-time is not going to be able to dedicate a solid, lengthy time frame to a home program, but intervals of exercise might work. Utilize the patients' changing environments to assist you in achieving their rehabilitation goals.

Theory of Planned Behavior

Ajzen's[11] theory of planned behavior incorporates the concept of social influence and intention in addition to self-efficacy. This theory uses 3 elements to explain individual behavior: (1) behavioral intentions, which reflect an individual's attitude (consequences and desirability) about the behavior; (2) the individual's perceptions of the subjective norms (attitudes of important others, such as family, friends, and society) about the performance of the behavior; and (3) the individual's perceptions of control (difficulty) over performance of the behavior. Ajzen's theory can be used to understand diverse and complex health behaviors, such as refraining from alcohol use and adherence to a recommended exercise program. The planned behavior approach takes into account that our behavior is influenced by our intentions and our beliefs about the attitudes of others, in addition to our perceptions of self-efficacy.

Health Promotion Model

Pender[12] built upon some of these ideas and identified modifying factors (demographic, biologic characteristics, interpersonal influences, situational and behavioral factors) that may influence perceptions of self-efficacy, health status, perceived benefits, and barriers. Pender's model also incorporates internal and external cues to action, further increasing the likelihood of engaging in health promoting behaviors.

	TABLE 15-2	
TRANSTHEORETICAL MODEL OF CHANGE: PATIENT EDUCATION IMPLICATIONS		
STAGE	PATIENT-CHANGE READINESS	IMPLICATIONS FOR PATIENT EDUCATION
Precontemplation	Not intending to change	Help client identify personal priorities and lifestyle goals. Establish trust and rapport to eventually provide insight into negative risk behaviors.
Contemplation	Intend to change within **6 months**	Provide motivational messages of pros and cons of risk behavior. Tie into goals. Support decision making and help clients evaluate pros/cons of the behavioral change.
Preparation	Actively planning to change in **next 30 days**	Seek commitment to risk behavior change and starting date. Support decision to take action with discussion of resources and coping skills.
Action	Has initiated change within the **past 6 months**	Support behavioral change and adaptive replacement of risk behaviors with new lifestyle practices. Provide information about social and medical resources that facilitate change. Teach self-management strategies to prevent relapse.
Maintenance	Has successfully modified behavior **for greater than 6 months**	Prevent relapse and encourage long-term change. Review skills for managing situations triggering relapse to prior behaviors. Reinforce new lifestyle habits and achievement of goals.

Adapted from Basler HD. Patient education with reference to the process of behavioral change. *Patient Educ Couns.* 1995;26:93-98; and Nolan RP. How can we help patients to initiate change? *Can J Cardio.* 1995;11(suppl):16A-19A.

Educational messages may serve as external cues to influence an individual to continue a behavior. For example, the use of internal cues, such as "I feel much better when I exercise," or external cues, such as "heart-healthy" symbols on a restaurant menu or health information on the evening news increase the likelihood of our continuing these beneficial behaviors.

Transtheoretical Model

The transtheoretical model[13] describes stages that individuals progress through as they change health behaviors. The model includes 5 stages of change[13,14]—precontemplation, contemplation, preparation, action, and maintenance—which allow for a nonlinear, or even cyclical, progression through the 5 stages before sustained behavior change can occur (Table 15-2). This integrative transformation model is particularly helpful in understanding change, such as starting an exercise routine or stopping smoking. With this orientation to patient education, a health care professional is aware of the activities that would support the patient in various stages of the change process and able to identify the stage(s) in which the patient/client presents in real-time.[14,15]

Let's look at how this applies.

Jeanette, a health care professions student, feels that she should begin an exercise program after a class on cardiovascular risk factors. She visits her physician to have her cholesterol checked. She looks through American Heart Association literature, reviews the American College of Sports Medicine guidelines, and scores more than 90% on her class test on the material 2 weeks later. Her friends talk about stopping at the gym almost daily; however, she has yet to go with them and join in the gym exercise activities.

One of the main messages that this model proposes is that if education is introduced when someone is in a precontemplative phase, it does not result in a behavior change. The transtheoretical model[13,14] is very important when considering the implementation of programs for major changes in life habits, smoking cessation, weight loss, and exercise programs. Health care professionals must emphasize readiness and give the patient responsibility and control. Also important to keep in mind when using this orientation is that the health behavior may be cyclical; therefore, we could often expect to see progress, setbacks, and periods of high and low compliance. Tolerance of those ups and downs with a general commitment to get back on track seems to be the key to incorporating the health behavior in one's life on a regular basis (see Table 15-2).

Motivational Interviewing

Motivational interviewing[16] is a cognitive-behavioral approach that uses the stages of change mentioned previously as a framework. Health care professionals use motivational interviewing to help an individual to identify and change behavior related to health issues. The approach includes techniques to promote understanding of one's thought processes and emotional reactions to a health problem and how those thoughts and feelings result in common behavior patterns. The key to behavior change using motivational interviewing is to challenge habitual thought patterns and encourage and support alternative behaviors. This approach has been used effectively to institute interventions to overcome addictive behaviors, practice safer sex, and promote healthier behaviors with chronic disease management.

WHICH APPROACH TO TAKE?

Given the variety of approaches that health behavior theorists[5-16] have taken to explain why patients choose or don't choose to take recommended action, health care professionals have quite a few things to consider. How can we incorporate this information into good patient education? What educational activities are needed?

PRINCIPLES OF EFFECTIVE PATIENT EDUCATION

Patient education skills are just as critical to our success as the discipline-specific skills and activities that we learn as part of our professional training. Health care professional–patient education, instructional skills, and strategies take practice and development. Just as not all patient care skills are applicable to all patients, not all patient education skills are applicable either. However, in general, the following assist to positively influence patient behavior:

- Build rapport with the patient, an essential ingredient for all other aspects of the process.
- Set the agenda for change with the patient. The patient's priorities, the difficulties he or she perceives, and realities of resource limitations are critical to this process.
- Communicate clearly and effectively. Focus on the message you want to send.
- Evaluate the patient's readiness to learn or intention for behavior change.
- Assess the patient's language skills, beliefs, cultural background, environment, coping skills, and abilities that will help or hinder the change process.
- Customize your approach to the patient, his or her readiness, and associated needs.
- Assess barriers (cognitive, emotional, physical, social, or support systems) to carrying out recommendations.
- Problem solve with patients to generate solutions to apparent problems and concerns.
- Use appropriate teaching resources (videos, web-based resources, written materials, peer support, family/caregivers, active learning approaches, and other health care professionals) to facilitate the learning process.

Notice that this list does not include giving the patient a poorly visible photocopy of something you found in the files or even a computer-generated, custom-made list of exercises. Understanding the process of individualized behavior change is the key to effective patient education. Once you have assessed that the patient is ready, willing, and able to make the recommended change, there is sufficient time to introduce the appropriate instructional materials as reinforcements of the change process. Assess where the patient is in the change process and proceed with appropriate interventions. Now, how can you deliver your message in the most effective manner?

	PASSIVE	ACTIVE
	TABLE 15-3	
	COMPARISON OF PASSIVE AND ACTIVE LEARNING APPROACHES	
Examples	Lectures, reading assignments, demonstrations, watching videos	Problem solving, feedback, peer support, discussion, experiments, role-play, journaling, writing, interactive participation, debate
Advantages	o Can present a large volume of information in short time period o Easier for teacher and learner o Teacher and learner expectations are simpler and easier to meet o Aligned with traditional testing and assessment techniques	o Relevant and action oriented o Incorporates learner feedback and increases relevancy to culture and environment o Encourages learner to problem solve and apply to individual circumstances o Encourages innovation and transfer of knowledge or the experiences of others to a new situations
Disadvantages	o Does not prepare learner for application or provide instructor with feedback of learner understanding and ability to use information o Lower level rote processing of information is unlikely to lead to innovation, new discoveries, or adherence to treatment recommendations	o Learners may be uncomfortable using active learning strategies, especially if they are accustomed to passive strategies o May be more time consuming o May require flexibility and more interaction by instructor or provider

ACTIVE AND PASSIVE APPROACHES TO LEARNING

Consider how to engage the patient as a partner in their education and best use of active, instead of passive, learning strategies. Passive learning approaches require the learner to acquire the information through listening, reading, or watching others. In contrast, active learning strategies require learners to process information, solve problems and respond, or take action.[17] Recent evidence confirms that high frequency contact through team-based interactive approaches encouraging patient participation and including feedback were associated with a higher effectiveness of lifestyle change in metabolic syndrome.[18] Examples of differences between passive and active learning are provided in Table 15-3.

INSTRUCTIONAL PLANNING GUIDELINES

Let's look at some ideas used by leading instructional designers. The key elements of any instructional sequence answer the following questions:

- What is the problem and what are the patient's (learner's) goals?
- What is the learner's state of readiness for the recommended action?
- What do you want the learner to know, feel, or do? When? How often? Where? With whom?
- What is the key content that must be presented to accomplish these outcomes?
- What learning experiences will help to transmit this content and teach these skills?
- What key steps, decisions, and activities must the learner do to follow the recommendations?
- What materials can reinforce, supplement, or draw attention to the content or process?
- How will you know that you have been successful in teaching?
- How can you evaluate that the learner has learned what you were trying to teach?

Refer to these instructional planning guidelines and respond to the questions with respect to the following case:

> Our patient has returned seeking treatment for a recurrent skin infection. The patient has already failed to take medication consistently on one occasion. The patient must now undergo a complicated, prolonged course of antibiotic treatment using medications with high potential for toxicity and will not be allowed to work in the hospital due to the possibility of spreading this antibiotic-resistant infection.

PRESENTATION TIPS AND EDUCATIONAL ACTIVITIES

Whether you are teaching one-on-one or in a group situation, you may find it useful to incorporate the following ideas in your presentation:

- Present the most important content first. ("First, I am going to teach you how to get out of bed.")
- Be brief and emphasize the main point. ("Bend forward as you begin to stand up.")
- Organize the information into topics, clusters, or categories. ("There are 3 steps to this process.")
- Give specific 1- to 2-step instructions. ("Test your blood sugar 1 hour prior to meals.")
- Repeat important information in a variety of ways. ("You can see it again here—you have to bend your knees, not your back.")
- Use a variety of instructional cues by considering visual, auditory, and kinesthetic prompts to address all varieties and types of ways in which learners prefer to receive information. Reinforce key principles by repeating in a way that addresses all potential learning styles through a variety of instructional modalities of dissemination. (Verbally explain good body mechanics and provide auditory cues; physically demonstrate proper body mechanics, implementing visual cues; guide the learner in physically performing an activity of daily living, such as lifting a box or vacuuming, using good body mechanics; implementing one activity with learning reinforcements.)
- Present at the comprehension level of the learner. ("We'll review some anatomy terms first before we get into the specifics of the technique.")

Now consider the Slujis **Checklist for Educational Activities**[19] in Table 15-4. The checklist was developed and validated by physical therapists, but the elements could be adapted and applied across multiple professions.[19] The checklist is helpful when you are providing home programming activities for patients/clients, caregivers, and their families. Examining the checklist, are there elements that you found surprising or unexpected? How would you choose to prioritize these elements for the aforementioned case? How might your approach be different if you were instructing a caregiver? Would you include all elements in every situation? Why are the various elements relevant?

CULTURE, LANGUAGE, AND LITERACY IN PATIENT EDUCATION

In *Unequal Treatment: Confronting Racial and Ethnic Disparities in Health Care*, Smedley et al[20] reported that regardless of a patient's insurance status or income, individuals from racial and ethnic minority groups tend to receive a lower quality of health care than do members of nonminority groups. The study documented that stereotyping, biases, and uncertainty on the part of health care professionals all contribute to unequal treatment.[20]

A failure to recognize the influence of language or culture can easily lead to undesirable health outcomes. Smedley et al[20] documented numerous examples of poor outcomes related to language barriers and cultural misunderstandings. For example, findings indicated that patients with limited English proficiency were less likely to visit physicians and receive preventive services, regardless of economic status, source of care, literacy, health status, or insurance status.[20] Patients with limited English proficiency also reported lower rates of satisfaction with their care. Researchers have found that patients who did not speak the same language as their health care professional were more likely to miss appointments or drop out of treatment. Findings indicated that using interpreters seemed to eliminate the likelihood of missed appointments.[20] The 2001 National Standards for Culturally and Linguistically Appropriate Services in Health Care mandate that health care organizations "ensure that patients/consumers receive from all staff members effective, understandable, and respectful care that is provided in a manner compatible with their cultural health beliefs and practices and preferred language, including access to interpreter services."[21]

TABLE 15-4

CHECKLIST FOR EDUCATIONAL ACTIVITIES

TEACHING AND PROVIDING INFORMATION ABOUT DIAGNOSIS

- About diagnosis and complaints
- About the cause of diagnosis/illness/pathology
- About the prognosis, health-related quality of life, and psychosocial implications
- Illustrative materials to clarify
- Miscellaneous or additional related/relevant topics
- Assessment of patient's/client's understanding

INSTRUCTIONS FOR HOME EXERCISES/ACTIVITIES

- Explaining home exercises/activities
- Frequency of each exercise/activity
- Number of sessions per day
- Exercise/activity specific instructions
- The build-up of the exercise/activity program
- The build-up of each exercise/activity
- Exercise/activity information—precautions/contraindications/indications/risk
- Instructions written by the health care professional and documented properly
- Integrating exercises and daily activities
- Motivating the patient to comply
- Monitoring the patient's compliance
- Resolving compliance problems
- Miscellaneous or remaining topics

ADVICE AND INFORMATION

- Rest intervals and expectations/outcomes
- Self-care activities
- Safety precautions/concerns
- Correct posture and movement
- General health education
- Stress management
- Caregiver/family member education
- Explanation of treatment, benefits
- Relating goals and outcomes
- Incorporating patient's/client's values and beliefs
- Support from current evidence
- Any referral needs and/or follow-up
- Contact information

Adapted from Sluijs EM. A checklist to assess patient education in physical therapy practice: development and reliability. *Phys Ther.* 1991;71(8):561-569.

COMMUNICATING WITH THE NON-ENGLISH-SPEAKING PATIENT

Developing sensitivity to verbal and nonverbal language, speech patterns, and communication styles is an important skill for health care professionals. Incorporating sensitivity to the potential influence of psychological, social, biological, physiological, cultural, political, spiritual, and environmental aspects of the patient's or client's experience is the obligation of health care professionals for appropriate patient-practitioner interactions.

Services for non-English-speaking patients should include informing them that they have the right to receive no-cost interpreter services. Signs and commonly used written patient education materials should be translated for the predominant language groups in a service area.

Try to use the patient's/client's preferred language whenever possible. Use interpreters as needed when bilingual clinicians are not available. Interpreters and bilingual staff should have bilingual proficiency and be trained in interpreting. They should have knowledge in both languages of the terms and concepts needed in the clinical encounter. Family members are not considered suitable substitutes for trained interpreters because they usually lack these skills and knowledge. Avoid using patients' children or grandchildren as interpreters.

The Provider's Guide to Quality and Culture, a joint project with the US Department of Health and Human Services, Management Sciences Health, Health Resources and Services Administration, and the Bureau of Primary Health Care, was developed to help to address life-threatening errors in health care for health care professionals. The Providers Guide to Quality and Culture website provides several rich examples on the topic of working with interpreters (http://erc.msh.org/mainpage.cfm?file=4.5.0.htm&module=provider&language=English). View these examples of clinical experiences with persons with limited English proficiency and the use of interpreters. Reflect on the queries posed in the videos and consider how you will effectively utilize interpreters.

BRIDGING THE HEALTH LITERACY GAP

Poor health literacy can lead to life-threatening accidents and errors from misunderstandings about dosages or methods of administering medication. It may keep a patient from accessing key services for screening or seeking effective intervention for treatable illnesses. Health literacy has especially serious implications for our older adult populations because older age has been shown to be strongly associated with limited health literacy, including reading, comprehension, reasoning, and numeracy skills.[22]

Approaches to patient education in conditions when individuals may face literacy issues should incorporate interactive techniques and a careful selection of written and online materials. For example, a return demonstration, in which the patient teaches the content back to the educator, may maximize recall. Written materials for low-literacy users serve to illustrate key concepts and aid memory. Follow-up telephone calls, random reminders, email and/or texts, and return visits also serve as a check for understanding. Random reminders for all patients are helpful, and even more so with limited English proficiency. Additional techniques, such as verbal quizzing, repetition, interactive games, individual coaching with concept mapping, theatrical productions, films, music, and radio, have all been used to reach low-literacy populations. The Partnership for Clear Health Communication at the National Patient Safety Foundation[23]—a coalition of national organizations that are working together to promote awareness and solutions around the issue of low health literacy and its effect on safe care and health outcomes—has developed a simple educational program called *Ask Me 3*[23] (http://www.npsf.org/?page=askme3).

This approach encourages individuals to ask their health care professionals 3 simple questions:

1. **What is my main problem?**
2. **What do I need to do?**
3. **Why is it important for me to do this?**

We invite you to view the video on the *Ask Me 3*[23] website and/or YouTube and reflect on the information to reinforce your learning of the method to improve communications as a health care professional.

USE OF TECHNOLOGY IN PATIENT EDUCATION

With the explosion of personal computer use and web-based information resources, many consumers turn to the internet for health information. Recent evidence shows that web-based interventions may be effective as a health information delivery system, especially for those with chronic conditions that can be self-managed and for those who lack health care access.[24] Evidence-based best practices for effective computer-based, health education includes use of engaging multimedia approaches, with voiceover and script messaging, opportunities for repetition, creation of a learning environment that allows privacy, designing questions and answers to reinforce key concepts, user control over sequence and information content, and careful integration with existing educational and preintervention procedures.[25]

Evidence supports the use of technology-specific interactive health communication applications to influence knowledge, social support, and clinical outcomes in chronic disease. Interactive health communication applications and web-based systems typically include a combination of health information, behavioral change support, social support, and decision-making support.[26] In addition, recent analyses report a positive effect of the use of social networking sites to share data and provide health and fitness messages, links, and videos to address health behavior–related outcomes.[27]

Be wary of relying solely on search engines for information because it is only as credible as the posting source(s). Table 15-5 lists some online resources that may enhance your patient education efforts.

EVALUATING WRITTEN MATERIAL

Written materials are important adjuncts to the patient education process, whether in print or online. They should be selected or written specifically for the population with whom you are working or the goals of the intervention. Start to collect or bookmark samples of good patient education materials when you see them. Your target audience should be able to read and understand the written materials you choose. Be sensitive to technical terms, long sentences, and complex

TABLE 15-5
HEALTH RESOURCES: NATIONAL ASSOCIATIONS, HEALTH CARE SOCIETIES, FOUNDATIONS, AND CORPORATIONS WEBSITES/APPS	
American Academy of Orthopaedic Surgeons	aaos.org/home.asp
American Cancer Society	cancer.org
American Diabetes Association	diabetes.org
American Heart Association	heart.org
American Lung Association	lung.org
American Physical Therapy Association	apta.org
American Physical Therapy Association Move Forward for Consumers	moveforwardpt.com
American Occupational Therapy Association	aota.org
American Red Cross First Aid, Blood, Emergency, etc apps	redcross.org/mobile-apps/
Arthritis Foundation	arthritis.org
Brain Injury Association of America	biausa.org
Brain Trauma Foundation	braintrauma.org
Centers for Disease Control and Prevention	cdc.gov
Health on the Net Foundation	hon.ch
Medscape and MedPulse app	medscape.com
MediBabble (translator app)	medibabble.com
National Association of Area Agencies on Aging	n4a.org
National Institute of Arthritis and Musculoskeletal and Skin Diseases	niams.nih.gov
National Institute of Diabetes and Digestive & Kidney Diseases	niddk.nih.gov
National Multiple Sclerosis Society	nationalmssociety.org
National Parkinson Foundation	parkinson.org
United Spinal Association	spinalcord.org
National Stroke Association	stroke.org
Parkinson's Disease Foundation	pdf.org/
WebMD	webmd.com

ideas. Watch the use of jargon and translation of medical language to lay terms. Materials should be written at a sixth- to eighth-grade reading level to reach the most people.

Examine the Flesch Reading Ease Readability Formula and the Gunning Fog Index Readability Formula for evaluating the reading level of written materials (Tables 15-6 to 15-8).

TABLE 15-6

THE FLESCH READING EASE READABILITY FORMULA

1. For short pieces, test the entire selection. For longer pieces, test at least 3 randomly selected samples of 100 words each. Do not use introductory paragraphs as part of the sample. Start each sample at the beginning of a paragraph.

2. Determine the average sentence length (SL) by counting the number of words in the sample and dividing by the number of sentences. Count as a sentence each independent unit of thought that is grammatically independent (ie, if its end is punctuated by a period, question mark, exclamation point, semicolon, or colon). In dialogue, count speech tags (eg, "he said") as part of the quoted sentence.

3. Determine the word length (WL) by counting all the syllables in the sample as if reading the words aloud. Divide the syllables by the number of words in the sample and multiply by 100.

4. These indices are then applied to the formula to compute the reading ease:

$$RE = 206.835 - (1.015 \times SL) - 0.846\ WL$$

where RE is the reading ease score, SL is the average sentence length in words, and WL is the average word length measured as syllables per 100 words.

Interpretation of the Flesch Reading Ease Score

Reading Ease	Grade	Description of Style	No. Syllables/ 100 Words	Average Sentence Length
90 to 100	5	Very easy	123	8
80 to 90	6	Easy	131	11
70 to 80	7	Fairly easy	139	14
60 to 70	8 to 9	Standard	147	17
50 to 60	10 to 12	Fairly difficult	155	21
30 to 50	College	Difficult	167	25
0 to 30	College graduate	Very difficult	192	29

You may also find it useful to use an online generator to test out the readability: http://www.readabilityformulas.com/free-readability-formula-tests.php

Adapted from Flesch R. *The Art of Readable Writing*. New York, NY: Harper & Row; 1974:184-186, 247-251.

PUTTING IT ALL TOGETHER

Health care professionals who educate patients join in a powerful partnership to achieve goals that each, separately, could not realize. Through understanding factors that influence attention, readiness for change, motivation, principles of instructional design and presentation, and the patient's desire for return to function,[28,29] we are better able to design and carry out effective patient education interventions.

TABLE 15-7

THE GUNNING FOG INDEX READABILITY FORMULA

1. Select a sample of writing 100 to 125 words long. If the piece is long, take several samples and average the results.
2. Calculate the average number of words per sentence. Treat independent clauses as separate sentences, "In school we studied: we learned: we improved" counts as 3 sentences.
3. Count the number of words of 3 syllables or more. In your count, omit capitalized words, combinations of short words such as bookkeeper or manpower, and verbs made into 3 syllables by adding "-es" or "-ed." Divide the count of long words by the passage length to get the percentage.
4. Add 2 (average sentence length) and 3 (percentage of long words). Multiply the sum by the factor 0.4, and ignore the digits following the decimal point. The result is the years of schooling needed to read the passage with ease. Few readers have more than 17 years of schooling, so any passage over 17 gets a Fog Index of "17-plus."

(0.4 x [words ÷ sentence]) + (100 x [complex words ÷ words]) = years of schooling needed

Adapted from Gunning R, Kallan R. *How to Take the Fog Out of Business Writing.* Chicago, IL: Dartnell Books; 1994.
The Fog Index Scale is a service mark licensed exclusively to RK Communication Consultants by D. and M. Mueller.
For comparison, you may also wish to utilize an online Gunning Fog Index Tool (http://gunning-fog-index.com/).

TABLE 15-8

SAMPLE PATIENT EDUCATION MATERIALS WRITTEN AT DIFFERENT GRADE LEVELS

WRITTEN AT THE 13TH GRADE LEVEL

The heart usually receives electrical signals from the sinoatrial node, an area in the top right chamber. In ventricular tachycardia, the signals that orchestrate the rhythm originate in the ventricle, located below the atrium. This area of origin results in an erratic beat or rhythm. The erratic beat disables the ventricles from contracting, thus blood is unable to be pumped out adequately. Inadequate blood supply affects all body parts because oxygen and nutrients are located in the blood. When the brain does not receive adequate blood supply, symptoms that include fainting, dizziness, and unconsciousness can occur. Stroke and death are also potential results.

With the knowledge that ventricular tachycardia is an erratic and potentially fatal rhythm that can occur at unpredictable times, physicians usually prescribe medications to control or prevent that rhythm. When medications are unable to keep the erratic beat dormant, the heart may require defibrillation. Defibrillation resets the electrical circuit, allowing the sinoatrial node to once again dominate.

REWRITTEN AT THE 6TH GRADE LEVEL

Electrical signals from the heart's pacemaker keep the heart beating in a normal way. The pacemaker is called the S-A node and is found in the top part of the heart. Signals can also come from the bottom part of the heart. If they come from the bottom part, an irregular or rapid beat results. Several rapid and irregular beats are called V Tach. V Tach means the heart is not able to pump blood. When this happens, the body is not able to get the blood it needs. Blood carries oxygen and food to the body. One of the body parts that needs blood most is the brain. When the brain does not get blood, it can make a person feel faint or dizzy. It can also cause a stroke or death.

Doctors order medicines to try to control or stop this irregular or rapid beat. The medicines usually control this type of beat. Sometimes they do not work. The heart may then need to be shocked. The shock is given by a machine called a defibrillator. The shock usually helps the heart to reset its signals. It then beats in a regular way. All parts of the body can then get the supply of blood they need.

Adapted from Evanoski CAM. Sample patient education materials written at different grade levels. *J Cardiovasc Nurs.* 1990;4(2):1-6.

REFERENCES

1. Brickman P, Rabinowitz VC, Karuza J Jr, Coates D, Cohn E, Kidder L. Models of helping and coping. *Am Psychol*. 1982;37(4):368-384.
2. Williams MV, Parker RM, Baker DW, et al. Inadequate functional health literacy among patients at two public hospitals. *JAMA*. 1995;274(21):1677-1682.
3. Kutner M, Greenberg E, Jin Y, Paulsen C. *The Health Literacy of America's Adults: Results From the 2003 National Assessment of Adult Literacy*. Washington, DC: US Department of Education, National Center for Education Statistics; 2006.
4. National Academy on an Aging Society. Fact sheet. Low health literacy skills increase annual health care expenditures by $73 billion. http://www.agingsociety.org/agingsociety/publications/fact/fact_low.html. Accessed June 11, 2015.
5. Rosenstock IM. Historical origins of the Health Belief Model. In: Becker MH, ed. *The Health Belief Model and Personal Health Behavior*. Thorofare, NJ: SLACK Incorporated; 1974:328-225.
6. Rotter JB. Generalized expectancies for internal versus external control of reinforcement. *Psychol Monogr*. 1966;80(1):1-28.
7. Arakelian M. Assessment and nursing applications of the concept of locus of control. *ANS Adv Nurs Sci*. 1980;3(25):25-42.
8. Johnston M, Gilbert P, Partridge C, Collins J. Changing perceived control in patients with physical disabilities: an intervention study with patients receiving rehabilitation. *Br J Clin Psychol*. 1992;31(pt 1):89-94.
9. Bandura A. Self-efficacy: toward a unifying theory of behavioral change. *Psychol Rev*. 1977;84(2):199-215.
10. Bandura A. Human agency in cognitive theory. *Am Psychol*. 1989;44(9):1175-1184.
11. Ajzen I. The theory of planned behavior. *Organ Behav Hum Decis Process*. 1991;50:179-211.
12. Pender NJ. *Health Promotion in Nursing Practice*. East Norwalk, CT: Appleton and Lange; 1982.
13. Prochaska JO, DiClemente CC. Transtheoretical therapy: toward a more integrative model of change. *Psychother Theory Res Pract*. 1982;19:276-288.
14. Basler HD. Patient education with reference to the process of behavioral change. *Patient Educ Couns*. 1995;26:93-98.
15. Nolan RP. How can we help patients to initiate change? *Can J Cardiol*. 1995;11(suppl):16A-19A.
16. Bundy C. Changing behaviour: using motivational interviewing techniques. *J R Soc Med*. 2004;97(suppl 44):43-47.
17. Russell AT, Comello RJ, Wright DL. Teaching strategies promoting active learning in healthcare education. *Journal of Education and Human Development*. 2007;1(1):1-12.
18. Bassi N, Karagodin I, Wang S, et al. Lifestyle modification for metabolic syndrome: a systematic review. *Am J Med*. 2014;127(12):1242.e1-1242.e10.
19. Sluijs EM. A checklist to assess patient education in physical therapy practice: development and reliability. *Phys Ther*. 1991;71(8):561-569.
20. Smedley BD, Stith AY, Nelson AR, eds. *Unequal Treatment: Confronting Racial and Ethnic Disparities in Health Care*. Washington, DC: The National Academies Press; 2002.
21. US Department of Health and Human Services. *National Standards for Culturally and Linguistically Appropriate Services in Health Care*. Washington, DC: US Department of Health and Human Services, Office of Minority Health; 2001.
22. Kobayashi LC, Wardle J, Wolf MS, von Wagner C. Aging and functional health literacy: a systematic review and meta-analysis [published online ahead of print December 11, 2014]. *J Gerontol B Psychol Sci Soc Sci*.
23. National Patient Safety Foundation. Ask Me 3. http://www.npsf.org/?page=askme3. Accessed June 13, 2015.
24. Kirsch SE, Lewis FM. Using the World Wide Web in health-related intervention research: a review of controlled trials. *Comput Inform Nurs*. 2004;22(1):8-18.
25. Fox MP. A systematic review of the literature reporting on studies that examined the impact of interactive, computer-based patient education programs. *Patient Educ Couns*. 2009;77(1):6-13.
26. Murray E, Burns J, See TS, Lai R, Nazareth I. Interactive health communication applications for people with chronic disease. *Cochrane Database Syst Rev*. 2005;19(4):CD004274.
27. Laranjo L, Arguel A, Neves AL, et al. The influence of social networking sites on health behavior change: a systematic review and meta-analysis. *J Am Med Inform Assoc*. 2015;22(1):243-256.
28. Randall KE, McEwen IR. Writing patient-centered functional goals. *Phys Ther*. 2000;80(12):1197-1203.
29. O'Neill DL, Harris SR. Developing goals and objectives for handicapped children. *Phys Ther*. 1982;62(3):295-98.

EXERCISES

EXERCISE 1: EXPLORING PROVIDER PERCEPTIONS OF RESPONSIBILITY

For what types of problems do you hold most patients responsible? List a few of these problems below.

EXERCISE 2: USING THEORY TO UNDERSTAND HEALTH BEHAVIOR CHOICES

1. Identify a health behavior that you put off, don't do, or do too much of on a daily basis (sleep, dentist, safe sex, healthy nutrition, physical activity, social media, recreational video gaming, etc). What are your beliefs about these behaviors?

2. Enter the answers to these in your journal (or here) and be prepared to discuss in class.

    a. Susceptibility to the health threat? (ie, How likely is it that I will have this problem?)

    b. Severity of the health threat? (ie, How serious is this problem?)

    c. Benefits of the recommended behavior? (ie, What will I gain by doing this?)

    d. Barriers or costs of the recommended behavior? (ie, What are the obstacles that stand in my way or the costs to me of taking this action?)

    e. What environmental cues influence you?

    f. What have you seen and learned from others?

    g. In what stage (transtheoretical model of change[13]) would you place yourself at this moment? Have you moved through various stages recently?

    h. What can you do to influence your own behavior?

    i. What beliefs must you change?

    j. What cues would make it more likely that you'll make the behavior change?

    k. What forms of social support or decision support would be helpful to you to make this change?

3. Now, make an action plan. Include your personal behavior change goal (in the ABCD format) and specifically include the following:

    - A—Audience or Who? (You in this case, or "I"):

    - B—Behavior or What? (Behavior you wish to change):

    - C—Condition or When? (By when will you complete the short- and long-term goals?):

    - D—Degree or How well? (How will you measure how well you are doing or your success and track your progress?):

    ABCD—Goal Statement:

    Then, develop your plan for action, and include the following: What steps will you take to make the change? What rewards might you build in to reinforce your efforts? How will you employ those who influence you (or not) to assist you in your goal achievement?

    Once you have formulated your goal and specific action plan on how you shall achieve your goal, identify a behavior change partner and work together to monitor, coach, and track each other's progress. Discover how your stage in the transtheoretical model of change[13] is impacting your or your partner's progress. Consider how you can each facilitate each other based upon the stage and progress (or regression) to date.

EXERCISE 3: EXPLORING THE PERCEPTIONS OF OTHERS

Identify a health behavior topic relevant to your field (eg, repetitive stress disorders for computer users, preventing low back pain, preventing sexually transmitted diseases, low-fat diet). Do a mini-survey of 10 people on campus, in your community, or at your facility about their beliefs on this topic (the cause, the severity of the problem, the effectiveness, and ease of prevention or treatment). You can do this as an in-class activity if the instructor assigns it.

1. List your chosen health behavior.

2. Prepare some questions (open-ended) to gather information.

3. Summarize your results (using data charts and summarizing feedback) and discuss in class.

4. Based on your results, how might your approach differ next time or how will you build upon the exploration? Discuss, as a health care professional, how you might address the outcomes in your community of service.

EXERCISE 4: DEVELOPING EFFECTIVE INTERVENTIONS TO PROMOTE HEALTHY CHOICES

Identify a health behavior topic relevant to your profession. You can choose the same topic on which you did a needs assessment in Exercise 2 or 3.

1. How would you organize a patient education approach?

2. What is the problem and your goals?

3. What is the learner's state of readiness for the recommended action?

4. What do you want the learner to know, feel, or do? When? How often? Where? With whom?

5. What is the key content that must be presented to accomplish these outcomes?

6. What learning experiences will help to transmit this content and teach these skills?

7. What key steps, decisions, and activities must the learner do to follow recommendations?

8. What materials can reinforce, supplement, or draw attention to the content or process?

9. How will you know that you've been successful in teaching? How can you evaluate that the learner has learned what you were trying to teach?

EXERCISE 5: EVALUATING WRITTEN PATIENT EDUCATION MATERIALS

Select a patient education pamphlet, brochure, or consumer education website with at least 30 sentences and analyze its reading level using the Flesch Reading Ease Readability Formula (see Table 15-6) and the Gunning Fog Index (see Table 15-7). Be prepared to talk about your pamphlet in a small group.

1. What messages specifically influence the reader's perceptions of the following:

    a. The cause of the problem and his or her susceptibility to the problem?

    b. The severity of the problem?

    c. The effectiveness of his or her actions?

    d. Ease of taking those actions?

    e. Barriers to those actions?

2. How would you improve the brochure?

The exercises at the end of this chapter are also available online.
Please refer to the sticker in the front of the book and enter the access code provided.

COMMUNICATING WITH PERSONS WHO HAVE DISABILITIES

Kathleen A. Curtis, PT, PhD

"We know that equality of individual ability has never existed and never will, but we do insist that equality of opportunity still must be sought." –Franklin D. Roosevelt

OBJECTIVES

- To emphasize the power of language and the use of words that reflect our innermost values, feelings, and thoughts.

- To explore the negative results of labeling people with disabilities.

- To distinguish between descriptors often used inappropriately (eg, disability and handicap).

- To explore models of disability and how our concepts of disability influence our actions.

- To advocate for people-first language as the humane choice that makes a difference in how we view people with disabilities.

- To emphasize that individuals with disabilities are human—no more, no less—and to emphasize what an inspiration they are often serves to dehumanize them as paragons of virtue.

- To emphasize that a person with a disability experiences a problem in context, and the meaning that any problem has to an individual may differ markedly from person to person.

- To explore how we might identify and counter our ingrained prejudices and/or biases from our culture.

Recent estimates indicate that approximately 1 in 5 Americans, numbering more than 56 million people, report a disability.[1] This may be a chronic disease process, such as heart disease, sickle cell anemia, epilepsy, or cancer; a sensory disability, such as a hearing or visual impairment; a physical disability, such as an amputation, paralysis, or problem with pain or movement; a learning disability, such as dyslexia or attention deficit disorder; a cognitive disability, such as confusion or poor memory; or a disability related to mental health, such as schizophrenia or bipolar disorder. Some disabilities are not visible to the casual observer; others are obvious. Some disabilities are stable; some are progressive or intermittent in nature.

How many members of your family have a disability? Rates of disability increase with age,[2] with an estimated 49.8% of older adults aged 65 years and older reporting a disability during the 2010 United States Census.[3] Disorders of the musculoskeletal, circulatory, and respiratory systems are the 3 leading causes of disability, accounting for more than 40% of all disabilities.[2] Regardless of the type of disability, individuals with disabilities share some common experiences

Davis CM, Musolino GM. *Patient Practitioner Interaction: An Experiential Manual for Developing the Art of Health Care, Sixth Edition* (pp 285-299).
© 2016 SLACK Incorporated.

and challenges in their lives. Even in writing a chapter about persons with disabilities, I am making an assumption that all, most, or some people with disabilities have some common characteristics. That assumption is as wrong as assuming that all people of Italian descent like spaghetti or that people who are tall must be good at basketball.

My attempt to provide guidelines is intended to enlighten and stimulate you to examine your attitudes, beliefs, and the subtle and not-so-subtle limitations that you may inadvertently place on the value of a person and his or her rights, privileges, and potential contribution to the world, based on the diagnosis or problems he or she presents to you.

Labels—The Power of Words

Health care professionals (HCPs) spend many years of education and training studying the characteristics of diagnoses, pathologies, and their typical signs and symptoms. In the seemingly endless task to master the extensive classification of diagnostic categories and subcategories, sometimes we lose sight of the fact that real people have these disorders.

Language is a powerful symbol of our understanding of these complex concepts. Our knowledge, attitudes, beliefs, and values determine what we pay attention to and the thoughts we have about what we hear, read, or experience. The language we use reflects, as well as influences, our thoughts and feelings. Our thoughts and feelings determine, to a large extent, how we act. Moreover, language is not just an issue of political correctness; it influences beliefs, attitudes, expectations, and the course of events.

The Results of Labeling

The experience of persons with disabilities throughout time has been largely negative. Summarily, people with disabilities undergo experiences that stigmatize, dehumanize, disempower, and generally discount their needs. Not only do individuals with disabilities face the discrimination of physical barriers in housing, schools, business, and health care, they often face staggering obstacles in overt and covert discrimination in the job market.

In 2010, US Census figures showed that the employment rate of working-age people (aged 21 to 64 years) with disabilities in the United States was 41.1%, compared with 79.1% of those without disabilities.[1] Furthermore, for people aged 21 to 64 years with severe disabilities, the employment rate was only 27.5%.[1] With the lower likelihood of employment, 10.8% of those with severe disabilities also reported persistent poverty (> 24 months).[3] Compared with the current national unemployment rates, these figures are staggering. Recent evidence indicated that unemployment has not markedly improved in the past decade for people with disabilities. Let's look at some of the beliefs that may underlie these statistics.

What's in a Name?

Let's consider verbs first. Look at the difference between the active and passive tense. In describing an individual's relationship to an assistive device, one can draw a marked distinction in the meaning of "being confined to a wheelchair" and "using a wheelchair."

There is also an essential distinction between being and having. Can you sense the difference between being a "quadriplegic" and being a "person who has quadriplegia"? Bottom line—describing a person as the attributes of his or her disability connotes an identity solely as the disability. In addition, the emphasis on the disability draws attention to our perception of difference, which most often increases psychological and social distance. We feel less at one with those we perceive to be most different.

Many terms have been used over the years to refer to people with disabilities. We can also draw a distinction between the terms *disability* and *handicap*. A disability has been defined as a condition of the person. The term *disability* has been debated, in that by pure definition it connotes a problem with ability. Some persons with disabilities prefer to define a disability as meaning "a person may do something a little differently from a person who does not have a disability, but with equal participation and equal results,"[4] hence, differently abled.

Another term, *handicap*, has been used to connote the accrued result of multiple barriers (emotional, physical, social, environmental) imposed by society that prevent an individual who has a disability from assuming a desired role in society. For example, the characteristic that a person cannot walk quickly from place to place is a feature of a disability. The employer who hires a less qualified applicant who walks more quickly, the landlord who rents to another tenant, the university classroom layout that requires a half-mile walk in the 10-minute break between classes—all help to create the handicaps associated with disability.

TABLE 16-1
MODELS OF DISABILITY

MODEL	CHARACTERISTICS OF MODEL	WHAT HEALTH CARE PROVIDERS SHOULD KNOW
Medical	This model denotes a medical etiology that emphasizes the cause of disability as a medical condition or disorder. Disabilities are treated as diagnostic categories. Individuals with disabilities assume a sick role.	Many providers assume that the cause of a disability is a medical condition. Instead, consider how the individual's social or emotional life affects his or her physical health. How do our social expectations or the environment influence the individual's experience of disability? The medical model also minimizes consideration of the social sources of disability, such as stigma, prejudice, and public policy.
Economic	The economic model relates to the individual's inability or limited ability to work. Medical evaluations of disability are used to predict the likelihood of employment. Links functional physical capacity with employment.	Research indicates that employment of persons with disabilities is influenced largely by social and economic trends, not by the nature of their disabilities or their functional capacities.
Functional-limitation paradigm	Pathology and impairment refer to an individual's medical condition and the related limitations. In contrast, the term disability refers to social function. It is the interaction of an individual's physical or mental limitations with environmental and social factors that determines disability.	Individuals with physical or mental impairments and functional limitations do not necessarily experience disability in the same ways. Individuals may have a disability in one environment and not in another.
Sociopolitical	At the heart of the disability rights movement is the common understanding that disability is an acceptable form of human variation. In this context, disability is viewed as a policy and civil rights issue, with individuals with disabilities considered an oppressed minority, facing daily prejudice and discrimination. Individuals with disabilities experience architectural, sensory, attitudinal, cognitive, and economic barriers, limiting their full participation in society.	Many health providers see their role as helping individuals with disabilities adapt to the demands of society. Instead, consider the role of policy to alter the barriers of the social, cultural, economic, and political environments in which persons with disabilities live. Facilitate environmental, societal, and political adjustment to accommodate the needs of individuals with disabilities and ensure their full participation.
Adapted from Hubbard S. Disability studies and health care curriculum: the great divide. *J Allied Health*. 2004;33(3):184-188.		

Various models have been proposed over the years to define the concepts surrounding disability (Table 16-1).[5] Notice the distinction between problems at the body organ level, the economic level, the functional activity or performance level, and the level of the cultural or social environment. Health care professionals often focus on factors at the body organ and functional level; the person with a disability experiences most life problems because of factors in the economic, cultural, political, and social environment.

The International Classification of Functioning, Disability and Health (ICF)[6] is perhaps the most prevalent framework used today. It incorporates health conditions and their effects as well as environmental factors. The ICF interactive model focuses on the concept of participation (involvement in a life situation), rather than the disorder or disease, impairment, or deviation.

Pay attention to whether your focus is on the disease or impairment or the life experience of the individual with a disability. Be sure to acknowledge individual differences. Few people with similar impairments experience the same degree of disability, activity limitation, or participation restriction. Similarly, the cultural, social, political, and physical

TABLE 16-2	
EXAMPLES OF EMPOWERING LANGUAGE	
USE THIS	**INSTEAD OF THIS**
Persons who have disabilities	Disabled people
Child without a disability	Normal child (in comparing with a child with a disability)
People who have visual impairments	The blind
Uses a wheelchair, crutches, or braces	Confined to a wheelchair, has to use crutches, unable to walk without braces
Individual or person who has (name of the problem)	Language such as: ◦ Victim of… ◦ Stricken ◦ Poor ◦ Suffers from… ◦ Crippled ◦ Unfortunate ◦ Afflicted with… Diseased ◦ Sick ◦ Burdened with… ◦ Disabled ◦ Tragic
Individual who has (describe what the person has accomplished)	◦ Courageous ◦ Heroic ◦ Inspirational ◦ Special
Use people-first language in verbal and written communication, professional journals, laws, and statutes (eg, a person who has epilepsy)	Referring to the disability as an adjective (the blind man), a noun (paraplegics, epileptics), or a passive form (help the handicapped)
Ms., Mrs., Mr., Dr., or preferred name—ask	First names or terms of endearment such as "Dear" or "Honey" or "Babe" in nonromantic or professional relationships (see Chapter 8)

Adapted from United Cerebral Palsy. *Watch Your Language Fact Sheet.* New York, NY: United Cerebral Palsy Association; 1991.

environment in which a person with a disability lives may vary widely and strongly influences the individual's activities and participation in society.

PEOPLE-FIRST LANGUAGE

An established standard of good writing, *people-first language*, requires that the writer identifies the person—the man, woman, child, professor, student, client, physician, receptionist, mother—and then refers to the attribute of having a disability (if it is applicable at all to the discussion; eg, the man with epilepsy) rather than using the disability as either an adjective (eg, the epileptic driver) or a noun (eg, an epileptic). This distinction, although subtle, makes a profound difference in our focus and perceptions. It empowers and provides information rather than stigmatizing and labeling (Table 16-2).[7] Language is one conscious choice we can make that makes a big difference. Let's look at some other typical beliefs about people with disabilities.

You Poor Thing!

Persons who have disabilities are often characterized by the uncontrollable nature of their problem, which leads the potential helper to feel pity for the person. The connotation of the "crippled child," for example, not only breaks some of the people-first language rules but immediately connotes a poster-child image intended to elicit donations to a well-meaning charitable organization. Social scientists and fundraisers have known for years that our perception that another person has a problem that is out of his or her control stimulates our desires to help. However, pity turns out to be an emotion that tends to marginalize people with disabilities and interferes with our ability to see them as people who share our aspirations and disappointments, with equal rights and responsibilities to take social and political action.

Health care professionals often choose to enter these professions out of their desire to help individuals who have experienced misfortune, disabilities, family problems, poverty, and similar challenges in their lives. Not all health care professionals agree on the nature of or the kind of help that will effect change in the lives of those they help, however (discussed in Chapter 6). Even health care professionals want to help most of those clients whom they see as least capable, least responsible, and least in control of their lives (see Chapters 8 and 15).[8,9]

None of these characteristics are consistent with the image of a healthy, competent, empowered, responsible member of society. As we learned in Chapter 2, health care professionals often want to "fix it" for their clients, an insurmountable and undesirable task given the complexity of our educational, social, and health care systems and the more lofty goal of empowering clients or patients to fix it for themselves. In contrast, when health care professionals are faced with persistent, unrelenting demands for medication, better care, benefits, equal access to opportunity, or legal rights, they often feel powerless or threatened and may be less likely to help.

When health care professionals feel angry at their clients, it actually may be an indication that they consider their clients to be competent and in control, albeit demanding or intrusive. Unfortunately, it may also cause withdrawal of needed services or less energy spent in moving the client in a positive direction that could further help or empower the client.[8] This is an interesting dilemma and one that is up to health care professionals, not patients and clients, to resolve for the good of the patients or clients.

Our professional help should be offered in accordance with our perceptions of how likely the client's situation is to benefit from that help. Ask yourself the question, "What type of help would be of greatest benefit and in what ways is this help likely to effect change?" Or, "How will my action change the individual's ability to participate in society?" Ask the client, "What would be most helpful? What are your goals?" and then listen. Recognize that some of those goals relate to the ways you have been educated to help and some do not. Be clear about what falls within your realm of professional expertise and what must be left for others or the individual to resolve (see Chapters 5, 10, and 14).

You Are Such an Inspiration!

At the awards banquet of a national track and field championship for athletes with disabilities, a famous sports figure rises to the podium to give an after-dinner speech. The speech follows: "You people … are such an inspiration. The courage I have seen is remarkable. You have faced the challenges and overcome them. You are all heroes today. You are all winners."

Although well intended, the speaker has distanced the group by immediately emphasizing the distinction of "you people." Furthermore, instead of complimenting the group on their athletic accomplishments, world record performances, or victories, the speaker has essentially created different standards for recognition of achievement in this group of athletes with disabilities. In reality, not everyone is a winner. Athletic competition is serious business; it requires long training hours, dedication, commitment, hard work, perseverance, and skill.

Of course, there may be a role for courage and inspiration somewhere in the mix, but the point is that athletes who have disabilities share the common experience of commitment, training, successes, and failures with all athletes. Individuals who have disabilities are human—no more, no less. A person with a disability is not a paragon of virtue, not an exceptional human being, not a person who has overcome adversity just because he or she happens to have a disability.

When we recognize persons who have disabilities for what they have accomplished, for their achievements and victories, using standards that are used for everyone, then we empower them, educate society, and change attitudes about disability. When we overdo it on praise for minimal achievements, it infers low ability of the achiever. When you are not held to the same standards that everyone else is, it is usually because the evaluator does not feel that you have the capacity to achieve those standards. This is not a good message to give and certainly a worse one to receive. Instead, give positive messages that emphasize what was accomplished and what standards you are using to judge this accomplishment. Indicate where the person stands in progress toward a goal and the endpoints to be reached if you are using a different standard to evaluate success.

What Happened to You? Tell Me About Your Disability

In Chapter 13, you learned how to interview patients and clients as part of your professional training. You learned how to ask specific questions that are intended to focus your professional attention on a problem at hand. Your questions assume a clinical orientation, describing the signs, symptoms, onset, and severity of problems. Although helpful for providing information for a specific diagnosis or planning a treatment, these questions might ignore the one essential factor that will determine the importance of all the information you seek—context.

A person who has a disability experiences a problem in context: in a family; on a wheelchair basketball team; as a student in school; as a colleague, supervisor, or supervisee in a work setting. The client may be with or without social support, financial resources, adequate health care, or housing. Focusing on the clinical aspects of the disability alone in the interview negates the importance of the context but, more important, may assume that the same common symptoms or problems have the same meaning to all people who have a similar disability.

The meaning that any problem has to an individual may differ markedly. One individual may be mortified by unexpected urinary incontinence; another may consider it a minor inconvenience and have strategies in place to deal with the problem quickly and without great emotional cost. Questions such as "How have you handled similar situations in the past?" or "How important is this to you to take care of?" associate competence and ability with the current issues. Never make assumptions about what a problem means to your patient or client. Ask him or her. Treat the individual as a "culture of one" (see Chapter 12). Avoid reference to disability groups to which some individuals belong, such as "Many of my clients who have quadriplegia have skin problems; is this a problem for you?" Instead, ask open-ended, empowering questions, such as "What strategies do you use to prevent pressure sores?" Use active listening instead of a relentless list of questions, and, most important, talk with the person who has the disability. Listen carefully to his or her story. You've never heard it before, and as you listen, the uniqueness of this particular person and his or her meanings will emerge to assist you in your role as an effective helper.

THE EFFECT OF BIASES AND STIGMATIZATION

Cultural beliefs—the way our lenses are set—including our values, practices, conceptions of illness, and acceptable behavior, greatly influence our perceptions of disability. The context in which we live determines the meaning of a disability. For example, as we realized in Chapter 14, Western practitioners tend to conceptualize medicine in a reductionistic and despiritualized fashion, searching for cause-and-effect relationships that can be explained and controlled.[10] In contrast, Eastern philosophies that may be based in concepts of a life force, such as energy or chi, defy Western scientific explanation yet may be just as valid to a practitioner of Eastern medicine. Similarly, an individual's illness or disability is understood and given significance based on the culture in which it occurs. It is important to understand that we take on social roles to meet the behavioral expectations of influential others. Consider the behavior-shaping influence of the environment on prisoners, institutionalized children, and people who have lived in situations of physical and emotional abuse.

People who do not have disabilities often hold attitudes and perceptions that separate them from individuals who have disabilities. For example, a study of more than 200 Spanish university students showed that they perceived individuals with hearing and visual impairments to be less communicative, less intelligent, less independent, slower, and less active than individuals with no sensory impairment.[9] In comparison of the descriptors of individuals with hearing impairments to those with visual impairments, these students perceived that those with hearing impairments were more reserved, less calm, less sociable, less attentive, less prudent, less sure, and less thoughtful than those with visual impairments.[10] Some researchers in other areas of the world have found that women tend to hold more positive perceptions of individuals with disabilities than men.[11,12] Interestingly, some studies of the perceptions of individuals who work in medical settings fail to show that their attitudes are more positive toward individuals with disabilities than those of the general public.[13,14]

In other words, those who often work with people with disabilities may hold the same prejudices as do laypeople. So, how do we influence attitudes and eliminate negative stereotypes? Some authors argue that even sensitivity training, intentionally provided in professional training programs, may overly emphasize negative perceptions of the difficulties encountered by persons with physical disabilities, rather than providing trainees with a positive perspective of ability.[14]

For example, the experiences of students using a wheelchair as a first-time simulation experience may provide some awareness of the physical barriers encountered but do not seem to reflect the overall generally positive quality of life experienced by persons who use wheelchairs. The apparent paradox of creating negative attitudes by focusing on the salient differences in the experience of persons with disabilities creates a dilemma for the education of human service professionals, such as teachers, health care professionals, and social workers, people who we want to be sensitive to the needs of and to recognize and foster the abilities of their students, patients, and clients.[15]

How Can We Counter Our Biases?

Recognition of sameness is a key factor. Social psychology tells us that rather than focusing on our differences, it is probably more productive to emphasize our similarities. What do we have in common with a person who has a disability? His or her age, educational objective, vocational choice, parenthood, daughterhood, brotherhood, status as a student, automobile owner, bus user, or technology user is often a more unifying characteristic than the apparent (or often unapparent) nature of his or her disability.

When health care professionals are providing services, they are often forced to focus on the disability or its effects. Don't forget that this person, with desires, aspirations, a family, a job, a living situation, is not defined by the nature of his or her disability. Be aware of the many limiting ideas and concepts that prevail in our culture, but also be aware that your cultural beliefs may not be shared by the patient. Today, the same is occurring with rapidly changing and evolving rehabilitation technology, such as with 3-dimensional printing of functional prosthetic upper extremities. One cannot be resistant to consider new technologies, while learning and incorporating lessons from the past.

Don't Be Afraid to Shift Your Paradigm!

Prior to the late 1970s, wheelchairs were all the same—chrome and exceptionally heavy, with black or blue upholstery. Due to the influence of young wheelchair users, wheelchair technology totally changed in the late 1970s, and innovative, lightweight wheelchair designs and colors became available as expressions of one's personality and activity, rather than the stigma of inability and confinement. Now the wheelchair market has become competitive; even the wheelchair manufacturers who once produced the heavy, chrome wheelchairs are happy to join in more creative ways of looking at the needs of wheelchair users in order to stay afloat in the market. Even though the old school eventually shifted, they lost a significant portion of the lightweight wheelchair market. Moral of the story: listen, believe, and don't allow yourself to be limited by stereotypes and expectations.

LEGISLATIVE AND ECONOMIC ASPECTS OF DISABILITY

In the past 30 years, we have seen many legislative acts that affect the quality of life of individuals with disabilities. Table 16-3 lists a few examples of the major pieces of legislation that provide the basis for the rights of persons with disabilities in the United States. Unfortunately, although there is legal protection in many situations, we still have a long way to go in changing public beliefs that it serves all people to make entrances to buildings barrier free, to actively foster opportunities for employment for individuals with disabilities, and to provide diagnostic and treatment services to the millions of children and adults with disabilities who live in poverty.

Fostering economic opportunity is not only the right thing to do, it is also good business. On a personal note, for example, I was struck by the experience I had at the 1996 Atlanta Paralympic Games, which followed the Olympic Games by several weeks. At the beginning of the Paralympic Games, there were many leftover Olympic souvenirs on sale and many street vendors who were profiting from the influx of thousands of competitors with disabilities and their coaches and sport organizers, friends, families, and spectators from more than 100 countries. Paradoxically, the Olympic pavilion, which housed many large companies and exhibitions, decided to close and tear down their exhibits and stores while the Paralympic Games opened, creating an eyesore and a racket. Not only did a lost opportunity to sell millions of dollars of merchandise occur; they also missed the chance to influence the international market and reap the benefits of the economic power of thousands of individuals with disabilities from all over the world.

STILL A LONG WAY TO GO

Although legislation (see Table 16-3) has protected some of the rights of individuals with disabilities, we still live largely in a world that does not yet meet the needs of those with disabilities, nor recognize their potential power as a group. Adequate income, education, health insurance, housing, and employment still largely remain challenges for members of our community who have disabilities (Table 16-4).[16]

AGING WITH A DISABILITY

The life expectancy for persons with disabilities has increased markedly, resulting in many people with severe disabilities reaching middle-age and older age groups. Age-related changes, when combined with preexisting impairments, often create secondary disabilities, which, if left unrecognized or untreated, may impair quality of life and independence.[17] Health care professionals must be aware of screening for recent loss of function in individuals with long-term disabilities. Routinely asking questions such as the following may identify a secondary problem before it becomes a serious health threat. Have you noticed the following:

- Any increased fatigue or pain during daily activities?
- A change in your posture?
- Difficulty sleeping?
- Any change in your weight?
- Any change in your sensation?
- Any shift in your abilities to perform the tasks, hobbies and recreational activities you enjoy?

Table 16-3

KEY LEGISLATIVE ACTIVITY AND DISABILITY ISSUES

LEGISLATION AFFECTING PERSONS WITH DISABILITIES

- **Rehabilitation Act of 1973:** Mandated no discrimination by federally funded agencies against workers and students with disabilities and affirmative action requirements for federally funded employers.

- **Americans With Disabilities Act of 1990:** Mandated reasonable accommodations to ensure the integration of people with disabilities in the private sector, including employment, telecommunications, transportation and public services, and accommodations.

- **The Workforce Investment Act of 1998:** Focuses on training, educating, and employing skilled workers to meet the needs of businesses. One-stop career centers (workforce centers) serve to meet job seekers' needs by providing an integrated service model to offer many work-related programs.

- **2001 New Freedom Initiative 2001:** Part of a nationwide effort to remove barriers and facilitate full participation in community life for people with disabilities. The initiative increased access to assistive and universally designed technologies, expanded educational and employment opportunities, and promoted increased access into daily community life. The act supported the integration of people with disabilities into the workforce through implementation of the Ticket to Work and Work Incentives Improvement Act of 1999 (TWWIIA); and the New Freedom Commission on Mental Health.

- **Americans With Disabilities Act Amendments Act of 2008:** Emphasizes the definition of disability should be recast to make it easier for an individual seeking protection under the ADA to establish disability. The ADA defines disability as an impairment that substantially limits one or more major life activities, a record of such an impairment, or being regarded as having such an impairment.

- **2013 Jimmo v. Sebelius:** A settlement to a class action lawsuit that determined that Medicare coverage for skilled services, to maintain an individual's condition, cannot be improperly denied or discontinued regardless of the individual's potential to improve.

- **2014 IMPACT Act:** Provides for establishing standardized postacute care assessment data, which can be shared by providers for quality, payment, and discharge planning to facilitate coordinated care and improved Medicare beneficiary outcomes.

LEGISLATION AFFECTING CHILDREN WITH DISABILITIES

- **PL 94-142 (Education for All Handicapped Children Act of 1975):** Mandated a free and appropriate education and the least restrictive environment (ie, mainstreaming) Annual Individual Educational Plans are developed for all children with disabilities.

- **PL 101-476:** Revised provisions of PL 94-142 to include children with autism and brain injury and included training and technology provisions for education of children with disabilities

- **Individuals With Disabilities Education Act of 1997:** Gave parents and school districts more autonomy in determining children's needs for special education services through a mediation process, further defines services available to infants and toddlers, and provides disciplinary sanctions for students who engage in criminal misconduct, unrelated to disability.

- **Individuals With Disabilities Education Improvement Act of 2004:** Four parts: (A) administrative aspects of the Office of Special Education Programs; (B) educational requirements of the Act; (C) guidelines for children with special needs who are less than 2 years of age, includes Early Intervention Programs; and (D) creates national grants and resources for implementation and established Child Find to identify those with disabilities in school districts and requirements for Individual Education Plans (IEPs) with annual review, with inclusion of needed treatments (including therapies) and assistive technology.

(continued)

TABLE 16-3 (CONTINUED)
KEY LEGISLATIVE ACTIVITY AND DISABILITY ISSUES

LEGISLATION AFFECTING OLDER ADULTS

- **PL 101-234 (The Omnibus Reconciliation Act [OBRA] of 1987):** A major piece of legislation that set standards for nursing home personnel; the rights of nursing home residents and set standards for home health agencies.
- **1990 Nursing Home Reform Amendments of OBRA:** Nursing homes required by law to focus on each resident's highest potential for physical, mental, and psychosocial well-being by assessing these abilities and developing individualized care plans. These care plans must be reassessed for any change in function at least quarterly. This created numerous employment opportunities for therapists in the nursing home setting.
- **Health Care and Education Affordability Reconciliation Act of 2010:** This legislation reformed Medicare payment policy so it more equitably reimburses those who care for older adults. In addition, it will support mechanisms to develop new payment and promising models of care, including comprehensive geriatric assessments and care coordination for older patients with multiple chronic illnesses and cognitive impairment. It supports the expansion of geriatrics training programs, including those designed to prepare specialists to meet the needs of the most complex, frailest older patients, as well education for the direct-care workers and family caregivers who provide day-to-day care for millions of America's seniors.

SECONDARY CONDITIONS

Although disability and health are 2 distinct phenomena, people with disabilities are 30% more likely to report a poor health status than are people without disabilities.[18-20] People with disabilities are at increased risk for secondary problems, impairments, and limitations to participation from a host of medical, social, emotional, family, or community issues.

A study of more than 1000 persons with disabilities showed that almost 9 in 10 persons with disabilities self-reported at least 1 secondary condition, with an average of 4.1 conditions. In addition to disability-specific medical issues, such as muscle spasms, bowel and bladder problems, falls and injuries, respiratory infections, asthma, and skin problems; the most common conditions reported by adults with disabilities included chronic pain, sleep disorders, fatigue, weight problems, depression and anxiety, difficulty getting out, feelings of isolation, and problems with making/seeing friends.[21] In addition to higher rates of these conditions, evidence supports that individuals with disabilities, in comparison with individuals without disabilities, are likely to have lower levels of education[22]; lower rates of employment[23]; higher rates of poverty[24]; problems finding safe, accessible, and affordable housing[24-26]; higher likelihood of being a victim of crime of domestic violence[27]; higher rates of being overweight and obese[22]; and higher rates of tobacco use.[22]

Individuals with disabilities experience high rates of disadvantages relating to the personal, social, economic, and environmental determinants of health that have been recognized by the Secretary's Advisory Committee on National Health Promotion and Disease Prevention Objectives for 2020.[28] In 10-year cycles, the US Department of Health and Human Services uses available evidence and experience to establish goals, action steps, and indicators for the nation's health. Using available evidence of the issues faced by persons with disabilities, Healthy People 2020 addresses targets for action to achieve better health by the year 2020,[28] including risks to health and wellness, emerging public health priorities, and critical issues related to preparedness and prevention. Clearly, the serious issues reported by persons with disabilities diminish their sense of health and well-being. Strategies to identify, address, and ameliorate these commonly experienced conditions are key to reducing disability-related health disparities.

WOMEN WITH DISABILITIES

More than 20 million women with disabilities experience unique challenges. Women with disabilities have been documented to have limited access to medical services, education, and vocational opportunities. These issues influence their health because they often lack information, financial resources, and health services to meet their unique needs. Despite the needs, there are many barriers that reduce the quality and accessibility of services for women with disabilities. Physical and communication barriers often limit access to health care settings, despite the requirements of the Americans with Disabilities Act. In many cases, women also lack adequate transportation and support services to get to health care appointments. Statistical differences exist with men with disabilities and women without disabilities in that they have

TABLE 16-4

NEEDS AND ISSUES FOR INDIVIDUALS WITH DISABILITIES	
MAJOR PROBLEMS IDENTIFIED BY AMERICANS WITH DISABILITIES[a]	**DETAILS**
Affordability and availability of assistive devices	Wheelchairs, prosthetic and orthotic devices, walking aids, home equipment are all very expensive to purchase and/or repair and are largely unavailable to rent. Because these devices mean independence to many persons with disabilities, lack of access to limits functional potential.
Accessibility of commercial services, facilities, restrooms, parking	Private businesses, restrooms, and parking are largely inaccessible in many areas. This may include the lack of curb cuts, snow removal, gravel, sand, and rough terrain.
Legal rights to public housing, transportation, social support agencies, programs, and systems	Despite legal rights to these services, lack of information, prejudices, institutional barriers, and shortages prevent many individuals with disabilities from accessing these services.
Employment accommodations, discrimination	Although the ADA has improved employer understanding of their responsibilities to provide reasonable accommodations, it does not keep the employer from discriminating against potential employees with disabilities in the hiring process.
Health care insurance and services inadequate for needs	Many HCPs refuse to treat Medicaid or Medicare patients. Respite care and attendant care are largely unfunded. Many individuals cannot buy health care insurance because of their disability or affordability.
Auto, life, and liability insurance costs	Insurance companies often discriminate based on disability, offering more expensive premiums or limit for preexisting.
Stigmatization, asexualization, grouping	The media portray individuals with disabilities in a negative, asexual, and unrealistic way. People with disabilities are often not portrayed as individuals who exist beyond the definition of their disability.
Fixed incomes, poverty	Many individuals with disabilities (mental and physical) exist on supplemental security income and live below the poverty level.

[a]Summarized from the results of a survey of 13,000 individuals with disabilities in 10 states.

Adapted from Suarez De Balcazar YS, Bradford B, Fawcett S. Common concerns of disabled Americans: issues and options. *Soc Policy.* 1988;19(2):29-35.

increased social isolation and less access to higher education. In comparison with men with disabilities, they also have higher unemployment rates, and even those employed earn lower incomes.[29]

A women's perspective on disability can be appreciated, in the words of Nancy Mairs, who wrote about body image and disability perceptions[30]:

The "her" I never was and am not now and never will become. In order to function as the body I am, I must forswear her, seductive though she may be, or make myself mad with self-loathing. In this project, I get virtually no cultural encouragement. Illness and deformity, instead of being thought of as human variants, the consequence of cosmic bad luck, have invariably been portrayed as deviations from the fully human condition, brought on by personal failing or by divine judgment.

Women with disabilities often have less access to breast health services than any other group of women. Women with disabilities are at a higher risk for delayed diagnosis of breast and cervical cancer, primarily for reasons of environmental, attitudinal, and information barriers, including reported difficulties receiving women's health services (eg, mammograms and Pap smears, reproductive health/birth control, sexually transmitted diseases screening, and services to address specific issues of aging). In addition to reproductive health needs, women with disabilities frequently experience a lack of privacy and autonomy while receiving health care, high rates of violence and abuse, and unmet mental health needs.[31]

Strategies that eliminate barriers to care include providing education to women and their health care professionals and identifying solutions, such as appropriate communication techniques, accessible equipment, and available services. Health care professionals can make a difference treating women with disabilities as women first, with health needs, perspectives, and issues that they share with all women.

What Can You Do to Make a Difference?

The chapter exercises are designed to help you raise your awareness to recognize the perceptions and biases you hold about individuals with disabilities. You are morally obliged to make an active effort to recognize the abilities of all people. Be aware of the influence of your language. Set a personal goal to empower individuals with whom you have contact and support access to health care, educational opportunities, employment, housing, and transportation. Do not be satisfied with being only an 8-hour-a-day advocate for people with disabilities!

References

1. Brault MW. *Americans with Disabilities: 2010. Current Population Reports.* July 2012. US Census Bureau. www.census.gov/prod/2012pubs/p70-131.pdf. Accessed June 15, 2015.
2. Kraus L, Stoddard S, Gilmartin D. *Chartbook on Disability in the United States, 1996. An InfoUse Report.* Washington, DC: US National Institute on Disability and Rehabilitation Research. www.infouse.com/disabilitydata/disability/index.php. Accessed June 15, 2015.
3. United States Census Bureau. Nearly 1 in 5 people have a disability in the US, Census Bureau reports. *Newsroom Archive.* July 25, 2012. www.census.gov/newsroom/releases/archives/miscellaneous/cb12-134.html. Accessed May 1, 2015.
4. Kailes J. Watch your language, please! *J Rehabil.* 1985;51:68-69.
5. Hubbard S. Disability studies and health care curriculum: the great divide. *J Allied Health.* 2004;33(3):184-188.
6. Centers for Disease Control and Prevention. The ICF: an overview. www.cdc.gov/nchs/data/icd/ICFoverview_FINALforWHO 10Sept.pdf. Accessed May 1, 2015.
7. United Cerebral Palsy Association. *Watch Your Language Fact Sheet.* New York, NY: United Cerebral Palsy Association; 1991.
8. Curtis KA. Role satisfaction of the physical therapist in the treatment of the spinal cord-injured person. *Phys Ther.* 1985;65(2):197-200.
9. Kahan M. *Physician Assistants' Models of Helping Behavior and Their Relationship to Perceived Responsibility, Attributions and Patient Education* [dissertation]. Los Angeles, CA: University of California; 1988.
10. Banja JD. Ethics, values, and world culture: the impact on rehabilitation. *Disabil Rehabil.* 1996;18(6):279-284.
11. Cambra C. A comparative study of personality descriptors attributed to the deaf, the blind, and individuals with no sensory disability. *Am Ann Deaf.* 1996;141(1):24-28.
12. Gannon PM, MacLean D. Attitudes toward disability and beliefs regarding support for a university student with quadriplegia. *Int J Rehabil Res.* 1996;19(2):163-169.
13. Lys K, Pernice R. Perceptions of positive attitudes toward people with spinal cord injury. *Int J Rehabil Res.* 1995;18(1):35-43.
14. Eberhardt K, Mayberry W. Factors influencing entry-level occupational therapists' attitudes toward persons with disabilities. *Am J Occup Ther.* 1995;49(7):629-636.
15. Grayson E, Marini I. Simulated disability exercises and their impact on attitudes toward persons with disabilities. *Int J Rehabil Res.* 1996;19(2):123-131.
16. Suarez De Balcazar Y, Bradford B, Fawcett SB. Common concerns of disabled Americans: issues and options. *Soc Policy.* 1988;19(2):29-35.
17. Klingbeil H, Baer HR, Wilson PE. Aging with a disability. *Arch Phys Med Rehabil.* 2004;85(7 suppl 3):S68-S73.
18. US Department of Health and Human Services. *The Surgeon General's Call to Action to Improve the Health and Wellness of Persons with Disabilities.* Washington, DC: US Department of Health and Human Services, Office of the Surgeon General; 2005.
19. Centers for Disease Control and Prevention. Racial/ethnic disparities in self-rated health status among adults with and without disabilities—United States, 2004-2006. *MMWR Morb Mortal Wkly Rep.* 2008;57(39):1069-1073.
20. Havercamp SM, Scandlin D, Roth M. Health disparities among adults with developmental disabilities, adults with other disabilities, and adults not reporting disability in North Carolina. *Public Health Rep.* 2004;119(4):418-426.
21. Kinne S. Distribution of secondary medical problems, impairments, and participation limitations among adults with disabilities and their relationship to health and other outcomes. *Disabil Health J.* 2008;1(1):42-50.
22. Iezzoni LI, O'Day BL. *More Than Ramps: A Guide to Improving Health Care Quality and Access for People With Disabilities.* New York, NY: Oxford University Press; 2006.

23. US Department of Labor, Bureau of Labor Statistics. Labor force statistics from the current population survey. www.bls.gov/cps/cpsdisability.htm. Accessed March 13, 2015.

24. Iezzoni LI. *When Walking Fails: Mobility Problems of Adults with Chronic Conditions.* Berkeley, CA: University of California Press; 2003.

25. Froehlich-Grobe K, Regan G, Reese-Smith JY, Heinrich KM, Lee RE. Physical access in urban public housing facilities. *Disabil Health J.* 2008;1(1):25-29.

26. Centers for Disease Control and Prevention. Environmental barriers to health care among persons with disabilities—Los Angeles County, California, 2002-2003. *MMWR Morb Mortal Wkly Rep.* 2006;55(48):1300-1303.

27. Brownridge DA. Partner violence against women with disabilities: prevalence, risk, and explanations. *Violence Against Women.* 2006;12(9):805-822.

28. Office of Disease Prevention and Health Promotion. Disability and health. Healthy People 2020 website. www.healthypeople.gov/2020/topics-objectives/topic/disability-and-health. Accessed May 1, 2015.

29. Jans L, Stoddard S. *Chartbook on Women and Disability.* Washington, DC: US National Institute on Disability and Rehabilitation Research; 1999. www.infouse.com/disabilitydata/womendisability. Accessed June 15, 2015.

30. Mairs N. *Waist-High in the World: A Life Among the Nondisabled.* Boston, MA: Beacon Press; 1997.

31. Nosek MA, Howland CA, Rintala DH, Young ME, Chanpong GF. *National Study of Women with Physical Disabilities 1992-1996: Final Report.* Houston, TX: Center for Research on Women with Disabilities; 1997.

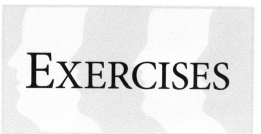

EXERCISES

EXERCISE 1: EXAMINING YOUR BELIEFS ABOUT DISABILITY

What beliefs do you have about the following conditions? What beliefs do you think most people have?

CONDITION	YOUR BELIEFS	OTHERS' BELIEFS
Epilepsy		
Cerebral palsy		
Quadriplegia		
Cataracts		
Cancer		
Brain injury		
HIV positive		
Congenital heart disease		

EXERCISE 2: USING PEOPLE-FIRST LANGUAGE

Replace each of the following phrases with people-first language:

1. He is a quadriplegic:

2. It is a fundraiser for the mentally retarded:

3. The blind man came in last:

4. The developmentally disabled children:

5. Congenitally dislocated baby hips:

6. Confined to a wheelchair:

7. Stroke victim:

8. Stricken with Lou Gehrig's disease (amyotrophic lateral sclerosis):

9. Cystic fibrosis kids:

EXERCISE 3: FILMS PORTRAYING PERSONS WITH DISABILITIES

Analyze the experience and portrayal of individuals with disabilities in one or more of the following films or documentaries:

- *A Beautiful Mind* (2001, Imagine Entertainment)
- *A Day in the Life of Bonnie Consolo* (1975, Independent Film, now on YouTube)
- *A Mile in His Shoes* (2011, MGN Productions)
- Attitude is Altitude.com/Life Without Limbs, Nick Vujicic (YouTube)
- *Children of a Lesser God* (1986, Paramount)
- *Do You Remember Love* (1985, CBS)
- *Home of the Brave* (2006, MGM)
- *I Am Sam* (2001, New Line Cinema)
- *King Gimp* (1999, HBO)
- *Love and Other Drugs* (2010, 20th Century Fox)
- *My Left Foot* (1989, Miramax)
- *Passion Fish* (1992, Miramax)
- *Rainman* (1988, United Artists)
- *Regarding Henry* (1991, Paramount)
- *Soul Surfer* (2011, Affirm Films)
- *Still Alice* (2014, Sony Pictures Classics)
- *The Diving Bell and the Butterfly* (*Le Scaphandre et le Papillon*) (2007, France, Miramax)
- *The Other Side of the Mountain* (Parts 1 and 2) (1975 and 1978, Universal)
- *The Other Sister* (1999, Touchstone)
- *The Normal Heart* (2014, HBO Films)
- *The Sea Inside* (*Mar Adentro*) (2004, Spain/France/Italy, Warner Home Video)
- *The Terry Fox Story* (1983, HBO)
- *The Wedding Gift* (1994, Miramax)
- *Whose Life Is It Anyway?* (1981, Warner Bros.)

The exercises at the end of this chapter are also available online.
Please refer to the sticker in the front of the book and enter the access code provided.

17

SEXUALITY AND DISABILITY

EFFECTIVE COMMUNICATION

Sherrill H. Hayes, PT, PhD

"Myths and misunderstandings often arise around groups of people who display three characteristics: (1) They are a minority; (2) members are clearly identifiable; and (3) society harbors fears or aversion toward them. Many physically disabled people meet all three criteria and thus become objects of social bias."[1] –T. M. Cole

OBJECTIVES

- To define sex, sex acts, and sexuality.
- To emphasize the importance of understanding one's own sexuality, values, and beliefs in order to communicate effectively in the clinical setting.
- To consider the negative effects of institutionalization on sexuality.
- To understand myths and misconceptions regarding sexuality and disability and how these may affect the patient's and practitioner's viewpoints and comfort levels.
- To introduce experiences of the patient that may compromise his or her image of self as asexual being and precipitate feelings of shame.
- To discuss the importance of self-esteem, self-image, and self-actualization with respect to rehabilitation.
- To review normal sexual arousal cycles for the male and female and the impact of certain disabilities on sexual functioning.
- To discuss the role of the rehabilitation professional with respect to sexuality and the disabled.
- To understand and utilize the principles of the permission, limited information, specific suggestions, and intensive therapy (PLISSIT) model as a structure for identifying one's knowledge base, comfort, and skills in sexuality and disability.
- To stress the importance of effective communication and therapeutic presence through case studies designed to prevent shaming experiences, maintain privacy, and promote the sexual integrity of the patient.

Davis CM, Musolino GM. *Patient Practitioner Interaction: An Experiential Manual for Developing the Art of Health Care, Sixth Edition* (pp 301-321).
© 2016 SLACK Incorporated.

PRECHECK EXERCISE

As a way of introducing you to this content, take a moment now and turn to Exercise 1 at the end of this chapter and complete the true-false precheck. Please first read the chapter before you check your answers. Then, review Exercise 1 once more as a postcheck. Check your answers as a last step in your learning process.

INTRODUCTION

Over the past 70 years, there has been a virtual revolution in Western society pertaining to sexuality and roles of males and females. The "typical" family core of the male working outside the home and the female staying home with the children has changed to the more common scenario of both parents working outside the home. In addition, we have seen a large increase in single-parent families; same-sex relationships, civil unions, and marriages; and same-sex parents raising children. Sexual behaviors have also changed, from relatively little premarital sex to the "free love" of the 1960s and 1970s to the current trend of more of a series of longer-lasting relationships or "serial monogamy," which is largely due to the HIV/AIDS epidemic beginning in the 1980s. These relationships may be heterosexual, homosexual, or bisexual in nature. Concomitantly, there has also been an increase in the number of people with disabilities due to improved medical interventions and technologies, providing for increased survival for injured persons or persons with chronic disabling conditions.

In the past 20 years, more research relating to sexual function and sexual counseling has ensued, albeit not the large volume as in the 1970s and 1980s. Sexual function and counseling research is predominantly published in medical journals, especially relating to cancer, spinal cord injury (SCI), Parkinson's disease, multiple sclerosis, and psychological issues and cognitive disabilities. In 2000, *Physical Therapy Journal* devoted a special series to SCI examining issues related to sexuality and disability, including challenges due to musculoskeletal, neuromuscular, and cardiopulmonary issues; seating and mobility; and chronic pain (see the Suggested Readings at the end of this chapter). Finally, there have been major advancements in the field of sexual dysfunction and infertility, which have dramatically improved the lives of able-bodied persons and persons with disabilities or chronic illnesses. For example, treatments for erectile dysfunction (ED) are widely known and advertised in the mainstream media, in vitro fertilization is common, and electrovibration and electroejaculation techniques have dramatically improved fertility in males with SCI.

Let's begin with 3 important definitions:

1. **Sex:** Maleness/femaleness; one of the 4 primary drives (along with hunger, thirst, and avoidance of pain) that originate in the subcortex and are modified by learned responses in the cortex.

2. **Sex acts:** Any behaviors involving the secondary erogenous zones and genitalia, such as kissing, hugging, caressing, and fondling, with sexual intercourse being only one kind of sex act.

3. **Sexuality:** The combination of sex drive, sex acts, and all those aspects of personality concerned with learned communications and relationship patterns. There are many levels to sexuality: conversation, shared activities and interests, various expressions of affection and intimacy, and sexual intercourse. Some persons equate sexuality with intimacy. Everyone is capable of intimacy—young or old, male or female, able-bodied or disabled.

Any discussion regarding sexuality should consider the broad picture and note that definitions of sexuality vary. Common thoughts regarding sexuality often focus on what happens in bed—or the sex acts—as the essence of sexuality. Some see sexuality as being "the major way people define and present themselves to others as people, and as men and women."[2] Another definition of sexuality involves "the way one dresses, the way one carries oneself, the way one looks at others and oneself, the way one speaks to other people, the way one touches other people and oneself."[3] Yet another definition includes "the many facets of an individual's personality, including affection, companionship, intimacy, and love."[4]

What all of these definitions display is the universality of the emotional importance of sexuality, whether someone is disabled or able-bodied. Some also feel that because of the relationship of sexuality to self-esteem and body image, it is an important part of rehabilitation.[5] Because self-esteem is so important to a person's psychological well-being and because disability affects the way a person feels about him- or herself, it is logical to see that a damaged self-esteem will also affect his or her sexuality. Self-image and self-efficacy are also important considerations and are affected by disability. In addition, disability and illness affect the injured person and his or her partner, which is dealt with in more detail later in this chapter.

In previous chapters, the importance of developing listening skills and effective communication in the patient-practitioner interaction (PPI) was presented. Identification of who owns the problem and communicating about emotion-laden topics is evident with issues of sexuality and self-image in the rehabilitation process. According to Sipski and Alexander,[6] communication within the health care system should have 6 goals, all of which are essential when addressing the topic of sexuality and disability:

1. To establish rapport

2. To determine a basic medical and interpersonal history

3. To assess the role and nature of relationships in the patient's life

4. To identify what changes have occurred since the onset of the disability or illness

5. To determine how those changes have been explained to the patient and how the changes have affected quality of life

6. To communicate in such a way so that questions are encouraged

Sexuality continues to be a sensitive topic that most clinicians are uncomfortable addressing with their patients. There are at least 2 major reasons for this discomfort: (1) lack of training and knowledge in the area of sexuality; and (2) the subject of sexuality being an area where the health care professional's (HCP's) own personal values and biases are based on their own upbringing, values, and life experiences. Thus, rehabilitation professionals often feel they lack competence to provide information, and they are unsure of their roles in providing this information to their patients. For many professionals, it is difficult to separate their own values and attitudes on sexuality from those of their patients in order to be objective. Therefore, it is not surprising that the subject of sexuality is rarely addressed, addressed inappropriately, or simply dismissed.

Attitudes of health care professionals toward sexuality have been studied, but most of these studies have been with nurses and few have been with physical or occupational therapists. In studies of nursing students, it has been found that they are less knowledgeable and more conservative than other students.[7] In rehabilitation nurses, increased religiosity was correlated with decreased knowledge of sexuality and more conservative sexual values.[8] Nursing faculty have been found to be unprepared to teach this content; thus, it was ignored or limited in content.[9] Although studies of health care professionals are limited and not current, one could assume that many of these health care professionals have similar origins and values. In one of the few studies of rehabilitation professionals, it was found that the majority (79%) thought that sexuality was as important as other aspects of rehabilitation, but few (7%) were comfortable addressing sexuality with their patients.[10]

A more recent study found that the majority of patients (73%), patients' partners (59%), and rehabilitation professionals (67%) thought that sexuality was an important issue to be addressed in the rehab setting.[11] However, the study also found that 93% of physicians, psychologists, and social workers felt it was within their domain of practice, as well as 87% of nurses, whereas only 48% of physical therapists felt it was within their practice domain. For something that is obviously important to patients, rehabilitation professionals shall need to increase their knowledge and comfort levels, at least to that of nurses and physicians. Physical and occupational therapists provide for rehabilitation to address movement and skills for the job of living; sex is in fact an activity of living, which involves movement! Sex is a valued function for many patients/clients, and many impairments, functional limitations, disabilities, and handicaps have an effect on the ability to function, perform sex acts, express sexuality, and influence sex drive.

The reasons for health care professionals' discomfort with sexuality have been noted to be a lack of knowledge or an assumption that "someone else does it." Because sexual identity, self-concept, and self-worth are so strongly linked, if one is impaired, all are affected. In addition, impaired sexual function has a direct adverse effect on the medical, psychological, and vocational rehabilitation of an individual, and addressing this issue can have a positive effect on the overall rehabilitation of a patient with a disability or chronic illness. It is the job of the rehabilitation professional to increase the function of our patients in all domains. Knowledge building in the areas of anatomy and physiology is easily accomplished, as well as disability-specific effects and cultural variables. Other areas to be included in the common education of patients in a rehabilitation setting are human sexual response, religion and religious values, and dispelling of myths and stereotypes, along with physical health, mental health, well-being, quality of life, and the topic of sexuality. More specific training is necessary for rehabilitation professionals to feel confident, as well as to reflect on their own values and beliefs regarding sexuality.

Skills training should address effective and active listening (see Chapter 7), interviews and assessment skills (see Chapter 13), and values clarification (see Chapter 3); discussion and modeling of compassion, patience, perceptiveness, and integrity are also valuable. Because of the close bonds patients develop with rehabilitation professionals, especially therapists, due to the intensity of contacts and type of care, therapists are in a unique position to respond to their patients, often more so than physicians. The main objectives are to create a supportive and safe environment and to encourage active participation of the patient in increasing function in all aspects of his or her life.

The Permission, Limited Information, Specific Suggestions, and Intensive Therapy (PLISSIT) Model

The PLISSIT model[12] is ideally utilized by all members of the health care team in conversing with people with disabilities who are asking about sex and sexuality. In this model, all members of the team are educated to feel comfortable enough with their own sexuality and have enough knowledge to function at the first 2 levels of the model (ie, permitting discussion of the topic of sex and sexuality and having enough knowledge about sexuality and about various specific disabilities to provide limited information). Team members should also reflect on their own values and beliefs. For instance, knowing what topics create feelings of unease or embarrassment for themselves, such as sexual orientation. What brings them sexual pleasure? What would it mean for them to have their own sexual ability affected by illness or trauma?[13] Rehabilitation professionals will undoubtedly encounter patients with different values from their own. Thus, awareness of one's own biases helps to define topics or areas one is not comfortable with and which, therefore, should be referred to someone else on the team. In addition, they should know enough about their own limits, or "know what they do not know," in order to properly refer the patient to a more knowledgeable health care professional. Each PLISSIT model[12] element will be briefly described here.

Permission

Permission is a valuable tool to help patients deal with basic issues of self-esteem, personal worth, and body image. At this first level, the health care professional gives overt and covert messages to the patient who inquires about sex, provides permission through his or her responses to the patient's questions, offers more information when the patient is ready, and introduces the topic in a nonthreatening manner (eg, using bridging statements, described later). Here, the health care professional is being open and accepting of the topic of sex and gives the patient permission to inquire without embarrassment. Although many rehabilitation professionals are not confident in discussing sexuality, most have adequate skills to perform at this level.

Limited Information

At this second level in the model, the health care professional provides general and basic education, such as anatomy and physiology, dispelling of myths, and describing general ways in which others in similar situations have resolved their own problems. At this level, it is important that the health care professional know his or her own **limitations** (in knowledge, skill, and comfort) and refer the patient to others when the patient's needs exceed his or her own limits.

Specific Suggestions

In this third level, the health care professional assists the patient with more specific needs or concerns by suggesting or providing specific ways to resolve a problem (eg, specific adapted positions for sexual intercourse, ED, and management of bowel or bladder problems) or **specific** effects of medications or surgeries. At this stage, discussion of sexual boundaries and roles that are acceptable to the patient and his or her partner would be appropriate. Depending on the injury, helping the patient redefine his or her personal definition of sexuality, including attitude change and broadening of views, may be included (eg, oral genital stimulation).[13] For functioning at this level, the health care professional should have additional education, expertise, or experience in sexuality and disability beyond others on the team and be astutely aware of his or her own limitations in knowledge, comfort, or skills.

Intensive Therapy

This level is usually beyond the rehabilitation setting and requires psychotherapy, relationship counseling, or surgical or invasive procedures (penile implants or injection therapy). **Referral** to these health care professionals for more intensive therapy is usually coordinated outside the inpatient setting.

Clearly, the PLISSIT model[12] provides a structure for an effective multidisciplinary team approach and for individuals to identify their own levels of appropriate practice or expertise, as well as a process that assists one to identify areas for future professional growth. Case presentations are particularly helpful in identifying options for management and problem solving, as well as mentoring opportunities for health care professionals (see Exercise 2).

SEXUALITY AND DISABILITY: HOSPITALIZATION—THE PROCESS OF *BECOMING* A PATIENT

Becoming a patient in today's medical care arena involves many processes that threaten one's independence and dignity and one's very sense of self-identity (see Table 12-1). The transformation of a person into a patient begins with several predictable events[14]:

- Answering the same seemingly innocuous questions from several people about personal information (name, address, Social Security number, insurance, age, weight, reason for admission)
- Undressing and donning the "neuter" hospital gown (affording little in the way of propriety)
- The surrendering of all personal effects
- The application of the familiar wristband for identification
- The transportation via wheelchair to a room with a bed and a chair, even when one is capable of walking unaided

Whether the hospitalization is for a minor procedure or life-threatening illness, the process remains the same. Even with the use of modern, electronic health records, much is unchanged as due to required reverifications. The point is that there is a **ubiquitous custom of forced dependence of individuals who have previously been in control of their lives outside the hospital but who are forced to lose their identities and senses of self when they become patients**. Suddenly, a person is no longer Mary Smith, CEO, or John Jones, Esq., but Mrs. Smith or Mr. Jones, or even worse, Mary and John. The ultimate insult occurs when he or she becomes "Room 22, Bed 2," and this process occurs in just about every inpatient setting in the country.

Following the initial round of the admission process and settling into the hospital routine is the process of myriad evaluations by different health care professionals assigned to the patient's care—nurses, physicians (including residents, interns, and medical students), and rehabilitation professionals and their assistants and students. All are asking similar questions about the patient's personal and medical history, doing physical examinations, and ordering invasive and non-invasive procedures in the process of establishing a diagnosis or treatment regimen.

All of these assessments are necessary and important in the process of diagnosis and treatment of the patient's problem. However, what is sometimes overlooked in this process is the privacy of the individual, and often there is a consistent lack of concern about personal modesty and humility as the patient is questioned, examined, prodded, and probed, often in intimate places. Significantly, the patient's problem may involve areas of the body that reflect one's sexuality, such as the breast, uterus, or prostate. When these areas of the body are the cause of the hospitalization, there is an inevitable increased sense of invasion accompanying the process of assessment. If surgery is imminent, whether a mastectomy, hysterectomy, or prostatectomy, there is a significant, unspoken fear about the patient's sense of self after the surgery.

"Loneliness and the feeling of being unwanted is the most terrible poverty." –Mother Teresa

BODY IMAGE

Any patient who experiences trauma, surgical removal of a body part, or treatment that results in disfigurement or loss of a body part experiences a disturbance of his or her body image. Body image disturbances may occur when there is a discrepancy between the way in which one had mentally pictured the body and the way the body is currently perceived. This conflict can arouse anxiety and fear of rejection. The response of loved ones is very important and thought to exert a significant influence on the patient's ability to reintegrate his or her new body image. Body image distortion may elicit feelings of unacceptability, thus negatively influencing the person's perception of self as a sexual being and, in turn, influencing sexual function.

EFFECTS OF ILLNESS ON SEXUALITY

Illness may influence one's sexuality in many different and diverse ways, as shown in Table 17-1. It is important for health care professionals to be aware of how various disease processes or drugs may affect their patients' physiological functioning, as well as their sense of self. There are several excellent and comprehensive resource textbooks for health care professionals (see Suggested Readings).

TABLE 17-1	
EFFECTS OF DISABILITIES ON SEXUALITY AND SELECT EXAMPLES	
EFFECT ON SEXUALITY	**SELECT EXAMPLE**
Interference with sexual function due to physiological changes or tissue damage	Spinal cord injury, diabetes, prostate cancer
Treatment may result in a change in body image, which may seem incompatible with maintaining a sexual relationship	Mastectomy, orchiectomy, ostomy, amputation
Pharmacological agents may interfere with sexual function	Antihypertensive medications, chemotherapy, insulin
Physical symptoms (fatigue) may interfere with or hamper sexual performance	Cancer patients on chemotherapy or radiation therapy, rheumatoid arthritis, multiple sclerosis
Anxiety related to illness may interfere with sexual response	Post-myocardial infarction, cancer, genital herpes, HIV
Depression or grief may be associated with impaired libido or sex drive	Post-myocardial infarction, hysterectomy, mastectomy, cancer, multiple sclerosis
Illness may necessitate physical separation from a partner	Spinal cord injury, post-stroke, accident, HIV, AIDS

ACTING OUT SEXUALLY

When patients consciously or unconsciously test the response of others to themselves as sexual beings, they may act out as a means of gaining control of a situation in which they feel dependent. For example, flirtatious behavior is often exhibited as a way to attract attention. What the patients may be expressing is the effect of sexual deprivation or separation from a sexual partner or significant other. Also, they may simply be seeking out validation of themselves as still being attractive or desirable. Chapter 11 on neurolinguistic psychology offers communication alternatives to help health care professionals set strong boundaries and break rapport if this acting out becomes sexual harassment (see also Chapter 8: Assertiveness Skills and Conflict Resolution).

CULTURAL VARIABLES

As described in Chapter 12, it is important for health care professionals to be aware of different cultural customs and beliefs in the patients they are treating. Often, without thinking of it consciously, different customs are considered odd or strange, when they should merely be considered different. Greater emphasis on cultural diversity is evident in most professional curricula, which is certainly needed in the multicultural environment encountered by practicing clinicians today. In many cultures, there are certain proscriptions that may modify an individual's response to hospitalization and treatment. For example, in certain Hispanic cultures, illness is believed to be a manifestation of weakness. Loss of blood is thought to impair sexual vigor. Protection of the wife's modesty is seen as a duty of a good husband during physical examinations. Any or all of these cultural dictates may be misinterpreted by uninformed health care professionals as stubbornness or stupidity, unless cultural differences are understood.

Likewise, if a health care professional is not accustomed to being in the presence of same-sex couples, they may find themselves acting in ways that are judgmental or unkind and not conducive to therapeutic presence. Because most studies regarding sexuality and disability do not distinguish between those who are heterosexual and those who are not, there is little information about potential sexual issues. Same-sex couples have similar needs and concerns as heterosexual couples, and efforts should be made to make them feel comfortable and understood, without judgment. When appropriate, safer sex options and practices should be discussed.

BASIC RULES FOR EFFECTIVE COMMUNICATION ABOUT SEXUALITY AND REHABILITATION

As a clinician, the following 3 basic rules will assist you in communicating with therapeutic sensitivity:

1. **Prevent shaming experiences.** Shame implies admitting to oneself that part or all of the self is unacceptable. Shaming experiences can be prevented by providing physical and psychological privacy, carefully reading body language, listening to words to avoid "touchy" areas, and explaining that the given situation is not intended to embarrass but is necessary for effective care.

2. **Maintain privacy.** During hospitalization, personal autonomy and the limitation and protection of information are usually jeopardized. In order to emphasize confidentiality, it is often wise to acknowledge to patients that you realize that some things are difficult to discuss; then provide some dimension of privacy and always show respect as a means to address this problem. Make use of curtains and closed doors whenever possible.

3. **Do not make judgments.** Chapters 2, 3, and 4 emphasize that we all have our own values, and there are some individuals whose values may be in conflict with our own. Accept that people are different and maintain a professional decorum without inflicting your own values on others, verbally or nonverbally. Be aware of whether you are a person who readily displays facial expressions that reveal dissatisfaction with different values than your own.

In sum, understanding oneself, understanding one's patient, and understanding the dysfunction or disability are all essential roles for rehabilitation professionals. Health care professionals should continually strive to continue their education and professional development and to address all aspects of being and knowing, for their patients' benefit and their own self-preservation, maintaining a humanistic approach to health care for all.

IMPROVING COMMUNICATION— BRIDGE AND BARNUM STATEMENTS

It is obvious to all health care professionals that not all questions are easy to ask, some questions need to be asked more than once, and not all answers will be the same to different health care professionals, and this holds especially true with the topic of sexuality. **Bridge statements** (including questions) facilitate the transition from easy, comfortable topics to those that are difficult or awkward. They move from the general to the specific, emphasize the professional relationship between the patient and the therapist, and focus on permission giving and permission seeking.

Some examples include the following:

- Has anyone talked to you about how your illness can affect your ability to have sex?
- How has your (multiple sclerosis, arthritis, stroke, Parkinson's disease) changed the kinds of things you and your partner do together?[6]
- Many people with amputations have concerns about their sexual attractiveness. Is this a concern of yours?[6]

Although bridge statements are a means to solicit information and improve communication, **Barnum statements** can hinder information and create anxiety. *Barnum statements* are overly general and empty of content, although fashioned to be encouraging or optimistic. Some examples include the following:

- You are in the best hospital for your condition (spoken to an anxious patient).
- Come on, smile—it's a wonderful day.[6]
- How is your love life?[6]

Barnum statements minimize and depersonalize the patient's problem and do **not** help the health care professional understand the problem from the patient's perspective. Although often heard in rehabilitation settings, they should be **avoided**.

MYTHS

As reflected in the quote from Cole[1] at the beginning of this chapter, people with disabilities fit the 3 criteria that would characterize them as being different from those in the general population. People with disabilities are a readily identifiable minority, and others often feel uncomfortable in their presence. Most people in ethnic or racial minorities have also experienced these 3 criteria at some point in their lives, and the similarities are striking.

Over the past 40 years, there have been numerous changes in behaviors and attitudes regarding disability and sexuality. During the 1970s and 1980s, there was a rash of medical, psychological, and behavioral investigations that added greatly to our body of knowledge about sexuality and disability. Prior to this period, there were many myths perpetuated by the media, as well as educational publications, which did little to explore the true realities and capabilities of sexual functioning in persons with disabilities. Furthermore, there was little in the medical literature regarding sexuality and disability, further perpetuating the myth of asexuality.

Prejudice against the disabled in our culture and others has existed for many years, often perpetuated by popular literature. Captain Ahab from *Moby Dick*; Quasimodo from *The Hunchback of Notre Dame*; and Dr. No, James Bond's arch rival, come readily to mind. Often these characters were referred to as "grotesquely deformed and evil." Is it any wonder that many of us have grown to harbor feelings of revulsion or pity for persons with a disability?

Similarly, many individuals with a traumatic disability, such as an amputation or SCI, may have themselves harbored feelings of revulsion toward the disabled prior to their own injury. In effect, these preconceived beliefs may result in considerable self-prejudice, hampering their own self-acceptance. This further complicates the acceptance of their new body image for their own self-esteem. In a society such as ours, with so much emphasis placed on beauty, health, and physical fitness, it is easy to see how physically disabled people may feel ostracized in today's sexual arena and low on a scale of sexual desirability. In an era of selfies, the visual perception may be even further magnified.

It is important to note that over the past 10 to 15 years, persons with visible disabilities have now been regularly featured in mainstream media in print and broadcast advertisements and as main characters in television shows. Social media and networking sites have also helped to provide increased opportunities for more interaction and education for persons with disabilities (yet some have also provided detrimental influences). Certain television shows have also utilized social and comedic satire to aid in changing perspectives, such as with the character Jimmy, a male fourth grader who is disabled, in the Comedy Central series *South Park*. Jimmy was first introduced in a "cripple fight" and has endless optimism, despite his disability. The episodes featuring Jimmy provide moral insights into the thoughts of the disabled, bringing forth important lessons, albeit in satirical comedy. Modern technology has also assisted in bringing about greater connectivity for all, and there are also online dating sites specific for persons with disabilities (eg, www.datedisabled.com, www.datingdisabled.net, www.whispers4u.com, and www.agreaterdate.com).[13] Fortunately, it would appear that at least some of these previously held attitudes and aversions may be changing in a positive manner.

To sum up, it is important for health care professionals to recognize that people are not "handicapped" intrinsically. As pointed out in Chapter 16, a person with a disability becomes handicapped when he or she is restrained from usual social interaction by barriers, social and architectural, that prohibit participation in normal daily activities.

SELF-ESTEEM

According to Abraham Maslow,[15] sex is one of the basic physiological needs that must be met, in addition to air, water, food, shelter, and sleep. All are needed in order for an individual to move toward self-esteem and self-actualization. Taking Maslow's theory to practical application, Anderson and Cole[16] did groundbreaking research with respect to examining the interrelationship of sexual success, work success (meaningful employment), and the self-esteem of an individual with a disability. They found that if there was perceived success in sexual activity, the person with a disability reported a higher self-esteem and fewer feelings of castration. If there was success in work life, there was less tolerance for dependency and thus a higher self-esteem. If there was success in both areas, the individual had a high self-esteem, fewer medical complaints, and less need for medical and social support. Many authors since Anderson and Cole[16] have stressed the importance of sexuality on self-esteem and self-image.[17-19]

Another meaningful point with respect to success in sexual relations relates to the importance and significance of the sexual partner or significant other. The significant other plays a pivotal role in the acceptance of a changed body image for a person with a disability. As Rosenbaum[20] so eloquently stated:

> *What becomes apparent when the direct genital urge toward physical release is lost, are the many other needs, that can be met or expressed through sexual activity—the need for touching, for reassuring body contact, to be held and to hold, to express love and caring through caressing and kissing. These become especially important when the body has been damaged and the individual is attempting to integrate and accept a new and altered body image. We all need the acceptance of another to make the image of ourselves whole and more loveable.*

Thus, the acceptance of the partner is important in allowing and assisting the reintegration of the disabled person in a new body image. Recent literature has emphasized the importance of the partner and the "couple relationship" because both persons (the person with the disability and his or her partner, if there was one prior to the disability) are affected.[18] Furthermore, a "couple" means 2 people in a committed relationship, regardless of whether the relationship is heterosexual or homosexual, married or cohabiting. Suffering a disability has a profound effect on the quality of life of an individual, as well as the life of his or her partner. Persons with disabilities, if married, also have higher divorce rates than persons with no disability.[18] Finally, it was also determined that partners of persons with disabilities have lower scores on all quality of life measures, presumably due to increased stress.[18] It has been postulated that the nondisabled partner often struggles in the role of caretaker, especially if it involves bowel and bladder care or management. On top of that, switching from caretaker to the role of intimate lover then becomes a major source of stress.

Besides the partner, the next most important person is the health care professional and his or her attitude toward his or her patients. Self-esteem and self-confidence depend on feedback from the environment and those around the patient. If the health care professional projects a sensitive, honest, and truthful attitude, with an openness to questions and concerns, the patient can be encouraged to discover a new sense of self without anxiety. If, however, the patient and his or her questions are not addressed openly and honestly or are brushed off in a shaming experience, the patient's adjustment and acceptance will be dealt a significant blow, and his or her recovery will be compromised.

NORMAL HUMAN SEXUAL RESPONSE—NEUROPHYSIOLOGY

In a culture and era when sexuality seems to scream from billboards, magazines, and movie theaters, it is amazing how little education those in the health care professions actually receive with respect to normal human sexuality. Understanding sexuality and disability, especially as it relates to the person with SCI, requires an understanding of the normal sexual response and its components. These components, and the male and female response cycles, are found in Table 17-2. In men, it is important to note the following facts regarding erection and ejaculation, based on neurophysiology. There are 2 centers for erection within the spinal cord:

1. **Psychogenic (T11-L2)**—Mental arousal, fantasizing, psychic stimuli (or "whatever turns you on")
2. **Reflexogenic (S2-S4)**—Local arousal, masturbation, rubbing the inside of the thigh, full bladder, catheter change (reflex sensorimotor feedback loop)

Ejaculation is mediated by the sympathetic nervous system (T11-L2), the parasympathetic nervous system (S2-S4), and the somatic nervous system. The 2 kinds of erection are not separate in the normal male response cycle but become important in understanding sexual function in men with SCI.

SEXUALITY AND SPINAL CORD INJURY

Sexuality is affected more with SCI than with any other disease or pathological condition. The patient's first question is usually, "Will I live?" The second question (often unexpressed) is, "How will this injury affect me sexually?"

There are far too many exceptions within each spinal cord level to state, with any certainty, what any one patient's sexual disability will be. What is known is that the majority of persons with SCI are satisfied (72%), although this is lower than able-bodied men and women.[21] In general, erection capability (whether reflexogenic or psychogenic) has been reported by 80% to 100% of males with SCI, and ejaculation occurs in 4% to 18%, with persons with quadriplegia being in the 0% to 4% range.[22] What should be emphasized is that sexual activity may or may not involve genital sensation. Ultimately, sexual satisfaction is a cerebral event and therefore can be achieved by everyone. Furthermore, sexual function has been found to be very important to the many patients with SCI (males and females) in several studies, in which the majority placed sexual functioning ahead of return of sensation, walking, or bowel and bladder function (and second only to hand function in persons with quadriplegia).[23]

SPINAL CORD INJURY—SEXUAL FUNCTION IN MEN

SCI is a devastating injury to anyone, but there are significant effects with respect to sexuality that affect men more than women (Table 17-3). For levels above the cauda equina, the ability to achieve and sustain an erection is generally maintained as long as there is local stimulation to activate the feedback loop for reflexogenic erection. Ejaculation is more rare, and fertility is a problem, although there have been recent major breakthroughs (eg, electrovibration and electroejaculation) in this area.

TABLE 17-2

THE NORMAL SEXUAL AROUSAL CYCLE: MALE AND FEMALE

1. EXCITATION: Develops from any source of bodily or psychic stimuli and, with adequate stimulation, leads to further excitation. The first phase may be interrupted, prolonged, or ended by distracting stimuli.

MALE	FEMALE
○ Rapid engorgement and erection of the penis	○ Clitoral glans enlarged
○ Tensing and thickening of the scrotal skin	○ Vaginal lubrication
○ Elevation of scrotal sac	○ Nipples become erect, breast size may enlarge
○ Occasional nipple erection	○ Sexual flush may be seen (rash on chest to breast)
○ Elevation of HR and BP	○ HR and BP increase

2. PLATEAU: Often called the consolidation period. A period of intensified sexual tension; also affected by distracting stimuli.

MALE	FEMALE
○ Increased penile circumference	○ Lower one-third of vagina constricts, upper two-thirds balloons (creates a squeezing action)
○ Increase in testes size	○ Clitoral glans retract
○ Continued increase in muscle tension, HR, RR, and BP	○ Uterus elevates
○ Sexual flush—rash over face, neck, and chest	○ Sexual flush may spread to entire body
	○ Increase in muscle tension, HR, RR, and BP

3. ORGASM: Involuntary climax of sexual tension increments; really only a few seconds of the sexual response cycle during which vasocongestion and myotonia are released; greater variety of intensity and duration in the female.

MALE	FEMALE
○ HR, RR, and BP increase further	○ Further increase in generalized muscle tone, HR, RR, and BP
○ Expulsive contraction of the penile urethra	○ Involuntary rhythmic muscle contraction in perineal muscles
○ Ejaculation (internal bladder sphincter closes, preventing retrograde ejaculation)	○ Involuntary contraction, spasm of muscle groups
○ Involuntary muscle contraction of perineal muscles	○ May be multiple orgasms (unlike males)

4. RESOLUTION: The period when involuntary changes occur that restore the individual to the pre-excitatory state.

MALE	FEMALE
○ Gradual reversal of anatomical and physiological changes	○ Gradual reversal of anatomical and physiological changes
○ Males require a refractory period before another cycle occurs	○ Females usually do not have a refractory period and may begin another cycle immediately

BP = blood pressure; HR = heart rate; RR = resting rate.

TABLE 17-3		
SPINAL CORD INJURY: EFFECTS OF SEXUAL FUNCTION IN MEN[a]		
QUADRIPLEGIA	**PARAPLEGIA[b]**	**CAUDA EQUINA LESIONS**
○ Reflexogenic—Intact ○ Psychogenic—Not intact ○ Ejaculation—Rare ○ Fertility[c]—Almost nil	○ Reflexogenic—Intact ○ Psychogenic—Not intact ○ Ejaculation—Rare ○ Fertility—Almost nil	○ Reflexogenic—Arc may be disturbed (below L2) ○ Psychogenic—Intact (T11-L2) ○ Ejaculation—Moderate chance ○ Fertility—May be present, but with sperm problems (retrograde ejaculation, temperature problems)
[a]There is a distinct difference between complete and incomplete lesions of the spinal cord, with effects from incomplete lesions being far less predictable than from complete lesions, although more positive with respect to ejaculation and orgasm in lower motor neuron lesions compared with upper motor neuron lesions. [b]Essentially, there is no difference between a male with quadriplegia or paraplegia with respect to sexual capability and fertility. The major difference is in the greater area of intact skin sensation and motor ability (trunk, arms, and abdomen). [c]Because ejaculation is rare, fertility is severely affected; however, fertility can be greatly assisted today with technological advances, such as electrovibration, electroejaculation, and artificial insemination.		

What is also important with respect to males with SCI is the entire socialization of males and masculinity in our culture. It is known that males are socialized very early into expected gender roles and behaviors. "Performing" is of primary importance, and strength, self-reliance, success, sexual interest and prowess, independence, aggressiveness, and dominance are all important male attributes. Their manhood is often tied to their penis, and having erections is directly related to masculinity. Sexual education and sexual comparisons go on all the time. With these messages, it is no surprise that if a male's ability to achieve an erection is impaired, as it certainly is in a man with SCI, this is a devastating blow to his manhood and his self-identity. It is yet another disability to contend with, in addition to the SCI, and one that must be addressed in the rehabilitation arena.

SPINAL CORD INJURY—SEXUAL FUNCTION IN WOMEN

There has been a sexual bias in the literature regarding female sexuality, although it is true that the majority of persons with traumatic SCI are young men. Women with SCI are often thought to be unaffected because their fertility remains intact; thus, many people mistakenly believe that they do not suffer the overt sexual disability that is seen with men. Often, they are told that their sexuality is unaffected, but women experience the same differences and inabilities, neurophysiologically, as do men. The female sexual cycle is similar to that of the male; thus, the lubrication, engorgement, and contraction components of the sexual response cycle are affected. Recent research has shown that women with complete SCIs with upper motor neuron lesions will have reflexogenic lubrication but not psychogenic lubrication, similar to their male counterparts with the same type of injuries.[24] Yet, because these problems are not as overt and obvious as when a man is unable to achieve erection or has difficulty doing so, women are mistakenly viewed as unaffected.

Immediately after a traumatic SCI, a woman's menses may be halted, but her menstrual cycles will usually return within 6 months, and fertility is therefore unaffected, unlike men. Pregnancy, if it occurs, can be problematic due to difficulties with movement and transfers due to the pregnant uterus, and there is an increased risk of autonomic dysreflexia. Labor and delivery also present complications due to the inability of a woman with SCI to sense labor contractions or to push during the expulsion phase of labor. Cesarean birth is usually not necessary because the uterus is an involuntary muscle capable of contracting despite loss of innervation. However, due to the inability of the woman to push and potential problems of emboli or autonomic dysreflexia, vaginal births are rare, although not impossible.

Sexuality is much more than childbearing for women and fertility for men, but information usually given in a rehabilitation setting is often overly clinical, focusing on bowel and bladder routines and stressing more on the physical act of intercourse, removed from the context of the entire relationship. Although it is true that the greatest concerns of men and women focus on the physical (autonomic dysreflexia and bowel or bladder accidents) and the psychological (satisfying the partner, being attractive), the latter usually diminishes over time, but the former persists, partially due to the emphasis placed by health care professionals who tell them to expect bowel and bladder accidents and other negative possibilities. If men and women with SCI are told repeatedly of the negative consequences during rehabilitation, a time when their self-esteem and self-confidence are already challenged, it is no wonder that many are not encouraged, or are scared, to face a relationship. Warnings about possible problems should be realistic but not overwhelming. Discussion of these issues should be done in a nonjudgmental way to promote self-confidence and self-acceptance.

With respect to the treatment of sexual difficulties, there are far more options and much more successful ones for men than for women. Various medications for sexual difficulties (eg, phosphodiesterase or topical prostaglandin) have not proven successful for disabled women or able-bodied women with sexual dysfunctions. Vibrostimulation and the use of vibrators have been helpful for many women, and there is some promise with new Food and Drug Administration– approved clitoral vacuum stimulation procedures.[25]

For men, current options include the common oral medications (Viagra [sildenafil], Levitra [vardenafil], and Cialis [tadalafil]), as well as injectable medications that relax the penile smooth muscle and cause an erection, topical agents, vacuum devices or penile rings, and surgical penile implants. Electroejaculation and artificial insemination have greatly aided fertility in males with SCI.

In the literature relating to the human sexual response, Masters and Johnson (see Suggested Readings) were pioneers and contributed greatly to our understanding of this basic human need of sexuality and sexual response. One of the things they noted is that the human sexual response is a total body response, rather than merely a pelvic phenomenon. There are changes in cardiovascular and respiratory function, as well as reactions of the skin, muscles, breasts, and rectal sphincter. This whole-body response is an important distinction because it is commonly reported that many individuals with SCI actually experience orgasm, although usually of a different type than they experienced prior to their injury. Individuals with SCI are often taught to use various methods of assignment, fantasy employment, memory, and recall and report that they experience a sensation that, although different, is nonetheless satisfying. In one study, sensory substitution techniques using training and neuroplasticity to map tongue sensations were successfully used to increase pleasure and orgasm in sexual experiences in men with SCI.[26] Orgasm can still remain elusive to men and women with SCI. They must undergo—accomplished much more easily with a partner—a process of learning to enhance their sexual responsiveness over time, and adjustment of their own values, through self-experimentation and openmindedness.

SEXUALITY AND MYOCARDIAL INFARCTION

Although a great volume of literature exists relating to sexuality and SCI, sexuality and myocardial infarction (MI) is the second most researched topic in the medical literature. With respect to sexuality and MI, there are still discrepancies in the literature. Either little information is given (and what is given is often too conservative) or conflicting information is given, making it difficult for patients to decide whether it is safe to resume sexual activity after an MI. Much of the discrepancy in the literature about sexuality and the post-MI patient is related to discrepancies in the maximal heart rate during sexual activity. In their studies of human sexual response, Masters and Johnson recorded couples' heart rates, respiratory rates, and other physiological responses during sexual intercourse and found that heart rates escalated to 180 bpm during intercourse. They therefore concluded that sexual activity is "heavy cardiac work."

Many cardiologists and other physicians, when asked by their patients, related these findings and cautioned against any excessive cardiac work for their post-MI patients (ie, resumption of sexual relations). What was missing in this information for cardiac patients was the fact that the Masters and Johnson studies were conducted on healthy, young college students in their early 20s. The average post-MI patient in the mid-1980s was a man in his 50s, married for 20 or more years to the same spouse. Hellerstein and Freidman[27] saw this discrepancy and pursued their own study, similar to that of Masters and Johnson, except using couples with a post-MI spouse in his or her 50s. Their results were dramatically different: They found the maximal heart rates to be 120 bpm, roughly the equivalent of climbing 2 flights of stairs, and lower than heart rates during a football game or during a heated argument in the office. They concluded that, for the "typical post-MI patient," with his or her spouse of 20 or more years and a frequency of sexual intercourse of 1 to 2 times per week, sexual activity was not the wild, amorous fit of passion seen often in the movies of today and did not constitute heavy cardiac work. Recent studies have shown promising results of a gradual return to sexual activity for most post-MI patients, although all studies have shown a reduction in the frequency of sexual activity when compared with the pre-MI state for males and females.[6]

Stratification of post-MI patients into high, intermediate, and low categories of cardiac risk appears to be the norm, with those in the low-risk category being the most ready to resume sexual activity and others dependent on results of exercise testing and other medications.[28] It was further presumed that patients without cardiac ischemia at exercise would

TABLE 17-4

OTHER CONDITIONS THAT MAY CAUSE PROBLEMS WITH SEXUAL INTERCOURSE

CONDITION	PROBLEM
Genital lesions	May cause difficulty with penetration or painful intercourse (dyspareunia)
Respiratory disease	May impair the ability to breathe adequately or limit positions used to engage in sexual intercourse
Cardiac disease	May involve poor circulation to the genital area, angina with exertion, or decreased libido due to medications; denial, anxiety, and depression
Neurological diseases (stroke, multiple sclerosis, Parkinson's)	May involve components of the nervous system, altering sensation or motor ability (erection, lubrication); may also have spasticity, impairing range of motion; decreased libido; language deficits or changes in affect
Amputations	May limit some positions due to inability to assume them; may be a physical turn-off or fetish for the partner, or body image
Arthritis	Limitations due to joint mobility and/or painful joints limiting activity
Ostomies	May limit some positions due to pressure on ostomy site; may be a physical turn-off to the partner, or body image
Severe burns	May be limited in joint range of motion, difficulty in assuming some positions due to limited mobility; may be a physical turn-off to the partner, or body image
Scleroderma	May be limited in joint range of motion, difficulty in assuming some positions due to limited mobility; loss of elasticity of skin may hamper intercourse or cause painful intercourse; may be a physical turn-off to the partner
Cancer	Physical and emotional disturbances; primary sexual organs may be affected (disfigurement, body image); treatment options (chemotherapy, radiation therapy, or surgery) may cause impairment; fatigue, nausea, vomiting; anxiety and depression; hormonal changes if early menopause as consequence (decreased lubrication, increased pain with intercourse)

not develop ischemia during sexual intercourse.[29] Finally, all episodes of ischemia were associated with increased heart rate; thus, therapeutic strategies to reduce heart rate and improve exercise threshold were preferred.[29]

The focus on SCI and post-MI patients in this chapter is largely due to the amount of literature in these areas, but almost any kind of disease process or treatment can have an effect on a person's sexuality (Table 17-4).

DRUGS THAT MAY INTERFERE WITH SEXUAL FUNCTION

Many pharmacological agents can affect sexual performance directly or indirectly, a factor that has been increasingly noted in the media today. Because most drugs affect the autonomic nervous system (sympathetic or parasympathetic), sexual function is commonly affected. Normal sexual function depends on multiple physiological mechanisms, including vascular, hormonal, neurologic, and psychological processes, all of which can be altered by medications. Again, there is a gender bias in much of the literature, with few studies evaluating adverse effects on female sexual response. The most common adverse side effect is erectile dysfunction (and presumably the female counterpart of inadequate lubrication during sexual intercourse). Some of the more common drug families and their effects are listed in Table 17-5.

CONCLUSION

Self-image and self-esteem are major considerations in the sexual rehabilitation of a person with a disability. When one's sense of self is seriously disrupted by the trauma of a SCI or any other disability, it is more important than ever

TABLE 17-5
DRUG FAMILIES

CARDIOVASCULAR DRUGS	PSYCHOTROPIC DRUGS	STIMULANTS/ANORECTICS (Weight control, ADD)
Antihypertensive agents	Antidepressants	
Sympatholytic	Tricyclic antidepressants	
Reserpine, beta-blockers	MAOIs	Anticonvulsants
Diuretics	SSRIs	
Thiazides	Lithium carbonate	Antiulcer drugs
Anticholesterolemic agents	Anti-anxiety agents	
(Statins)		
Digoxin	Neuroleptics	Anticancer drugs
Antiarrhythmic drugs	Phenothiazines	Glycemic control
	Butyrophenones	Insulin

ADD = attention deficit disorder; MAOIs = monoamine oxidase inhibitors; SSRIs = selective serotonin reuptake inhibitors.

to help the patient reestablish a positive self-concept. Responding to an individual's sexual concerns can go a long way toward reestablishing a feeling of self-worth, which is essential to rehabilitation in general. Rehabilitation has traditionally emphasized the comprehensive management of the total patient. The basic premise is to help each patient to use all of his or her strengths and assets to the maximum in forming a new self-image based on positive factors and to help the patient to focus on areas of worth instead of deficiency. It is unfortunate that the patient's sexuality, with its potential as a positive integrating force in building a new image of self and body, has been neglected for so long.

Many health care professionals do not volunteer information to the patient because the patient has not asked. Because the subject of sex is viewed with discomfort by the patient and the health care professional, they are caught in the dilemma of who will initiate the communication. It is easy to ask questions regarding the patient's home, family, number of stairs to climb, etc; it is not easy to ask questions about the patient's customary sex life. Hence, patients are afraid of asking, and health care professionals are not comfortable with asking or with answering when asked. Yet, it has been shown that increased knowledge about a subject enhances feelings of comfort about the subject matter. Perhaps by providing health care professionals with at least minimal information and suggesting where to look for more information, comfort levels in providing this necessary care will improve.

Physical and occupational therapists are in an excellent position to coordinate discussions about sexuality because they are members of the disciplines around which total rehabilitation evolves, especially for the individual with SCI. Therapists must be comfortable with their own sexuality, however, through adequate knowledge and an accepting, nonjudgmental attitude. In addition, because most previous studies never distinguished between differing sexual orientations (heterosexual, homosexual, bisexual), there is no specific information for persons with disabilities who are nonheterosexual. Responding to questions without judging is important, and an emphasis on safe sex practices is also vital.

Attitudes around sexual expression may communicate a message that encourages adjustment and growth or may accomplish the opposite and inhibit patients from taking positive avenues of action, thus discourage a desirable outcome. Harmful attitudes can, in effect, add a new disability to the preexisting one for the patient. If a therapist is uncomfortable with a patient's questions, at the very least he or she should refer the patient to another person on the rehabilitation team who could answer the patient's questions and render the assistance and advice that the patient is seeking. To ignore the subject or downplay it only further handicaps the patient, exposes him or her to a shaming behavior, and closes down any further communication regarding this important component in his or her self-esteem. All rehabilitation professionals should be comfortable communicating within the first 2 components of the PLISSIT model and should be knowledgeable about referring to other health care professionals if more specific information is requested that is beyond their knowledge or comfort levels.

Cole and Cole[30] perhaps said it best as they listed guidelines for health care professionals and patients in learning about the sexuality of physical disability:

> Absence of sensation does not mean absence of feelings … the presence of deformities does not mean absence of the desire … the inability to perform does not mean the inability to enjoy. … Sexual health cannot be separated from total health.

Thus, education and communication are key components in providing our patients with information regarding sexuality and disability. All rehabilitation professionals are educators to our patients, their partners, and their families and caregivers. In this value-laden topic of sexuality, education of the couple (the patient and the partner) about the disability itself, the prognosis, complications, sexual anatomy and physiology and function, fertility, pregnancy, contraception, bowel and bladder issues, safer sex, and dispelling of myths should all be done by the rehabilitation team. It matters little who is responsible for which content. It just matters that someone is there and listens to the patient.

The exercises following the chapter will assist you in understanding your knowledge and attitudes in order to facilitate your therapeutic presence in helping patients reconcile unwelcome changes in their ability to be sexual following injury or illness.

REFERENCES

1. Cole TM. Teaching for professionals in the sexuality of the physically disabled. In: Rosenzweig N, Pearsall FP, eds. *Sex Education for the Health Professional—A Curriculum Guide*. New York, NY: Grune & Stratton; 1978:88.
2. Chipouras S, Cornelius D, Daniels SM, Makas E. *Who Cares? A Handbook on Sex Education and Counseling Services for Disabled People*. Austin, TX: Pro-Ed; 1979.
3. Trieschmann RB. *Spinal Cord Injuries: Psychological, Social and Vocational Rehabilitation*. 2nd ed. New York, NY: Demos; 1988.
4. Rotberg A. An introduction to women, aging, and sexuality. *Phys Occup Ther Geri*. 1987;5(3):3-12.
5. Ducharme SH, Gill KM. *Sexuality After Spinal Cord Injury: Answers to Your Questions*. Baltimore, MD: Paul H. Brooks Publishing; 1997.
6. Sipski ML, Alexander CJ. *Sexual Function in People With Disability and Chronic Illness: A Health Professional's Guide*. Gaithersburg, MD: Aspen Publications; 1997.
7. Medlar T, Medlar J. Nursing management of sexuality issues. *J Head Trauma Rehabil*. 1990;5(2):46-51.
8. Wilson PS, Dibble SL. Rehabilitation nurses' knowledge and attitudes toward sexuality. *Rehabil Nurs Res*. 1993;2(2):69-74.
9. Gender AR. An overview of the nurse's role in dealing with sexuality. *Sex Disabil*. 1992;10(2):81-89.
10. Ducharme S, Gill KM. Sexual values, training, and professional roles. *J Head Trauma Rehabil*. 1990; 5(2):38-45.
11. Gianotten WL, Bender JL, Post MW, Hoing M. Training in sexology for medical and paramedical professionals: a model for the rehabilitation setting. *Sexual Relationship Ther*. 2006;21(3):303-317.
12. Annon J. The PLISSIT model: a proposed conceptual scheme for the behavioral treatment for sexual problems. *J Sex Educ Ther*. 1976;2:1-15.
13. Esmail S, Know H, Scott H. Sexuality and the role of the rehabilitation professional. In: Stone JH, Blouin M, eds. *International Encyclopedia of Rehabilitation*. http://cirrie.buffalo.edu/encyclopedia/en/article/29/. Accessed April 20, 2015.
14. Woods NF. *Human Sexuality in Health and Illness*. 2nd ed. St. Louis, MO: CV Mosby Co; 1979.
15. Maslow A. *The Further Reaches of the Mind*. New York, NY: Viking Press; 1971.
16. Anderson TP, Cole TM. Sexual counselling of the physically disabled. *Postgrad Med*. 1975;58:117-123.
17. Klein MJ, Merritt LM, Moberg-Wolff EA, Salcido R, Talavera F. *Sexuality and Disability*. Meier RH, ed. New York, NY: Medscape, LLC; 2015.
18. Esmail S, Esmail Y, Munro B. Sexuality and disability: the role of health care professionals in providing options and alternatives for couples. *Sexuality and Disability*. 2001;19(4):267-282.
19. Ganz PA, Rowland JH, Desmond K, Meyerowitz BE, Wyatt GE. Life after breast cancer: understanding women's health-related quality of life and sexual functioning. *J Clin Oncol*. 1998;16(2):501-514.
20. Rosenbaum M. Sexuality and the physically disabled: the role of the professional. *Bull NY Acad Med*. 1978;54:501-559.
21. Kennedy P, Lude P, Taylor N. Quality of life, social participation, appraisals and coping post spinal cord injury: a review of four community samples. *Spinal Cord*. 2006;44:94-105.
22. Courtois FJ, Charvier KF, Leriche A, Raymond DP. Sexual function in spinal cord injured men. I. Assessing sexual capacity. *Paraplegia*. 1993;31(12):771-784.
23. Anderson KD, Borisoff JF, Johnson RD, Stiens SA, Elliott SL. The impact of spinal cord injury on sexual function: concerns of the general population. *Spinal Cord*. 2007;45(5):328-337.
24. Sipski ML, Alexander CJ, Rosen RC. Physiological parameters associated with psychogenic arousal in women with complete spinal cord injuries. *Arch Phys Med Rehab*. 1995;76:811-818.
25. Elliott S. Sexuality after spinal cord injury. In: Field-Foote E, ed. *Spinal Cord Injury Rehabilitation*. Philadelphia, PA: FA Davis & Co; 2009.
26. Borosoff JF, Elliott SL, Hocaloski S, Birch GE. The development of a sensory substitution system for the sexual rehabilitation of men with chronic spinal cord injury. *J Sex Med*. 2010;7(11):3647-3658.
27. Hellerstein H, Friedman EH. Sexual activity and the post-coronary patient. *Medical Aspects of Human Sexuality*. 1969;3:70-96.
28. Drory Y, Shapiro I, Fisman EZ, Pines A. Myocardial ischemia during sexual activity in patients with coronary artery disease. *Am J Cardiol*. 1995;75(4):835-837.

29. DeBusk R, Drory Y, Goldstein I, et al. Management of sexual dysfunction in patients with cardiovascular disease: recommenda-tion of the Princeton Consensus Panel. *Am J Cardio.* 2000;86(2):175-181.

30. Cole TM, Cole SS. The handicapped and sexual health. In: Comfort A, ed. *Sexual Consequences of Disability.* Philadelphia, PA: George F. Stickley Co; 1978.

SUGGESTED READINGS

Abramson CE, McBride KE, Konnyu KJ, Elliott SL; SCIRE Research Team. Sexual health outcome measures for individuals with a spinal cord injury: a systematic review. *Spinal Cord.* 2008;46(5):320-324.

Alappattu MJ, Bishop MD. Psychological factors in chronic pelvic pain in women: relevance and application of the fear-avoidance model of pain. *Phys Ther.* 2011;91(10):1542-1550.

Alexander CJ, Sipski ML, Findley TW. Sexual activities, desire, and satisfaction in males pre- and post-spinal cord injury. *Arch Sex Behav.* 1993;22(3):217-228.

Benevento BT, Sipski ML. Neurogenic bladder, neurogenic bowel, and sexual dysfunction in people with spinal cord injury. *Phys Ther.* 2002;82(6):601-612.

Borisoff JF, Elliott SL, Hocaloski S, Birch GE. The development of a sensory substitution system for the sexual rehabilitation of men with chronic spinal cord injury. *J Sex Med.* 2010;7(11):3647-3658.

Brackett NL, Nash MS, Lynne CM. Male fertility following spinal cord injury: facts and fiction. *Phys Ther.* 1996;76(11):1221-1231.

Burch A. Health care providers' knowledge, attitudes, and self-efficacy for working with patients with spinal cord injury who have diverse sexual orientations. *Phys Ther.* 2008;88(2):191-198.

Carpenter C. The experience of spinal cord injury: the individual's perspective—implications for rehabilitation practice. *Phys Ther.* 1994;74(7):614-628.

Couldrick L. Sexual issues within occupational therapy, part 1: attitudes and practice. *Br J Occupational Ther.* 1998;61:493-496.

Craik RL. Spinal cord injury: the bridge between basic science and clinical practice. *Phys Ther.* 2000;80:671-672.

Derogatis LR, Edelson J, Jordan R, Greenberg S, Portman DJ. Bremelanotide for female sexual dysfunctions: responder analyses from a phase 2B dose-ranging study. *Obstet Gynecol.* 2014;123(suppl 1):26S.

Ducharme SH, Gill KM. *Sexuality After Spinal Cord Injury: Answers to Your Questions.* Baltimore, MD: Paul H. Brooks Publishing; 1997.

Dumolin, Davis S, Taylor B. From PLISSIT to ExPLISSIT. In: Davis S, ed. *Rehabilitation: The Use of Theories and Models in Practice.* Edinburgh, United Kingdom: Elsevier Health Sciences, Churchill Livingstone; 2006:101-130.

Ferreiro-Velasco ME, Barca-Buyo A, de la Barrera SS, Montoto-Marqués A, Vázquez XM, Rodríguez-Sotillo A. Sexual issues in a sample of women with spinal cord injury. *Spinal Cord.* 2005;43(1):51-55.

Giaquinto S, Buzzelli S, Di Francesco L, et al. Evaluation of sexual changes after stroke. *J Clin Psychiatry.* 2003;64(3):302-307.

Hatzimouratidis K, Amar A, Eardley I, et al. Guidelines on male sexual dysfunction: erectile dysfunction and premature ejaculation. *European Urology.* 2010; 57:804-14. http://uroweb.org/wp-content/uploads/2010-Male-Sex-Dysfunction.pdf. Accessed December 23, 2015.

Hazeltine FP, Cole SS, Gray DB. *Reproductive Issues for Persons With Physical Disabilities.* Baltimore, MD: Paul H. Brooks Publishing; 1993.

Ide M. Sexuality in persons with limb amputation: a meaningful discussion of re-integration. *Disabil Rehabil.* 2004;26(14-15):939-943.

Kaufman M, Silverberg C, Odette F. *The Ultimate Guide to Sex and Disability: For All of Us Who Live With Disabilities, Chronic Pain, and Illness.* San Francisco, CA: Cleis Press; 2007.

Kingsberg SA, Woodard T. Female sexual dysfunction: focus on low desire. *Obstetr Gynecol.* 2015;125(2):477-486.

Krotoski DM, Nosek MA, Turk MA. *Women With Physical Disabilities—Achieving and Maintaining Health and Well Being.* Baltimore, MD: Paul H. Brooks Publishing; 1996.

Lavoisier P, Roy P, Dantony E, Watrelot A, Ruggeri J, Dumoulin S. Pelvic-floor muscle rehabilitation in erectile dysfunction and pre-mature ejaculation. *Phys Ther.* 2014;94(12):1731-1743.

Masters WH, Johnson V. *Human Sexuality.* Boston, MA: Little Brown & Co; 1966.

Nosek MA, Howland CA, Young ME, et al. Wellness models and sexuality among women with physical disabilities. *J Applied Rehabil Couns.* 1994;25:50-58.

Nosek MA, Rintala DH, Young ME, et al. Sexual functioning among women with physical disabilities. *Arch Phys Med Rehabil.* 1996;77(2):107-115.

Pynor R, Weerakoon P, Jones MK. A preliminary investigation of physiotherapy students' attitudes towards issues of sexuality in clini-cal practice. *Physiother.* 2005;91:42-48.

Rosenzweig N, Pearsall FP. *Sex Education for the Health Professional—A Curriculum Guide.* New York, NY: Grune & Stratton; 1978.

Sipski ML, Alexander, CJ. *Sexual Function in People With Disability and Chronic Illness: A Health Professional's Guide.* Gaithersburg, MD: Aspen; 1997.

Weerakoon P, Jones M, Kilburn-Watt E. Allied health professional students' perceived level of comfort in clinical situations that have sexual connotations. *J Allied Health.* 2004;33(3):189-193.

SUGGESTED VIEWING

Born on the Fourth of July (1989, Universal): Biography of Ron Kovic, a paralyzed Vietnam veteran who later becomes an anti-war and pro–human rights activist. It follows his travels and struggles adjusting to life post-Vietnam and explores issues of sexuality and disability.

Coming Home (1978, United Artists; 2004, MGM): Riveting drama about 3 people whose lives changed dramatically following the Vietnam War. It explores issues of sexuality, relationships, and disability.

Murderball (2005, MTV Films, Paramount Pictures): US Quadriplegic Rugby Team plays full-contact, fast-paced rugby in specialized wheelchairs, overcoming obstacles to compete in the Paralympic Games in Athens, Greece. It explores lives of wheelchair-abled athletes and their function. It blows away many stereotypes for those with disabilities and explores issues of bias, prejudice, sex, relationships, and disabilities.

The Waterdance (1993, The Samuel Goldwyn Company; 2001, Sony): Examines the struggles of dealing with paralysis following a cervical spine fracture from a hiking injury and explores issues of sexuality, relationships, and disability.

EDUCATIONAL RESOURCES

Christopher & Dana Reeve Foundation. Sexual health. http://www.christopherreeve.org/site/c.mtKZKgMWKwG/b.4453429/k.8982/Sexual_Health.htm.

Consortium for Spinal Cord Medicine. Sexuality and reproductive health in adults with spinal cord injury: a clinical practice guideline for health-care professionals. *J Spinal Cord Med.* 2010;33(3):281-336.

"This clinical practice guideline on sexuality and reproductive health was written for all health care professionals who care for individuals who have a SCI. In developing the guideline, the position was taken that all health care professionals have a role in promoting sexual health and that a positive attitude that encourages questions and education about sexuality must be conveyed by everyone who works with individuals with SCI. It is imperative that health care professionals be aware of their personal limitations and specific areas of expertise. Questions and concerns about sexuality should be referred to an appropriate specialist when a provider feels ill-equipped or uncomfortable answering a question or discussing a concern. Most important, discussion and education about sexuality needs to be tailored to each individual's specific needs and comfort level. Under all circumstances, ethical boundaries must remain the highest priority for everyone involved in the care of the people with SCI."

Decreased Sexual Desire Screener Brief Diagnostic Assessment for Generalized or Acquired HSDD. Boehringer Ingelheim Pharmaceuticals, Inc. 2010. www.obgynalliance.com/files/fsd/DSDS_Pocketcard.pdf. Accessed April 27, 2015.

Facing Disability: Expert Topics. http://www.facingdisability.com/expert-topics/what-is-the-first-thing-to-know-about-having-sex-after-a-spinal-cord-injury/diane-m-rowles-ms-np.

Facing Disability: Social Life and Sex After SCI. http://www.facingdisability.com/spinal-cord-injury-videos/social-life-and-sex.

McCollough L. Male sexual function after SCI. *Spinal Cord Injury SIG* newsletter. Winter 2014. http://www.neuropt.org/docs/sci-sig/sci-sig-winter-newsletter-2014.pdf.

The Miami Project to Cure Paralysis. http://www.miamiproject.miami.edu/.

Nahtail K, MacHattie E, Elliott SL, Krassloukov A. Pleasure ABLE: Sexual Device Manual for Persons With Disabilities. Disabilities Health Research Network. http://www.dhrn.ca/files/sexualhealthmanual_lowres_2010_0208.pdf.

National Rehabilitation Information Center. Sexuality, intimacy, and disability. http://www.naric.com/?q=en/node/80#Journal%20of%20Sexuality%20and%20Disability.

Explores sexuality, intimacy, and disability. The National Rehabilitation Information Center shares funded projects and research activities. Individuals with disabilities have the same emotional and physical sexual drives as people without disabilities. However, issues of sexual intimacy and disability remained unaddressed for many years. Individuals with disabilities seeking intimacy face psychosocial barriers such as stereotyping, a lack of adequate information, and negative societal and cultural attitudes regarding sexuality and disability and often lack the proper education and resources to prepare for intimate relationships. The National Rehabilitation Information Center shares funded projects and related research activities.

United Spinal Association. Sexuality for women with SCI. http://www.spinalcord.org/resource-center/askus/index.php?pg=kb.page&id=1579.

Sexuality Reborn (Kessler Foundation, Kessler Institute for Rehabilitation, West Orange, New Jersey; 1993). http://kesslerfoundation.org/consumers&families/resourcesandeducationalmaterials.php

In Sexuality Reborn, which was funded by the Paralyzed Veterans of America, 4 couples frankly discuss the physical and emotional effects of spinal cord injury. It was produced and narrated by Drs. Alexander and Sipski, with guest narrator, Ben Vereen. The couples demonstrate and share their personal experiences concerning: self-esteem, dating, bowel and bladder function, sexual response, and varying types of sexual activities. This video is 48 minutes in length and is an educational tool. This video is for spinal cord–injured and other physically disabled individuals. It can be viewed by individuals, their partners, or as part of a sexuality education session in rehabilitation. It contains sexually graphic content.

EXERCISES

EXERCISE 1: SEXUALITY AND DISABILITY

Respond to the following questions as a precheck and postcheck to your Chapter 17 learning.
Please check your answers following your chapter readings; answers for Exercise 1 follow Exercise 2.

Indicate **True** or **False**.

1. Sexual activity is more important than walking to some persons with paraplegia.   T   F

2. The menstrual period of a woman with a SCI will cease after the trauma and never resume.   T   F

3. Orgasm can be reached in men and women with SCI by stimulating parts of the body
    other than the genitals.   T   F

4. Erection in most men with SCI can be maintained as long as stimulation is present.   T   F

5. If the man with SCI can ejaculate, he is likely to be fertile.   T   F

6. Cesarean sections are necessary in women with SCI because their uterine muscles will
    no longer contract.   T   F

7. Fertility in men with SCI is low, but fertility is unaffected for women with SCI.   T   F

8. Sperm from a man with SCI can be obtained via electroejaculation and stored until there is
    enough for artificial insemination.   T   F

9. Muscle spasms in the extremities during sexual activity can result in either loss or
    facilitation of an erection.   T   F

10. The alteration in the body's heat regulatory mechanism could affect fertility of the man
    with SCI.   T   F

11. It is not appropriate for therapists/allied health care professionals to address sexual concerns
    of clients who have sustained a brain injury.   T   F

12. People who have had a brain injury and/or neurological injury should not be concerned with
    having a sexual relationship with their partner.   T   F

EXERCISE 2: PATIENT-PRACTITIONER INTERACTIONS

A series of case studies follow. Each involves an actual patient-practitioner scenario that may be encountered in the clinical setting. Divide into groups and discuss how you would handle the following PPIs. Discuss the case study as it is written among yourselves, but first write down how you would handle the patient's or other health care professional's requests before your discussion.

Use your understanding of the PLISSIT model in framing your response. Use your active listening skills and effective communication skills when presented with difficult and emotion-laden questions. Avoid using less-than-helpful responses, such as those mentioned in Chapter 7 (reassurance, judgmental responses, defensiveness), and remember that indifference is the most unhelpful response.

1. A 37-year-old divorced female with a complete C6-C7 lesion requests assistance from the sex counselor. She wishes to have sex with a male friend but is afraid that, "I won't be able to move my hips and clasp my legs around him." The sex counselor approaches you, the physical or occupational therapist, for specific information on the woman's hip movement capabilities and asks for possible assistance with pillow supports under her pelvis and legs and for some method of helping her hold her ankles together to clasp the male. What are your feelings as the sex counselor asks for this information?

2. A 49-year-old male with complete paraplegia and his 37-year-old wife expressed great concern about involuntary urinary and bowel discharge during sex play. The patient is on intermittent catheterization and uses a condom catheter during the daytime. The patient's wife approaches you for suggestions about alternate positions to avoid undue pressure or irritation for both partners. You verified the patient's sexual functioning status with the sex counselor before discussing these questions with the couple. How does this request make you feel? (Remember, feelings are one word.) What information must you have in order to respond to their request?

3. An 18-year-old female patient with spina bifida is engaged in a lighthearted conversation with a male physical therapy aide about the latest fashions and clothing styles while doing her exercises in the gym. Discussion focuses on the difference between "sexy" and "sensuous" clothing, and the patient turns to you for your opinion. What are you feeling? What would your response be? Does your code of ethics inform you on appropriate boundaries in this situation? If so, what are they?

4. A 21-year-old single male with quadriplegia turns to you, a female, to express his embarrassment over his constant erections (priapism), which are particularly noticeable while doing mat exercises. How would you feel? What would be an appropriate way to respond to him? Role-play this PPI in your group.

5. An 18-year-old female with complete T4 paraplegia is planning on going to her high school prom and then wants to spend the night afterward in a hotel with her boyfriend. She asks you, a female, for suggestions for different positions that she could use for sexual intercourse with her boyfriend. Before the accident, they were sexually active, and she is unsure what she is able to do now. Also, due to problems with thrombophlebitis, she is no longer able to take birth control pills and asks what other birth control method is possible. How would you feel? What would you respond? If you are a man, how would you tell your female colleagues to respond?

6. The wife of your 54-year-old patient with a previous MI asks to speak with you outside the physical therapy gym. Her husband is about to be discharged home, and she is uncertain about resumption of sexual activities due to his heart condition. Before his MI, they engaged in sexual intercourse 2 to 3 times per week for most of their 26-year marriage. She is afraid that he might have another heart attack if they resume sex. How would you feel? What advice would you give her?

7. A 57-year-old female patient with severe rheumatoid arthritis asks you about sexual activity now that her disease has progressed to severe joint immobility and pain. Previously, she and her husband had always favored the missionary position, but that has become impossible due to her lack of hip range of motion. How would you feel? Where would you direct her to go for the information she needs?

8. A 29-year-old female patient with severe low back pain approaches you with questions about positions for sexual intercourse that would not aggravate her back pain. You know that she has limited flexibility in her low back, either in flexion or extension. How would you feel? What would you do first to respond to her?

9. A 55-year-old male patient displays obvious discomfort as an older female nurse cares for him following complications of a cerebrovascular accident following prostate surgery. As head nurse in the intensive care unit, he asks to speak to you in private. He shares with you that he feels very uncomfortable being cared for by an older woman and he feels that his nurse is touching him inappropriately when caring for his surgical site. When you question him further, he tearfully tells you he is an adult survivor of sexual abuse. How would you feel? As the administrator of the unit, what are your duties and priorities? What would you say to the patient? What would you do to diminish his discomfort?

Exercise 3: Resource Reflections

Decades ago, the thought of addressing sexuality with patients during rehabilitation would have potentially been seen as taboo or controversial and infrequently accomplished by health care professionals. Today, health care professionals realize the importance and relevance of sexuality in the lives of their patients and must self-develop to not only be more comfortable in addressing the topic with their patients and clients, but also to serve as a resource in 3 specific areas: (1) educational information, (2) lending the "third ear" (see Chapter 13), and (3) appropriate interprofessional referral. With this in mind, please select 2 to 3 of the suggested additional readings, multimedia, and/or educational resources provided at the end of the chapter; review and provide your reflections, summarizing your self-learning and using the guiding questions which follow; and be prepared to share with your peers in roundtable discussions.

1. How did the additional resources specifically assist you in being more comfortable with aspects of sexuality and disability?

2. How do you feel now that you have completed the additional exploration of the topic for your self-learning? (Recall that feelings are one-word descriptors.) How has this resource changed your approach to practice?

3. How did each resource assist you in your health care professional role and abilities to do the following?:

   a. Provide educational information

   b. Enhance your skills in your ability to lend the "third ear" (see Chapter 13)

   c. Provide appropriate interprofessional referral

The exercises at the end of this chapter are also available online.
Please refer to the sticker in the front of the book and enter the access code provided.

COMMUNICATING WITH PEOPLE WHO ARE DYING AND THEIR FAMILIES

Carol M. Davis, DPT, EdD, MS, FAPTA and
Gina Maria Musolino, PT, MSEd, EdD

"The truth is that there is only one terminal dignity—love. And the story of a love is not important—what is important is that one is capable of love. It is perhaps the only glimpse we are permitted of eternity." –Helen Hayes

OBJECTIVES

- To clarify the importance of death and dying for the maturation of the health care professional (HCP).
- To emphasize the importance of the therapeutic communication skills of touch and active listening.
- To assist the reader to clarify current values around dying and death.
- To identify current values and current comfort around dying and death.
- To delineate the knowledge and skill needed to facilitate a life of quality for the dying patient.
- To describe the developmental stages health care professionals go through as they learn to cope with the anxiety of caring for dying patients.
- To emphasize the importance of a written living will and one's Five Wishes related to aging with dignity.

No one likes to contemplate death, except perhaps those for whom living has become entirely too painful. But to deny death totally throughout one's life, to refuse to reflect on the certainty that one day life will end for each one of us, is to avoid a wonderful opportunity for enriching the quality of one's life. You've heard the phrase, "The unexamined life is not worth living." Elisabeth Kübler-Ross wrote[1]:

> *It is the denial of death that is partially responsible for people living empty, purposeless lives; for when you live as if you'll live forever, it becomes too easy to postpone the things you know that you must do. You live your life in preparation for tomorrow or in remembrance of yesterday, and meanwhile, each today is lost. In contrast, when you fully understand that each day you awaken could be the last you have, you take the time that day to grow, to become more of who you really are to reach out to other human beings.*

Camus said, "There is only one liberty … to come to terms with death. After which, everything is possible."[2] Ernest Becker, in his Pulitzer prize-winning book, *The Denial of Death*,[2] wrote, "Of all the things that move men [and women],

Davis CM, Musolino GM. *Patient Practitioner Interaction: An Experiential Manual for Developing the Art of Health Care, Sixth Edition* (pp 323-338).
© 2016 SLACK Incorporated.

one of the principal ones is his [or her] death. … All historical religions address themselves to this same problem of how to bear the end of life."

This may seem like an unlikely chapter for a book aimed at facilitating professional socialization, but we believe that it deals with a topic that is most critical to the maturation of health care professionals. To grow into one's profession requires personal growth along with professional growth. To deal with death greatly enhances this life task. Some of you who have already lost a loved one will know what I mean when I say that this experience is unique in its ability to "grow one up" rapidly. James Agee, in *A Death in the Family*,[3] recounted a tale of fresh grief as experienced by several members of one family following the sudden death of the husband and father in a car accident. Mary, the victim's wife, stands in front of a mirror ready to place the mourning veil over her face as she dresses for the funeral. She thinks to herself:

I am carrying a heavier weight than I could have dreamed it possible for a human being to carry, yet I am living through it. … She thought: this is simply what living is; I never realized before what it is … now I am more nearly a grown member of the human race; bearing children, which has seemed so much, was just so much apprenticeship. She thought that she has never before had a chance to realize the strength that human beings have to endure.

THE EXISTENTIAL FEAR OF DEATH

Children are not born with a fear of death. At about age 3 years, children begin to deal with object loss and experience fear at the disappearance of a parent and joy at playing peek-a-boo. It is not until age 10 or so that we begin to realize what it means for "life to disappear forever."[2] In fact, if fear of death were held constantly conscious, we would be unable to function normally, so we repress it, and by adulthood, the common thought is, "I know I'll die one day, but I'm having too much fun living to worry about it."[2]

We can ignore our fears of death, or we can carefully absorb them and repress them in what Becker[2] described as our "life-expanding process." With each victory in life comes a feeling of indestructibility, of proven power. Each time we notice the strength of our bodies, recover from the flu, avoid an automobile accident, or narrowly escape an injury—or, more phenomenal yet, escape death—we further prove that we are indestructible. In addition, as we grow into secure and loving relationships with partners, parents, and children, we feel secure support and appreciation for our existence, and a warmly enhanced sense of self acts to further repress the fear of our inevitable death. A healthy self-esteem doesn't have time to ponder death, we believe.

Only when death confronts us in remarkable ways do we even consider our own mortality. Besides near-death experiences, perhaps the deepest assault to our repression of the fear of death as health care professionals is to care for a patient or a cherished family member who is close to the moment of death. If we pay close attention, an indescribable glimpse into the soul is possible.

WHY CONCERN OURSELVES WITH DEATH AND DYING IN HEALTH CARE?

To come to terms with imminent death is one of the most difficult tasks human beings ever have to face, and we face it absolutely alone. No one can take our death away from us or give us the courage to die. However, the role others play at our side during this intense time can be tremendously helpful or cruelly fragmenting and hurtful.

The quality of the help we render to those who are dying and their families has everything to do with our own ideas, values, and fears about death, and until we clarify those ideas and values and confront our fears, we will be apt to increase the burden that is already almost too great to bear.

When death is imminent, we will be governed by what is deep inside of us, and our patients or loved ones will either benefit or suffer. If our fears of death predominate, we will deny the inevitable or defend fiercely against it. Out of our inner anxiety will emanate denial statements such as, "Oh hogwash! You're healthier than I am! You're going to live forever!" or, "Don't talk like that, silly. It makes me depressed." If our fears get stirred up too much and our denial starts to break, we can expect anger and aggressive and passive-aggressive assaults against those who are suffering.

Just before we took my father home from the hospital to die (he was given 6 to 8 weeks more to live after fighting cancer of the larynx with brain metastasis for the greater part of 2 years), the young nurse came to my father's hospital room and harshly asked, "Are you the daughter?" When I replied, "Yes, I'm John's daughter," he cautioned me as he flipped a vial of pills in front of my face, my father's medication for pain: "Now, don't give this to him when he asks for it, give it like the label says. I can't help it if he's in pain; he has to learn to endure it. If you give him medication every time he asks for it and he comes back here to my unit, I'll have to be in his room every hour or so, and I have 30 other people who need me just as much as he does."

I felt frightened and assaulted in that moment by a person who had supposedly studied to be a healing professional. The more our behavior is governed by our denial and fear of death, the greater the chance that we will add to the already overwhelming burdens of the patient and the family as they struggle with one of life's deepest pains. As health care professionals, we should work hard to never lose touch with our feelings and emotions about all matters of life and death. When needed, we should not hesitate to seek our own counseling and debriefing to work on our own coping strategies and abilities so that we can best serve our patients. Trauma and loss abound in health care, and debriefing from critical incident stressors is vital for effective coping and not becoming numb and insensitive. Follow-up counseling is certainly utilized by the healthiest of health care professionals to maintain psychological well-being. It takes courage and strength to cope and not just push the feelings aside or suppress them and later have them resurface inappropriately or at the expense of our patients and their families and caregivers.

Author and dancer Isadora Duncan lost both of her young children in a tragic accident in which a taxicab carrying them both fell in the water and they drowned. After the accident, she fled to her friend, the Italian actress Eleanora Duse, at her villa in Italy. Her friend knew how to help her grieve and did not offer platitudes or sit with her in embarrassed silence, offering her ideas and activities to "take her mind off her worries." She allowed Duncan to feel what had happened to her, to experience her loss. Duncan wrote in *My Life*[4]:

> *The next morning I drove out to see Duse. … She took me in her arms and her wonderful eyes beamed upon me such love and tenderness that I felt just as Dante must have felt when, in "Paradisio," he encounters the Divine Beatrice. From then on I lived at Biareggio, finding courage from the radiance of Eleanora's eyes. She used to rock me in her arms, consoling my pain, but not only consoling me, for she seemed to take my sorrow to her own breast, and I realized that if I had not been able to bear the society of other people, it was because they all played the comedy of trying to cheer me with forgetfulness. Whereas Eleanora said: "Tell me about Deidre and Patrick," and made me repeat to her all their little sayings and ways, and show her their photos, which she kissed and cried over. She never said, "Cease to grieve," but she grieved with me, for the first time since their death, I felt I was not alone.*

As a health care professional, you will not be called upon to provide this level of support and caring. However, once people have matured and confronted their innate fears of death, we find that their ability to comfort and support the dying in whatever way is needed in the moment develops into quite profound skill and sensitivity. Susan Block and Andrew Billings,[5] physician educators, wrote in the *New England Journal of Medicine* about teaching a course to first-year medical students called "Living With a Life-Threatening Illness." Students visited critically ill patients in their homes and interviewed them, asking them about their lives, focusing on how different patients and families deal with dying, truth telling, decision making, and after-death rituals. When asked how this course helped to prepare students for providing end-of-life care, they reported[5]:

> *[The students'] tendency to avoid the sadness, hopelessness, and helplessness they had associated with a dying person is replaced by a sense of the approachability of the dying, an interest in the medical, psychosocial, and spiritual aspects of "the case," and a belief in the possibility of doing good work through such encounters.*

They learned to value the patient's perspective and to understand that each person's approach to dealing with illness is unique.[5]

When we get beyond our defenses about death, we can then learn how to be therapeutically present for the dying. Life affirmation replaces death denial, and our actions are characterized by an intrinsic belief that life, moment to moment, is good and that we have the power to do something about the quality of a person's life, moment to moment. We realize that, even in the face of inevitable death, the support and comfort of family and mature health care professionals can actually help the patient transform his or her last days into some of the most rich and meaningful of his or her entire life.

Confronting our fears of death is not easy, and we reflexively avoid it. But when we face this task with courage, we experience a quality of growth that is unparalleled in our development, personally and professionally.

QUALITY OF LIFE IS MORE IMPORTANT THAN QUANTITY

Each one of us will die. We're only here for a short time on earth. The average life expectancy is about 76 to 81 years (78.8 years average in United States), which may seem like forever to us when we are young, but as we approach that age, we will wonder where the years went. Dying is a holistic experience. All of a person is involved—the physical part of us "gives up the ghost," the intellectual often struggles with meaning, the emotional with the deep feelings of the inevitability of this moment, and the spirit is released to continue on in a journey that we can only speculate about.

The lucky ones among us will have time to prepare for death. We believe this preparation time is a cherished gift, not just because it feels good to be able to tie up loose ends, to tell our dear friends how much life with them has meant to us, and to make final arrangements. In most cases, when you know your time is very limited and you accept the inevitability of your death, the quality of that time increases exponentially. You become as liberated as a 4-year-old child in your intentions and in your communication. You ask for what you want and you say what you really feel without the concern for whether someone will think ill of you or not like you. This is a tremendously freeing experience. Commonly felt anxieties are replaced with living each moment just as you wish because these are your last moments here on earth, and they are very precious because few of us feel that we really know what lies beyond death. Genuine, heartfelt feelings are expressed. There is no time for superficialities or small talk unless one chooses. Every conversation reflects deeply held thoughts and values. Great wisdom is passed along without fear of being accused of egocentrism. In fact, the predominant feeling becomes, "What is to be feared now?" The ultimate fear has been confronted. The goal becomes how to live well the remaining time, rather than how to avoid death. This acceptance does not happen all at once but takes place in stages over time, as we'll discuss in a moment.

When we, as health care professionals, take the opportunity to work with the dying, the quality of our lives can also improve. However, we find it far easier to be present to the dying, who have accepted the inevitability of their imminent death, than to work with patients and families, who refuse to face inevitable death and live each day working furiously to maintain denial or controlling the anxiety of the inevitable. There are few worse situations in life than to try to be present, in a therapeutic way, to a patient or family who is denying imminent death. This situation most often develops out of a mistaken fear that the patient (or family) will lose hope and the patient will give up the will to live. Studies reveal the opposite.[6] Depression and the loss of hope may appear as part of the coping of dealing with dying, but these feelings usually do not last long and are replaced by hope for more realistic things. For example, patients will maintain their hope for a miracle, all the while accepting the inevitability of death. Then, more pragmatically, they will shift their emphasis to, for example, the hope to live long enough to see a child be married or return home to see loved ones or pets.[6]

STAGES OF LOSS

Elisabeth Kübler-Ross, in her well-known book *On Death and Dying*,[6] described what we can expect to experience as we go through the loss of a loved one or experience our own dying. People initially experience a **denial** at the news of impending or actual death of a loved one. The most extreme forms of denial include total repression of the news or actually losing consciousness. Denial is often followed by **anger**. Once we allow the news to begin to penetrate, intense feelings of anger can be expected to emerge. Health care professionals must take care not to personalize this anger, but to allow patients to fully experience it and express it. This is made more difficult in a society that does not tolerate emotional outbursts of any kind.

Following anger, the patient often experiences a brief **bargaining** phase in which a kind of deal is cut with life, with fate, or with God. For example, one will hear such thoughts as, "Okay, I know I'm going to die soon, but please let me live long enough to see my children get married." Or, "If I can live, I'll never smoke another cigarette again."

Often the next stage that emerges is **depression**. Patients become quiet and more lethargic, reacting to the undeniability of this news, as they live with it, day after day. They keep to themselves, often refusing to see visitors or speak to certain family members. Reactive depression then leads into a preparatory depression in which patients quietly reflect on the sadness of their fate and prepare for inevitable death.

Finally, patients move into **acceptance** of their fate and begin to live life as a precious gift. Not everyone reaches this stage before dying, and very often these stages do not occur in a linear sequence. It is quite common to hear a patient who seems to have worked through the stages into acceptance say, for example, "Next year I'm going to plant a different garden. I'm tired of the same old flowers. I'm going to rethink the whole layout and do it the way I always wanted to."

Thus, the dynamics of coping with inevitable death take on a certain predictable rhythm and character, **but each person copes in his or her unique way**.[5-7] It would be wrong to suggest that each and every person follows the same identical linear pattern of coping stages. Likewise, family members go through their own unique stage processes, and it can become quite complex just trying to keep track of where each person is in the process of accepting one person's imminent death. The patient may be in acceptance, but her husband may still be angry. Children may need to deny until the end. It takes great sensitivity and acceptance to be willing to be therapeutically present to each of these people and requires that we choose to believe that each one is doing the very best he or she can, at the moment, to cope. It is not our role to force reality onto them.

Most important, be careful not to use this knowledge of the various stages as a way of diminishing the importance of certain statements and removing them from the context of their meaning. For example, to say, "Oh, he's just in the anger stage. He'll get over that" as a way to avoid meaningful interaction is not a wise use of this knowledge.

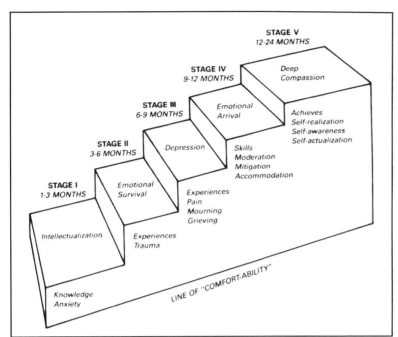

Figure 18-1. Coping with professional anxiety in terminal illness. (Reprinted with permission from Harper B. *Death: The Coping Mechanism of the Health Professional.* Greenville, SC: Southeastern University Press; 1977.)

PREDICTABLE RESPONSES FROM CAREGIVERS

Working with the dying can become a great challenge, depending on the extent to which we have confronted our own fears and the extent to which the patient and family have accepted the inevitability of the imminent death. What data exist to help us understand our natural responses to this caregiving challenge? How can we be guided to offer a healing response no matter the atmosphere surrounding the patient?

Beatrice Harper[7] has studied the development of health care professionals' ability to cope with the anxiety surrounding the death of their patients. Figure 18-1 illustrates the 5 stages of coping she observed in social workers as they dealt with their anxiety about dying patients. She observed that the nature and intensity of anxiety of caregivers shifted in a developmentally predictable way from stage I (intellectualization, characterized by the need to deny and intellectualize death) to the inevitable stage V (deep compassion, characterized by the development of the ability to give of oneself and a feeling of comfort in relation to oneself, the patient, the family, and the tasks of caregiving).

Figure 18-1 can help you anticipate and analyze your responses when you first confront a patient who is dying. We offer it to assure you that your therapeutic skill in caring for the dying will develop and improve and to remind you that caregiving for the ill involves a personal as well as professional growth process. You should not expect yourself to be an expert in this area from the very start. Here is a good example:

In a 2-year study, residents in the intensive care units at the University of Washington and University of Utah hospitals participated in "death rounds" once each month.[8] They met regularly to debrief and to respond to 3 questions following the deaths of patients in their intensive care unit: (1) Did you have any concerns about how care was provided?; (2) What could have been done differently?; and (3) How did it feel? The study, reported in the *Journal of Critical Care*,[8] found that the residents who attended death rounds regularly became increasingly more at ease with dealing with dying and death and appreciated the opportunity to discuss their feelings about how they and the staff responded to situations, as they unfolded, that led to the deaths of their patients. The residents felt that this experience, over time, helped improve their ability to care for dying patients, and even the more introverted residents were eventually able to express emotions around this experience, which they felt was beneficial in their ability to help others.

THERAPEUTIC PRESENCE IN THE ATMOSPHERE OF DENIAL OF IMMINENT DEATH

The atmosphere of death denial is very uncomfortable. As mentioned earlier, there seems to be an aura of fear surrounding the patient and family member; a false cheerfulness pervades that is edged with an iciness of the need to control every situation and every conversation. Instead of feelings of liberation, genuineness, and authenticity, we feel surrounded by paranoia, fear, defensiveness, and nervous chatter. Silence is often avoided, as is warm eye contact.

When we contribute to the conspiracy of silence, we condemn a patient to the pain of facing death alone.[7] Our task is not to judge those who need to deny death or to contribute to that conspiracy. Rather, we can help more by accepting his or her fear and by realizing that his or her need to deny is very likely well intentioned. Active listening skills are imperative, as is the use of touch.[9] The health care professional would do well to find out what the patient has been told and what the patient's response has been to what he or she has been told. Knowing what the patient has been told allows the health care professional to support and interpret the health care team's plan of treatment. How the patient feels dictates the main thrust of the treatment approach.

Whether the patient has accepted the imminence of death or not, our approach to caring remains essentially the same. Debra Flomenhoft,[9] a physical therapist who died of cancer, wrote the following important suggestions after having undergone treatment for more than a year:

- Don't be afraid to say the wrong thing, and don't keep silent out of that fear. Silence is often interpreted as avoidance and rejection. Instead of worrying about the content of your response, reach out to the patient and show your support by actively listening and allowing the patient to talk.

- Learn to recognize your feelings and the effect these feelings may have on the communication process. Direct your predictable anger at something other than the patient.

- When patients ask the hard questions (eg, "Why me?"), don't respond by trying to fix it. Patients aren't looking for answers as much as they are expressing grief and anger. Allow that expression. Supportive listening is the best response.

- Recognize the importance of touch, even as simple as a handshake or a touch on the shoulder. Communicate with touch and eye contact that you care and that you are there to listen and to do whatever you can to maintain or improve the quality of the patient's life.

- Don't assume that patients want to talk about their illness. Ask the patient if he or she wants to talk about his or her illness before initiating a discussion.

- Never assume that you know what the patient is feeling. Ask instead, "Am I right that you are feeling...?"

- Communicate confidence in your therapeutic skills both verbally and nonverbally. This is essential for patient trust. Answer the patient with authority and no hesitation, and if you don't know the answer, simply say, "I can't answer that, but I will find out who can."

- Don't try to anticipate which stage of coping patients are in, or that they will progress through the stages in exact linear sequence. Accept patients where they are, each day, with caring and understanding. Try to view the impending death from the patient's perspective, not from the "theory" of dealing with loss.

- Take care not to contribute to isolation of the patient as death nears. Once a relationship has been established, work to maintain it, even if the required therapy is minimal or the patient has been discharged from your service. Stopping in to say hello, no matter how busy you are, will mean a great deal.

- Help patients maintain hope at all costs. Maintaining hope is not in direct conflict with being realistic. The value of hope far exceeds the need to face the truth of the inevitable. One can feel hope in spite of imminent death, and it is important to nurture and sustain it, being both realistic and hopeful at the same time. Learn to communicate honestly and frankly, always with hope.

- Take care of your own emotional needs to prevent professional burnout so that you can continue to communicate care, sympathy, and support to the patient and family. If you need help in dealing with your feelings, get it. Your patient can't wait for you to grow at your own pace.

What do dying patients want and deserve to have with regard to care? Table 18-1 illustrates the Dying Person's Bill of Rights, which was developed by the Southwestern Michigan Inservice Education Council.[10] Read each item carefully. Each right represents the minimal goals for care by which we all should be guided.

PALLIATIVE CARE

Many patients would like to be able to die at home, but for those for whom that is not possible, palliative care programs are offered in institutions to provide pain control and simple quality of life measures similar to hospice care. The growth of palliative care programs in hospitals in the United States has been documented to be significant. Between 2000 and

TABLE 18-1
THE DYING PERSON'S BILL OF RIGHTS
○ I have the right to be treated as a living human being until I die.
○ I have the right to maintain a sense of hopefulness, however changing its focus may be.
○ I have the right to be cared for by those who can maintain a sense of hopefulness, however changing this might be.
○ I have the right to express my feelings and emotions about my approaching death, in my own way.
○ I have the right to participate in decisions concerning my case.
○ I have the right to expect continuing medical and nursing attention even though "cure" goals must be changed to "comfort" goals.
○ I have the right not to die alone.
○ I have the right to be free from pain.
○ I have the right to have my questions answered honestly.
○ I have the right not to be deceived.
○ I have the right to have help from and for my family in accepting my death.
○ I have the right to die in peace and dignity.
○ I have the right to retain my individuality and not be judged for my decisions, which may be contrary to the beliefs of others.
○ I have the right to expect that the sanctity of the human body will be respected after death.
○ I have the right to be cared for by caring, sensitive, knowledgeable people who will attempt to understand my needs and will be able to gain some satisfaction.
Adapted from Barbus A. The Dying Person's Bill of Rights. Presented at: The Terminally Ill Patient and the Helping Person. Southwestern Michigan In-service Education Council. Lansing, MI; 1975.

2003, the number of palliative care programs grew from 15% to 25% of hospitals surveyed by the American Hospital Association.[11] Once the family agrees, physicians and health care staff do all they can to keep patients comfortable, control pain, and allow family to be present. Do-not-resuscitate orders are firmly agreed to and hopefully determined in advance of the final stage of life.[11]

HOSPICE CARE

An effective way of helping to ensure therapeutic effectiveness in caring for the dying is the hospice movement. Hospice is not a building but a philosophy of care that promises that the patient will die with pain controlled to the greatest possible extent and that the quality of life will become the primary focus of all treatment. Hospice is considered to be the model for quality, compassionate care for people facing life-limiting illness or injury and involves a team to manage medical care, pain management, and emotional and spiritual support. Interdisciplinary team members each contribute to the care of the patient through direct services, often in the home, and by teaching family members and volunteers how to ensure that the quality of life for the patient remains as high as possible. Pain is controlled while maintaining alertness. Death is accepted as inevitable, and family members are encouraged to talk openly with patients in preparation for the time of death. In addition to effective control of pain, it is important for the physical and occupational therapists to teach the patient and family how to keep the lived world of the patient as large as possible, for as long as possible. By lived world, we mean the world that is accessible for the patient to live in.

Traditionally, our lived world shrinks from almost limitless possibilities (given funds and opportunity to travel) to confinement to a chair or bed in one room as we age and become unable to move about. Range of motion, ambulation with support, bed mobility, getting up for meals, even placing the bed in the living room in front of a window, all help to prevent the lived world of the patient from shrinking to a circle on the ceiling above the bed, as some patients have reported. Family members have utilized technology to project images (in a user-friendly format) of a person's life and family for their recollection, reliving, and reflection. If the patient wishes, the time to celebrate his or her life is a welcome opportunity to share and for you to learn and appreciate your patient more too. The health care professional can help by learning the patient's life story and incorporating it with his or her care. The quality of life has every bit to do with how much of the world is available for us to experience.

Family members are encouraged to be around the patient as the patient requests. Pets are allowed to be close by for comfort. The atmosphere becomes one of living life fully. Pain control is made possible through finely titrated narcotics, massage and exercise to the patient's tolerance, and the use of transcutaneous electrical stimulation (TENS) to the nervous system. Patients often respond very favorably to TENS, especially in the presence of severe, intractable pain, often accompanying imminent death.[12]

Importance of a Living Will—The Schiavo Case

Throughout the latter part of 2004 and early 2005, the media in the United States detailed the struggle of Terri Schiavo, a young woman in Florida who had been in an irreversible coma for more than 10 years and was being cared for in a hospice.[13] Her husband wanted to honor her verbal wishes to not have her life extended by extraordinary means under these circumstances, but because Ms. Schiavo never wrote down her wishes in a living will or end-of-life document, her parents contested her husband's decision to remove her feeding tube and allow her to die and took their case to the Florida Supreme Court. The court ruled that her husband had the final authority, not her parents, and ruled in favor of the husband. The parents appealed but lost in court, and Terri Schiavo died peacefully a week after removal of the feeding tube, with her husband at her side.

There were many lessons learned from this case. Primary is the importance of writing down and sharing with close family members your wishes for end-of-life care, as specifically as you can. This is an ethical dilemma between beneficence and autonomy. It seemed as though everyone wanted to do for Terri Schiavo what they felt she wanted, but no written instructions were made to help them. The court ruled that her husband had more recent and intimate knowledge of her wishes than her parents, but her parents had been caring for her for the better part of the last decade of her life and found great meaning in that process. They held out hope that one day she would wake up and heal from this crisis.

Unfortunately, the main fact that the media failed to mention in many of the debates was that those who believed that Terri Schiavo would wake up one day and be back to her old self didn't know or chose to ignore, for personal reasons, that this was impossible given the magnetic resonance images of her brain. Her ventricles had expanded to the point that the greater percentage of her cranium was filled with fluid; insufficient gray matter existed to support meaningful cognition.

Terri Schiavo went into cardiac arrest as a result of a metabolic electrolyte imbalance in her early 20s, most likely due to a lifelong struggle with anorexia. When young people are doing their best to be approved of and loved by others, the last thing on their minds would be to create a living will. The fear of death, or the superstition that thinking about one's death will bring it on, must be faced to confront this issue in a mature way. Perhaps Terri Schiavo's gift to others will be to point out the extreme dangers of anorexia and to emphasize the critical importance of creating a living will and communicating to your loved ones your wishes, if you should lapse into irreversible coma or brain death. It is important to share your choices for advance directives and let others know your wishes so they don't have to make hard choices without your input if you become very ill or have a bad accident. Today, as a gift to our own family and friends, we can complete our Five Wishes for aging with dignity, at any age, and voice our choices online, print and sign them, and encourage our patients, clients, family members, and colleagues to do the same (http://www.fivewishes.org/).

Other Issues

This chapter does not have the space to deal with several important issues that accompany a consideration of death. The moral issues of "mercy killing" or euthanasia (active and passive), suicide, the unique needs of persons around the world who are dying from AIDS, and the fascination with past lives as described by Dr. Brian L. Weiss[14] are just 4 issues that would require greater attention than this chapter can give them. After the fear of death is confronted, it becomes easier to read and study such topics independently. All are critically important to one's development as a health care professional.

Finally, there exists some controversy around the topic of near-death experiences as researched by Moody[15] and around the person of Elisabeth Kübler-Ross.[16] Any consideration of death must, by necessity, incorporate the spiritual because to ask, "Why have I lived?" is a spiritual question (see Chapter 14). It is within this category of awareness that much criticism was leveled at Kübler-Ross. I would encourage you to read about this controversy and form your own opinions. Once you have experienced the death of one who resides in your innermost circles of self, these readings—indeed, this entire chapter—will likely assume new meaning. For now, deal with this material seriously and as best you can. You may wish to revisit the chapter at a later point in your life journey and as you gain additional experiences with direct patient care.

Victor Frankl,[17] a survivor of 2 Nazi death camps, said, "Everything can be taken from a man [or woman] but one thing: The last of the human freedoms—to choose one's attitude in any given set of circumstances, to choose one's own way." To accept death as a necessary part of life is not resignation; it is surrender to an opportunity to grow into one's own complete humanness. I conclude with the following thoughts from Elisabeth Kübler-Ross[1]:

> *We are living in a time of uncertainty, anxiety, fear, and despair. It is essential that you become aware of the light, power, and strength within each of you, and that you learn to use those inner resources in service of your own and others' growth. The world is in desperate need of human beings whose own level of growth is sufficient to enable them to learn to live and work with others cooperatively and lovingly, to care for others—not for what those others can do for you or for what they think of you, but rather in terms of what you can do for them. If you send forth love to others, you will receive in return the reflection of that love; because of your loving behavior, you will grow, and you will shine a light that will brighten the darkness of the time we live in—whether it is in a sickroom of a dying patient, on the corner of a ghetto street in Harlem, or in your own home. Humankind will survive only through the commitment and involvement of individuals in their own and others' growth and development as human beings. [Through this commitment will come] … the evolution of the whole species to become all that humankind can and is meant to be. Death is the key to that evolution. For only when we understand the real meaning of death to human existence will we have the courage to become what we are destined to be.*

CONCLUSION

This text is devoted to helping you, as health care professionals, grow to be mature and healing in your very nature, so that your actions with those needing your help will be healing and therapeutically whole. The goals for this chapter are for you to confront your own fears about death at whatever level you can at this time in order for you to become more aware of whom you are to be. By way of reflection on this content and completing the exercises, you will conduct a current values clarification about death, recognizing your experiences of death-denying rather than life-affirming ways.

What should our goals be with persons who are facing imminent death? In sum, what we want to achieve with dying patients includes the following:

- Assist the patient to remain in control of most decisions concerning daily life for as long as possible and serve as the advocate for his or her wishes when called upon.

- Keep the patient's lived world (the world available for the patient to move about) as large as possible for as long as possible by helping the family learn to transfer or assist with ambulation or wheelchair management, assist with transfers out of bed, or move the bed to an appropriate place to avoid isolation, and work to incorporate the patient's life stories in the provision of health care.

- Control pain with medication, activity, imagery, and TENS, yet allow maximum alertness.

- Along with other health care professionals, perform professional skills with self-confidence and patience, being sure to include the patient and family in the therapeutic process.

- Provide support for loved ones and family, realizing that each is in different stages of coping with the impending loss of a loved one.

- Utilize active listening skills and touch as our primary forms of communication, allowing the dying person to have control over the topics and length of conversations.

- Avoid the desire to want to fix anything.

- Be willing to stand by, to touch, to reach out, and to risk in the face of our own fears.

- Clarify in writing (see Exercise 2), your wishes at the end of your life.

This is not an easy task. Stanley Kellerman, in *Living Your Dying*,[18] said, "There's big dying and there's little dying." As health care professionals, we confront loss of health and mobility as a "little death" rather regularly. In your day-to-day patient care, always remember that people cope with little deaths similarly to big deaths.

Now move on to the exercises, and don't forget to journal about what you're feeling and about what you've learned.

References

1. Kübler-Ross E. *Death—The Final Stage of Growth.* Englewood Cliffs, NJ: Prentice Hall; 1975.
2. Becker E. *The Denial of Death.* New York, NY: Free Press; 1973.
3. Agee J. *A Death in the Family.* New York, NY: Grosset and Dunlap; 1957.
4. Duncan I. *My Life.* New York, NY: Liveright Publishing Corp; 1955.
5. Block SD, Billings JA. Becoming a physician—learning from the dying. *N Engl J Med.* 2005;353:1313-1315.
6. Kübler-Ross E. *On Death and Dying.* New York, NY: Macmillan; 1969.
7. Harper B. *Death: The Coping Mechanisms of the Health Professional.* Greenville, SC: Southeastern University Press; 1977.
8. Hough CL, Hudson LD, Salud A, Lahey T, Curtis JR. Death rounds: end of life discussions among medical residents in the intensive care unit. *J Crit Care.* 2005;20:20-25.
9. Flomenhoft DA. Understanding and helping people who have cancer. *Phys Ther.* 1984;4:1232-1234.
10. Barbus A. The Dying Person's Bill of Rights. Paper presented at: The Terminally Ill Patient and the Helping Person. Southwestern Michigan In-service Education Council. Lansing, MI; 1975.
11. Morrison RS, Maroney-Galin C, Kralovec PD, Meier DE. The growth of palliative care programs in United States hospitals. *J Palliat Med.* 2005;8:1127-1134.
12. Reuss R. Hospice: one PT's personal account. *Clin Manage.* 1985;4(6):28-37.
13. Quill T. Terri Schiavo—a tragedy compounded. *N Engl J Med.* 2005;352:1630-1634.
14. Weiss BL. *Many Lives, Many Master.* New York, NY: Simon and Schuster; 1990.
15. Moody R. The light beyond. *New Age J.* 1988;May-June:55-67.
16. Nietzke A. The miracle of Kübler-Ross. *Hum Behav.* 1977;206-211,254.
17. Frankl V. *Man's Search for Meaning.* New York, NY: Washington Square Press; 1963.
18. Kellerman S. *Living Your Dying.* New York, NY: Random House; 1974.

EXERCISES

EXERCISE 1: PERSONAL DEATH HISTORY

Answer the following history questions.

1. The first death I ever experienced was the death of:

2. I was _____ years old.

3. At that time I felt:

4. I was most curious about:

5. The things that frightened me most were:

6. The feelings I have now as I think of that death are:

7. The first funeral I ever attended was for:

8. The most intriguing thing about the funeral was:

9. I was most scared or upset at the funeral by:

10. The first personal acquaintance of my own age who died was:

11. I remember thinking:

12. I lost my first parent when I was:

13. The death of this parent was especially significant because:

14. The most recent death I experienced was when _____ died _____ years ago.

15. The most traumatic death I ever experienced was:

16. At age _____ I personally came closest to death when:

17. The most significant loss I have ever had to endure was:

Because:

What insights come to you as you review your answers or as you discuss your answers with a classmate? What do these answers have to do with your current ideas about death? The next exercise will help you clarify your current ideas.

(Adapted from Worden JW, Proctor W. *Personal Death Awareness.* Englewood Cliffs, NJ: Prentice Hall; 1976.)

EXERCISE 2: VALUES AROUND DEATH AND DYING

In order to better clarify your current feelings, attitudes, and beliefs concerning death and dying, please reflect on and respond to the following questions:

1. When I die, I believe that... (What will happen?):

2. I would rather die... (Suddenly and without warning or after being given a period of time in which to say goodbye to loved ones? What beliefs make me say this?):

3. When I die, I'd like the following to be done. (Be as specific as possible. Make a list.):

4. The person I want to be in charge of this process is:

    Because:

5. The worst possible thing that could happen to me around my dying and death is:

6. As a health care professional, the best thing I can do for my dying patients and their families is:

    Because:

EXERCISE 3: HOPE AND HOSPICE

You are working with a John, a 59-year-old White male patient who was referred from hospice to keep his endurance and activity levels as high as possible and to assist with his ability to complete activities of daily living (ADLs.) You have come to know the patient as a formerly thriving engineer, and, due to his cancer, he is unable to return to work because of fatigue from radiation therapy. The 1920s building he works in has his office on the second floor. There is no elevator, and the first floor is the machinery production floor. Your patient does not anticipate returning to work and reports he does not have the mental stamina for the job any longer. He enjoys classical music, problem solving, and spending time with his wife of 40 years. John understands that his cancer is terminal and that he has been given a prognosis of 2 to 4 months to live. His goal is to be able to continue to get to the bathroom with assistance of the walker; to maintain, as he states, "his dignity"; to stay as strong and mobile as possible around the home; and to feed himself. He knows he does not have long to live and is realistic in his goals. He appreciates all the help of the hospice care providers. You have also met the patient's overbearing yet well-meaning and loving wife and homemaker, who is working with a lawyer, trying to get the company he worked for to install an elevator. She wants him to be able to walk more so he can return to work and attend church with her on Sundays. Each home visit, you continue to educate the hospice aides and the patient's wife in how they can assist him in his home program activities and the related precautions and contraindications to keep John as safe and comfortable as possible. Some of the aides are not following the home program because they don't see it as their job, and they express this to you. You have also educated the patient's wife and caregivers in the appropriate body mechanics and safe patient-handling skills; you consider aspects of the transtheoretical model of change (see Chapter 15) in your educational approach. You recommend some adaptive equipment to assist in his ADL functions.

In the course of your twice-weekly home visits, John has had varied and fluctuating abilities physically. As his condition and vitals tolerate, John has been able to walk short distances of 50 to 200 feet, endurance dependent, with a rolling walker and minimal to moderate assistance of one person, and he completes generalized strengthening and conditioning exercises to tolerance. Although John is more of a quiet man and deep thinker, he begins to share more of his life story. John shares some of his work accomplishments during rest periods while on your strolls and speaks with warmhearted remembrance of dates with his wife and of their vacation travels. John's wife is planning to have a bed brought in for the downstairs to the living room in the next few weeks just during his chemo time so he does not have to deal with the stairs at home, but she is not happy about the rearrangement because she will miss him at night. John tries to make light of the situation. Using the permission, limited information, specific suggestions, and intensive therapy (PLISSIT) model and some bridge statements (see Chapter 17), you recognize that the couple shares loving embraces and massages and pleasure each other with sexual activities but are no longer interested in sexual intercourse. John and his wife are careful not to overfatigue him in these sexual activities. No referral is needed.

As the first few weeks of care commence, on good days, John takes short strolls in the driveway to the sidewalk, picks up the mail from the mailbox, and completes 15 to 20 minutes of exercise activity. On bad days, John can barely walk to the bathroom due to the toll of the 3-times-weekly chemotherapy sessions and the related side effects. His recovery time following bouts of exercise and ADLs is becoming more prolonged. John has begun occasionally using a bedside commode and urinal when he is particularly fatigued. John has bouts of intense nausea, hair loss, and difficulties with bowel and bladder movements at times; is beginning to present with muscle atrophy; and at times has labored breathing.

In the third week, John is utilizing intravenous-drip morphine and a pain-control pump more regularly to control his pain. In the fourth week of care, he is unable to rise from the bed, so you complete all the care at the bedside. You turn on the patient's classical music to assist in his comfort during the therapy session. As you begin working with him at the bedside on light exercises and assisted range of motion activities while performing your skin integrity assessment, you and the patient hear his wife in the background speaking loudly with a neighbor about how therapy is here working with John to get him outside and walking today. As you assist him with his movements, you note that John is particularly dependent upon you today as the weight of his atrophied limbs becomes heavier in your hands. As you begin to work with John's arms while John is lying supine, he looks up at you despondently and asks, "How much longer are we going to do this?"

1.   How does this make you feel? How will you respond?

2. What additional information would you like to know from the patient? What aspects of culture and spirituality might be relevant (see Chapters 12 and 14)? What losses are John and his wife experiencing? Compare where you think the patient is vs where the wife is in the stages of acceptance.

3. What is your role for advocating for the patient's wishes in this case? How might you use your neurolinguistic psychology skills in pacing, leading, and matching and your describe, express, specify, and consequences (DESC) skills (see Chapters 8 and 11) to educate and advocate?

4. What aspects of the Patient's Bill of Rights apply? Do you need to make any specific referrals?

5. Select one aspect of the case to role-play, with a partner, the specific skill you would like to practice (describe, express, specify, and consequences; neurolinguistic psychology; etc). Share with your partner the specific skill you are practicing and open your text to the related skill information for reference during the practice session. Verbally role-play and then debrief about your abilities through peer and self-assessment.

(To learn more about hospice care and meaningful moments made possible by hospice in care for the dying, for all ages, view the families' stories shared to see the difference and impact of the person-centered care [http://www.momentsoflife.org/].)

EXERCISE 4: LIFE LINE

The line below represents your total life span. At the end of the line, mark the year and your age at the point of your death. Indicate the ups and downs of your life by labeling them with words and dates.

_____

1. Reflections:

   a. Is your line a straight line, or does it have curves and dips in it?

   b. How does it feel to consider the total span of your life? Remember, feelings are one word, such as "anxious" or "exciting," not "I feel like my life…"

   c. How would you characterize your life so far? More up than down, the reverse, or neutral?

   d. What are the major forces that have contributed to this assessment?

   e. Did you have difficulty actually marking the date of your death? Some people think this a difficult, if not impossible, task. If you did, why? Why not?

   f. Do you have certain life goals that you can identify? If so, identify them and comment on how well you feel you are progressing toward them. Indicate what goals you expect to have achieved at certain points along your lifeline.

2. Journal about this experience.

"Don't cry because it's over, smile because it happened." –Dr. Seuss

**The exercises at the end of this chapter are also available online.
Please refer to the sticker in the front of the book and enter the access code provided.**

AFTERWORD

Carol M. Davis, DPT, EdD, MS, FAPTA and
Gina Maria Musolino, PT, MSEd, EdD

OUR FINAL CONCLUSION, WITH BEST WISHES

One of the goals of this text is to help you grow in self-awareness to be less susceptible to professional burnout. Only you can evaluate your current world view, level of self-esteem, and ability to alter harmful perceptions that contribute to negative stress. Only you can change your self-esteem. And only you can alter the perceptions about yourself, the world, and other people to the end that you experience a deep sense of personal confidence and satisfaction in your self and in your work. That is our wish for you. You, your patients, and the world will benefit from the positive energy that you will convey.

You've got a start toward self-awareness and personal growth. Don't stop. Find ways to continue to take regular personal inventory of your self-esteem and stress levels. Use your journal to stay on top of feelings that would become buried in the overwhelming amount of work you've agreed to do. Make a personal commitment to ongoing growth in all 4 of your quadrants, and keep a check on the imbalances. You know the value of peer and self-assessment for professional growth as a reflective practitioner and will assist others in introspective development, peers, patients, and future protégés.

The Signs of Maturation

How will you know when you're succeeding at the maturation process? Someone very wise once offered this description: Life will become more enjoyable, and you will become less worried about making mistakes or not being liked. Relationships will become more important to you than things. You will accept criticism gratefully and graciously, glad for the opportunity to improve. You will not indulge in self-pity, but you will begin to see the marvelous opportunities for growth that misfortune and pain often bring. You will not expect special consideration from anyone. You will be aware of your emotions, and you will rarely feel the need to react impulsively in a tense situation. You will meet emergencies with poise; your feelings will not be hurt easily. You will accept responsibility for your own actions without needing to make excuses, readily acknowledging that you are still growing and learning.

You will have grown beyond dualistic, all-or-none, black-or-white thinking about the world, and you will be able to tolerate ambiguity. You will recognize that people are doing the best they can and that no one is all bad or all good. You will come to know that true humility is not feeling less important than others are, but believing that everyone else is every bit as important as you are. You will be present for your patients and colleagues, listening reflectively and reflexively.

Davis CM, Musolino GM. *Patient Practitioner Interaction: An Experiential Manual for Developing the Art of Health Care, Sixth Edition* (pp 339-340).
© 2016 SLACK Incorporated.

You will be less impatient with reasonable delay. You will be willing to adjust yourself to others and their needs. You will be a gracious loser and will endure defeat without whining or complaining. You will not worry about things you have no control over, and you will learn how to take control of appropriate things with confidence and sensitivity.

You will not need to boast or call attention to yourself. You will feel sincere joy at the success of others, outgrowing both jealousy and envy. And you will be open-minded enough to thoughtfully listen to the thoughts of others. In the future, as you begin to work with patients and clients as a health care professional, you will be more concerned about the successes and triumphs of the people you serve. Because you will be giving in service to others, you will not need to be egotistical or brag about the work that you do because your patient care—helping them to achieve their goals —will allow you to naturally achieve. Your patients shall be the grateful ones, and that is the most wonderful gift that you can provide in health care. Together with your interprofessional health care teams, you will ensure that expectations are clear, work to break down any barriers to communication, and address conflict assertively.

Above all, you will not tolerate the mistreatment of human beings, especially those who are ill, by those who are careless in their interactions. You will take personal responsibility to help people realize the negative effects of their fragmenting interactions on you and on others, and you will kindly ask them to change their behavior for the good of all concerned. Best of luck to you as you set out to make the world, and yourself, better than they were when you started. You are on your way to becoming a leader in health care, putting your patients' needs forward and advocating for those who are unable to do so for themselves.

FINANCIAL DISCLOSURES

Dr. Kathleen A. Curtis has no financial or proprietary interest in the materials presented herein.

Dr. Carol M. Davis has no financial or proprietary interest in the materials presented herein.

Dr. Sherrill H. Hayes has no financial or proprietary interest in the materials presented herein.

Dr. Helen L. Masin has no financial or proprietary interest in the materials presented herein.

Dr. Gina Maria Musolino has no financial or proprietary interest in the materials presented herein.

Dr. Shirley A. Sahrmann has no financial or proprietary interest in the materials presented herein.

Dr. Darina Sargeant has no financial or proprietary interest in the materials presented herein.

Index

2-Minute Clinical Instructor, 146

acceptance stage of loss, 326
accountability, 32, 58, 74, 143, 212
acquired immunodeficiency syndrome, 34, 294, 302, 306, 330
    sexuality, 302
action
    awareness through, 38–39, 98
    self-awareness through, 23
action stage of change, 268
active engagement model, 65
active learning, 270
    passive learning, compared, 270
active listening, 106–107, 111
ADD. *See* attention deficit disorder
adolescents, interviewing, 225
advocacy, 59–60, 159, 169–170, 176, 179
    advocacy in action exercise, 179
aggression, 117, 118, 121–123, 128
aging with disability, 291–293
AIDS. *See* acquired immunodeficiency syndrome
alcoholism, fear of, 20
altruism, 32, 58, 66, 73
ambiguity, 4, 81, 146, 210, 339
American Academy of Orthopaedic Surgeons, 274
American Cancer Society, 274
American Diabetes Association, 274
American Heart Association, 268, 274
American Lung Association, 274
American Occupational Therapy Association, 74, 142, 170, 175, 274
American Physical Therapy Association, 32, 59, 74, 142, 170, 175, 190, 203, 244, 274
American Speech-Language-Hearing Association, 170
Americans With Disabilities Act, 292, 293
amputation, 172, 285, 306, 307, 308, 313
anger
    dealing with, 126–127
    stage of loss, 326
anorectics, 314
anti-anxiety agents, 314

antiarrhythmic drugs, 314
anticancer drugs, 314
anticonvulsants, 314
antidepressants, 314
antihypertensive agents, 306, 314
antiulcer drugs, 314
anxiety, spiritual, 250
AOTA leadership resources, 175
apathy, 78–79, 79
APTA leadership resources, 175
arousal cycle, sexual, 310
arthritis, 76, 80, 274, 306, 307, 313
Arthritis Foundation, 274
assertiveness
    aggressive behavior, 122
    anger, dealing with, 126–127
    assertive action, 125
    assertive behavior, 122
    assertive response examples, 122
    attribution, 123–125
        exercise, 124
    benefits of, 128
    bullying behaviors, 119
    bullying in workplace, 118–119
    communication, 119
    cultural differences, 120
    DESC response, 126
    exercises, 131–137
    gender differences, 119–120
    hostility curve, 127–128
    myths about, 128
    nonassertive behavior, 121
    personal power, 120–121
    personal rights, 121
    response types, 123
    stress, situations causing, 120–121
    training in, 117–118
attention deficit disorder, 285, 314
attitude, in interview, 224
attribution, 123–125
    exercise, 124

autonomy, 16, 55
awareness of self, 1–12
 desire for self-awareness, 2
 example of self-awareness, 5
 exercises, 8–12
 nature of self, 3
 search for self, 5–6
 self, 2–4
  defining, 1–2
 self-awareness, 4
 signs of growth in self-awareness, 6

baby boomers, 19, 21, 22, 118, 189, 190
bargaining stage of loss, 326
behavior change, 60, 162, 263, 266, 268–269, 279–280
belief systems, 203
beliefs of effective helpers, 95–97, 96
beneficence, 55
Bennis's managers vs leaders, 165
beta-blockers, 314
biases, disability, 290–291
bill of rights, patient's, 329
biomedical ethics, 51–53
body of interview, 227
boundaries, 95
brain injury, 103, 292, 297, 318
Brain Injury Association of America, 274
Brain Trauma Foundation, 274
bridge and Barnum statements, 307
builders/traditionalists, 22
bullying behaviors, 118–119
burnout, 77–89, 78–79
 causes of, 81
 symptoms, 77–78
burns, 52, 208, 313
butyrophenones, 314

cancer, 313
cardiac disease, 313
cardiovascular drugs, 314
cardiovascular symptoms of stress, 80
care
 ethic of, 59
 models of, 59–60
cauda equina lesions, 311
 sexuality, 311
Centers for Disease Control and Prevention, 274
challenges of leadership, 164–167, 166
change
 readiness for, 268
 transtheoretical model, 268

character, moral, 54
characteristics of families, 15
chemotherapy, 249, 306, 313
chronic illnesses, 82, 225, 264, 302
clarification in active listening, 107
clarification of values, 34
CLAS standards, 212
closed families, 15, 18–19
codependence, 21–23
collaborative style, 141, 142
collaborator style, 169
collectivism, 204
 cultures associated with, 204
commitment to learning, 142, 169, 204
communication
 about disability, 301–321
 about sexuality, 301–321, 307
  improving, 307
 active listening, 106–107, 107
 adjustments, 184
 adolescents, interviewing, 225
 assertiveness, 126
 attitude, 224, 228
 belief systems, 203
 clarification, 107
 collectivism, 204
 communication form, 228
 conflict resolution, 126
 congruence, 108
 cultural competence, 202, 213–214
 cultural diversity, 201
 cultural sensitivity
  intercultural, 203
  nonverbal, 210–211
  self-respect, 205
 culture, health care, 203–204
 culture shock, 200–201
 digital communication, 189–190
 digital technologies, 105
 disability, 285–299
 with dying, 323–340
 emotion-laden interchanges, 105
 environments, 206–210
 eye movements, 188–189
 face, concept of, 205–206
 with family member of dying, 323–340
 format for assertive communication, 126
 generational differences, 189
 high-context cultures, 204–205
 "I" statements, 107–108, 108
 impact on therapeutic effectiveness, 202–203

implicit meanings in, 210
individualism, cultures associated with, 204
interactions, 223–224
intercultural, 203
interview, 227–228
    form, 228
    phrasing, 226
    stages, 227
    timing, 226
learning communication skills, 104–105
less-than-helpful responses, 106
low-context cultures, 204–205
mindfulness, 190
neurolinguistic psychology, 184, 185–187
with non-English-speaking patient, 272–273
nonverbal, 210–211, 227–228
older patients, interviewing, 225–226
perceptual filter, 191–192
positive descriptive statements, 189
positive psychology, 190–191
problem
    identifying, 104
    ownership of, identifying, 106
professional behaviors, 182
quantum perspective, 183
from quantum perspective, 183
questioning, 224
rapport, 185–187
    leading, 186–187
    matching, 185–186
    modeling movements, 185–186
    pacing, 186–187
reflection, 107
relationships, 201–202
representational systems, 187–188
restatement, 107
self-respect, 205
services standards, 212–213
somatization, 211
space, 206–210
spirituality, 213
stress reduction, mindfulness-based, 190
therapeutic, 93
therapeutic responses, values in, 106
time, 206–210
values in therapeutic responses, 106
compensatory model, 265
complacency, 143, 146
compulsive behavior, 20, 23, 77, 82
confidentiality, 55
conflict, fear of, 20

conflict resolution, 117–137
    anger, dealing with, 126–127
    assertive action, 125
    assertive response examples, 122
    assertiveness, 121–122, 123
        aggressive behavior, 122
        assertive behavior, 122
        nonassertive behavior, 121
        response types, 123
    assertiveness training, 117–118
    attribution, 123–125
        exercise, 124
    benefits of, 128
    bullying behaviors, 119
    bullying in workplace, 118–119
    communication, 119
    cultural differences, 120
    DESC response, 126
    exercises, 131–137
    gender differences, 119–120
    hostility curve, 127–128
    personal power, 120–121
    personal rights, 121
    stress, situations causing, 120–121
congruence, 108
constructed sounds, 188
contemplation stage of change, 268
core values, 32
cortisol, 247
courage, moral, 54
Covey's 7 Habits of Highly Effective People, 164
critical thinking, 29, 65, 161, 182
cultural competence, 146, 199, 202, 212–214
cultural differences in communication, 120
cultural sensitivity, 199–222
    belief systems, 203
    collectivism, cultures associated with, 204
    cultural competence, 202
    cultural diversity, 201
    culture, health care, 203–204
    culture shock, 200–201
    environments, 206–210
    exercises, 218–222
    face, concept of, 205–206
    high-context cultures, 204–205
    impact on therapeutic effectiveness, 202–203
    implicit meanings in, 210
    individualism, cultures associated with, 204
    intercultural, 203
    intercultural communication, 203
    low-context cultures, 204–205

nonverbal, 210–211
nonverbal communication, 210–211
relationships, 201–202
self-respect, 205
services standards, 212–213
somatization, 211
space, 206–210
spirituality, 213
time, 206–210

DATA model, 144
   exercise, 155
debriefing, 32, 129, 148, 325
decision making
   moral, 49–72
      active engagement model, 65
      biomedical ethics, 51–53
      care ethic, 59
      care models, 59–60
      decision making, principled, 56
      ethical action, components of, 53–54
      ethical decisions, 50
      ethical problems, 61–62
      ethical situations, 50–51
      exercises, 68–72
      individual process-situation conceptual analysis model, 60–61
      law, ethics and, 59
      manners, as moral behaviors, 50
      moral action, components of, 54
      moral decision, 54
      nondiscursive approach, 56–57, 57
      principle, utilization of, 56
      problem-solving method, 62–65
      professional codes of ethics, rules of, 55–56
      rationalistic discursive resolution, 51
      traditional biomedical ethics, 54–55
      uncertainty, 51
      virtue, discernment as, 58–59
      virtue ethics, 57–58
   principled, 56
defensiveness, 5, 105, 106, 200, 328
denial stage of loss, 326
dependency, fear of, 20
depression stage of loss, 326
desire for self-awareness, 2
despair, 17, 250, 251, 331
destabilization, 118, 119
diabetes, 76, 210, 225, 274, 306
digital technology, 105, 189–190
digoxin, 314
dimensions of listening, 248

disability
   aging with, 291–293
   biases, 290–291
   change, affecting, 295
   communication about, 301–321
   context, seeking, 289–290
   economic aspects, 291
   empowering language, 288
   exercises, 297–299
   health status, 293
   International Classification of Functioning, Disability and Health, 287
   labeling, results of, 286
   legislation, 291
   models of, 287
   non-distancing terms, 289
   paradigm shift, 291
   Paralymic Games, 291
   pity, 288–289
   secondary conditions, 293
   sexuality and, 301–321
   stigmatization, 290–291
   women with, 293–295
   words, power of, 286
dishonesty, 146
distress, spiritual, 250
diversity, cultural, 201
do-not-resuscitate orders, 329
drug dependency, fear of, 20
dying
   acquired immunodeficiency syndrome, 330
   bill of rights, 329
   death, 324–325
   do-not-resuscitate orders, 329
   exercises, 333–338
   fear of, 324
   hospice care, 329–330
   living will, 330
   mercy killing, 330
   pain control, 328
   palliative care, 328–329
   quality of life, 325–326
   stages of loss, 326–327
      acceptance, 326
      anger, 326
      bargaining, 326
      denial, 326
      depression, 326
   terminal illness, professional anxiety, 327
   therapeutic presence, 327–328
dysfunctional families, 15, 18–19

ECHOWS tool, 231
economic aspects of disability, 291
Education for All Handicapped Children Act, 292
educational activities, 271, 272
emotion-laden interchanges, 105
emotional listening, 248
empathy, 91–102
    action, awareness through, 98
    boundaries, 95
    effective helpers, beliefs of, 95–97
    empathy, 94–95
    exercises, 99–102
    interpersonal interaction processes, 93–94
    pity, distinguished, 91–102
    purpose of helping, 97–98
    therapeutic communication, 93
    therapeutic use of self, 92–93
empowering language, 288
encouragement, 168, 250, 294
energizer style, 169
enlightenment model, 265
enthusiasm, 19, 77–79
    as stress stage, 78–79
erection, 309–313
Erikson, Erik, stages of development, 16–17
ethical action, components of, 53–54
ethical consciousness, 34–35
ethical decisions, 50
ethical problems, 61–62
ethical relativism, 34
ethical situations, 50–51
ethical subjectivism, 34
euthanasia, 51, 330
example of self-awareness, 5
eye movements, in communication, 188–189

face, in communication, cultural concepts, 205–206
false self, 13, 19–21, 20
families, characteristics of, 15
family history, 13–28
    baby boomers, 22
    characteristics of families, 15
    codependence, 21–23
    dysfunctional families, 18–19
    Erikson, Erik, stages of development, 16–17
    exercises, 25–28
    false self, 20
    generation X, 22
    generation Y, 22
    generation Z, 22
    generations, defining, 22

health care professional, self-esteem, 19–21
    healthy families, 15, 18
    influence of family on self-esteem, 14–18
    millennial generation, parenting of, 19
    self-awareness through action, 23
    stages of development, 16–17, 17
    troubled families, 15
    unhealthy families, 15
fear of death, 324
feedback, 129, 145, 171, 182, 229
FICA, 251, 252
fidelity, 55
Flesch Reading Ease Readability Formula, 275
format for assertive communication, 126
frustration, stress stage, 78–79

gastrointestinal symptoms of stress, 80
gender differences in communication, 119–120
generation X, 21, 22
generation Y, 21, 22
generation Z, 21, 22
generational differences in communication, 189
generations, defining, 22
generativity vs stagnation, developmental stage, 17
genital herpes, 306
genital lesions, 313
glycemic control, 314
grief, 20, 63, 306, 324, 328
growth in self-awareness, signs of, 6
guilt, 20
Gunning Fog Index Readability Formula, 276

habits of leaders, 162–164
harmonizer style, 169
health behavior, 263–283
    active learning, 270
    change, transtheoretical model, 268
    culture, 271–272
    defining, 264
    educational activities, 271, 272
    exercises, 278–283
    Flesch Reading Ease Readability Formula, 275
    Gunning Fog Index Readability Formula, 276
    health literacy, 264, 273
    health resources, 274
    instructional planning, 270–271
    language, 271–272
    literacy, 271–272
    non-English-speaking patient, 272–273
    passive learning, 270
        active learning, compared, 270

patient education, 265
readiness for change, 268
responsibility, 264–266, 265–266
sample patient education materials, 276
technology, 273
theories, 266–269
    health belief model, 266
    health promotion model, 267–268
    locus of control, 266
    motivational interviewing, 269
    self-efficacy, 266–267
    theory of planned behavior, 267
    transtheoretical model, 268–269
written materials, evaluating, 273–275
health belief model, 266
health benefits of spiritual health care, 247
health care advocacy, 159–180
Health Care and Education Affordability Reconciliation Act, 293
health care professional, self-esteem, 19–21
health literacy, 264, 273
Health on Net Foundation, 274
health promotion activities, 264
health promotion model, 267–268
healthy families, 15, 18
helping, purpose of, 97–98
high-context cultures, 204–205
history, family, 13–28, 23. *See also* family history
HIV. *See* human immunodeficiency virus
home exercises, 244, 272
hospice care, 207, 249, 328–330
hostility curve, 127–128
human immunodeficiency virus, 34, 265, 302, 306
    sexuality, 302
humanity, 32, 253
humiliation, 118, 122
    as bullying, 118
hysterectomy, 306

"I" statements, 107–108, 108
ICF, 244, 245, 253, 287
identifying problem, 104
identifying problem's ownership, 106
identity diffusion, 17
identity vs identity diffusion, developmental stage, 17
immunity symptoms of stress, 80
IMPACT Act, 292
implicit meanings, 210
individual process-situation conceptual analysis model, 60–61
individualism, cultures associated with, 204

Individuals With Disabilities Education Act, 202, 292
industry vs inferiority, developmental stage, 16
inferiority, 17
initiative vs guilt, developmental stage, 16
instructional planning, 270–271
instrumental relativist orientation, 36, 37
insulin, 225, 306, 314
integrity, 38
integrity in practice, 89
integrity vs despair, developmental stage, 17
intellect, 7, 75, 83, 246, 248, 251, 325
intellectual listening, 248
intercourse, problems with, 313
intercultural communication, 203
internal dialogue, 187
internalization, 20, 33
International Classification of Functioning, Disability and Health, 244, 287
interpersonal concordance, 37
interpersonal interaction processes, 93–94
interpersonal skills, 59, 97, 166, 182
interview, 223–242, 226
    body of, 227
    form, 228
    interactions, 223–224
intimacy, 17, 20, 23, 36, 95, 302
    difficulties with, 20
intimacy vs isolation, developmental stage, 17
intimidation, as bullying, 118
isolation, 119, 293, 294, 328, 331

Jimmo v. Sebelius, 292
journaling, 1, 140, 142, 145, 148, 248, 270, 288
judgment, moral, 54
judgmental responses, 106
justice, 55

knowing-in-action, 141, 147, 148
Kouzes and Posner's leadership challenge, 166

labeling, results of, 286
law, ethics and, 59
leadership, 159–180
    advocacy, 169–170
    archetypes of, 169
    challenge, 164–167, 166
    exercises, 176–180
    frameworks, 167–169
    habits of, 162–164
    proactive reading, 161–162
    qualities, 164–167

reflection, 161–162
  signature, 169
  societal transformation, 170–173
  style inventories, 175
  team evaluation instruments, 168
  teaming, 167–169
  writing, 161–162
leading for rapport, 186–187
learning communication skills, 104–105
legislation affecting children with disabilities, 292
legislation affecting disability issues, 292–293
legislation affecting older adults, 293
legislation affecting persons with disabilities, 292
less-than-helpful responses, 106
listening, 226, 227
  dimensions of, 248
literacy, 271–272
lithium carbonate, 314
living will, 330
locus of control, 266
longevity, 247
loss, stages of, 326–327
loss of control, fear of, 20
low-context cultures, 204–205

maintenance of change, 268
manners, as moral behaviors, 50
MAOIs. *See* monoamine oxidase inhibitors
mastectomy, 305, 306
matching for rapport, 185–186
maturation, signs of, 339–340
MBSR. *See* mindfulness-based stress reduction
MediBabble, 212, 274
medical model, 82, 205, 265, 287
meditation, 4, 77, 82, 83, 190, 247, 248
Mental Measurements Yearbook, 231
mercy killing, 330
metabolic symptoms of stress, 80
millennial generation, parenting, 19
mindfulness-based stress reduction, 190
mistrust, 16
modeling movements for rapport, 185–186
models of disability, 287
models of illness, health, 244–245
monoamine oxidase inhibitors, 314
moral action, components of, 54
moral awareness vs moral consciousness, 37–38
moral courage, 49, 53, 54, 62
moral decision making, 35–37, 54
moral development model, Piaget, 36
moral development stages, Kohlberg, 36–37

moral dilemmas, 49–72
  active engagement model, 65
  biomedical ethics, 51–53
  care
    ethic of, 59
    models of, 59–60
  decision making, principled, 56
  ethical action, components of, 53–54
  ethical decisions, 50
  ethical problems, 61–62
  ethical situations, 50–51
  exercises, 68–72
  law, ethics and, 59
  manners, as moral behaviors, 50
  moral action, components of, 54
  moral decision, 54
  nondiscursive approach, 56–57
    individual's story, 57
  principle, utilization of, 56
  problem-solving method, 63–65
    decision, 64–65
  problem-solving process, 62–63
  process-situation conceptual analysis model, 60–61
  professional codes of ethics, rules of, 55–56
  rationalistic discursive resolution, 51
  traditional biomedical ethics, 54–55
  uncertainty, 51
  virtue, discernment as, 58–59
  virtue ethics, 57–58
moral judgment, 53, 62–64
moral model, 265
moral motivation, 53, 54, 62
moral principles, 32, 55, 57
moral sensitivity, 53, 54, 58, 59, 61–63
morals vs nonmoral values, 31
motivation, moral, 54
motivational interviewing, 269
Movement System, 244
multiple sclerosis, 274, 302, 307, 313
muscular symptoms of stress, 80
myocardial infarction, 251, 312
  sexuality with, 312–313

National Association of Area Agencies on Aging, 274
National Institute of Arthritis and Musculoskeletal and Skin Disease, 274
National Institute of Diabetes and Digestive and Kidney Diseases, 274
National Multiple Sclerosis Society, 274
National Parkinson Foundation, 274
National Stroke Association, 274

nature of self, 3
negativity, reducing, 181–198
networking, 146, 189, 207, 273, 308
neuroleptics, 314
neurolinguistic psychology, 184, 185–187
neurological diseases, 313
New Freedom Initiative, 292
non-distancing terms, in communication, 289
non-English-speaking patient, 272–273
    communication, 272–273
nonassertive behavior, 121
nondiscursive approach, 56–57
    individual's story, 57
nonmaleficence, 55
nonverbal communication, 210–211, 227–228
Nursing Home Reform Amendments of OBRA, 293

obedience orientation, 36, 37
objectivity, 94, 95, 143, 144, 146
OBRA. *See* Omnibus Reconciliation Act
older patients, interviewing, 225–226
Omnibus Reconciliation Act, 293
open families, 15, 18
orchiectomy, 306
ostomy, 306, 313
overachievement, 20
overwhelming feelings, fear of, 20
overwork, 82, 119, 229
ownership of problem, 106

pacing for rapport, 186–187
pain control, 208, 247, 328, 330
palliative care, 328–329
Paralymic Games, 291
paraplegia, sexuality with, 311
parasympathetic nervous system, 77, 247, 309
parenting of millennial generation, 19
Parkinson's disease, 249, 274, 302, 307, 313
Parkinson's Disease Foundation, 274
passive learning, 270
    active learning, compared, 270
patient education
    active learning, 270
    change, transtheoretical model, 268
    culture, 271–272
    educational activities, 271, 272
    exercises, 278–283
    Flesch Reading Ease Readability Formula, 275
    Gunning Fog Index Readability Formula, 276
    health behavior theories, 266–269
        health belief model, 266

    health promotion model, 267–268
    locus of control, 266
    motivational interviewing, 269
    self-efficacy, 266–267
    theory of planned behavior, 267
    transtheoretical model, 268–269
health literacy, 264, 273
health resources, 274
instructional planning, 270–271
language, 271–272
literacy, 271–272
non-English-speaking patient, 272–273
passive learning, 270
    active learning, compared, 270
readiness for change, 268
responsibility, 264–266, 265–266
sample patient education materials, 276
technology, 273
written materials, evaluating, 273–275
patient-family education plan, 180
patient-practitioner interactions, 113–115
peer assessment, 145
perceptual filter, 191–192
personal power, 120–121
personal rights, 121
phenothiazines, 314
phrasing, in interview, 226
physical effects of stress, 76
physical listening, 248
physical stress symptom scale, 78–80, 80
Piaget, Jean, 2, 14, 35, 36
pity, 91–102, 288–289
portfolios, 142, 146
positive descriptive statements, 189
positive psychology, 190–191
post-myocardial infarction, 306
post-stroke, 306
prayer, 247, 248, 251–253
precontemplation stage of change, 268
preparation stage of change, 268
prevention of stress, 82–83
principle, utilization of, 56
proactive reading, 161–162, 177
problem identification
    active listening, 106–107, 107
    assertiveness, 126
    clarification, 107
    conflict resolution, 126
    congruence, 108
    cultural sensitivity
        intercultural, 203

nonverbal, 210–211
   self-respect in, 205
digital, 189–190
digital technologies, 105
disability, 301–321
emotion-laden interchanges, 105
exercises, 110–116
format for assertive communication, 126
generational differences, 189
"I" statements, 107–108, 108
intercultural, 203
interview form, 228
learning communication skills, 104–105
less-than-helpful responses, 106
with non-English-speaking patient, 272–273
nonverbal, 227–228
ownership of problem, 106
quantum perspective, 183
reflection, 107
restatement, 107
sexuality, 301–321, 307
   improving, 307
therapeutic, 93
therapeutic responses, values in, 106
values in therapeutic responses, 106
problem-solving method, 63–65
   decision, 64–65
producer style, 169
Professional Behaviors for the 21st Century, 182
professional codes of ethics, rules of, 55–56
professional duty, 32
professional status, threat to, as bullying, 119
professional values, 32
professionalism, 32, 38, 143, 145, 191
prostate cancer, 306
Psych Congress Network, 231
psychogenics, 309, 311
psychotropic drugs, 314

quadriplegia, 64, 286, 290, 309, 311
   sexuality with, 311
qualities of leaders, 164–167
quality of life, 325–326
quantum physics, 183, 184, 201, 202
questioning, in interview, 224

rapport
   adjustments, 184
   digital communication, 189–190
   exercises, 194–198
   eye movements, 188–189

generational differences in, 189
   leading, 186–187
   matching, 185–186
   mindfulness, 190
   modeling movements, 185–186
   neurolinguistic psychology, 184, 185–187
   pacing, 186–187
   perceptual filter, 191–192
   positive descriptive statements, 189
   positive psychology, 190–191
   professional behaviors, 182
   from quantum perspective, 183
   representational systems, 187–188
rationalistic discursive resolution, 51
reassurances, 106
reflective practice
   in active listening, 107
   collaborative mode, 141
   exercises, 152–157
   feedback/networking, 146
   knowing-in-action, 141
   reflection-in-action, 141
   reflection-on-action, 141
   self-assessment, 139
     support for, 146
reflexogenic awareness, 309, 311
Rehabilitation Act, 292
relationships, cultural, 201–202
religion, spirituality, distinguished, 244
remembered sounds, 188
representational systems in communication, 187–188
reserpine, 314
respiratory disease, 313
respiratory symptoms of stress, 80
responsibility, 265–266
   overdeveloped sense of, 20
restatement in active listening, 107
role ambiguity, 81
   stress, 81
role conflict, 81
   stress, 81

Schiavo, Terri, 330
scleroderma, 313
search for self, 5–6
selective serotonin reuptake inhibitors, 314
self-assessment, 139, 146
   defined, 145
   barriers to, 146
   examples of, 147, 150–151, 156
   support for, 146

self-awareness
    defining self, 1–2
    desire for, 2
    example of, 5
    exercises, 8–12
    nature of self, 3
    search for self, 5–6
    signs of growth in, 6
    through action, 23
self-criticism, 20
self-efficacy, 247–248, 266–267
self-esteem
    of health care professional, 19–21
    influence of family on, 14–18
self-focus, 146
self-respect, 205
sensitivity, moral, 54
serotonin, 247, 314
severe burns, 313
sexual response, neurophysiology of, 309
sexuality
    acquired immunodeficiency syndrome, 302
    acting out sexually, 306
    body image, 305
    cauda equina lesions, 311
    communication about, 301–321, 307
    cultural variables, 306
    exercises, 318–321
    hospitalization-process, 305
    human immunodeficiency virus, 302
    illness, effect of, 305–306
    intercourse, problems with, 313
    medications, sexual function, 313, 314
    myocardial infarction, 312–313
    myths, 307–308
    neurophysiology of sexual response, 309
    paraplegia, 311
        PLISSIT model, 304
        intensive therapy, 304
        limited information, 304
        permission, 304
        specific suggestions, 304
    patient-practitioner interactions, 319–320
    quadriplegia, 311
    rehabilitation, communication about, 307
    self-esteem, 308–309
    sexual arousal cycle, 310
    spinal cord injury, 309–311, 311–312
        sexuality and, 309
shame, 16–20, 58, 206, 301, 307
skin symptoms of stress, 80

Slujis Checklist for Educational Activities, 271–272
social contract, 36, 37
social media, digital technologies, 105
social responsibility, 32
somatization, 211
spinal cord injury, 302, 306, 311–312
    sexuality, 309–311
spiritual anxiety, 250
spiritual listening, 248
spirituality
    challenges, 252–253
    discomfort, 250
    encouragement, 250
    exercises, 256–262
    health benefits, 247
    health care, 246
    impact of spiritual care, 247–249
    listening, dimensions of, 248
    models of illness, health, 244–245
    religion distinguished, 244
    spiritual anxiety, 250
    spiritual distress, 250
    spiritual domain, 250–251
SSRIs. *See* selective serotonin reuptake inhibitors
stages of development, 16–17, 17
stages of interview, 227
stages of loss, 326–327
    acceptance, 326
    anger, 326
    bargaining, 326
    denial, 326
    depression, 326
stagnation, stress stage, 78–79
statins, 314
stigmatization, with disability, 290–291
stimulants, 314
stress
    burnout, 77–89, 78–79
        causes of, 81
        symptoms, 77–78
    development model, 76
    exercises, 85–89
    health care professionals, 74–75
    intervention, 81–82
    misperceptions, 76–77
    physical effects, 76
    physical stress symptom scale, 78–80, 80
    prevention, 82–83
    role ambiguity, 81
    role conflict, 81
    situations causing, 120–121

students, 75–76
    work overload, 81
stress reduction, mindfulness-based, 190
stress-related illnesses, 20
stroke, 51, 173, 274, 307, 313
supportive environment, 18, 146
sympathetic nervous system, 76, 77, 247, 309
sympathy
    action, awareness through, 98
    boundaries, 95
    effective helpers, beliefs of, 95–97, 96
    empathy, 94–95
    exercises, 99–102
    interpersonal interaction processes, 93–94
    purpose of helping, 97–98
    therapeutic communication, 93
    therapeutic use of self, 92–93

team evaluation instruments, 168
teaming, 167–169
teamwork, 30, 32, 146, 164, 166–168
temperance, 32
terminal illness, professional anxiety regarding, 327
texting, 105
theory of planned behavior, 267
therapeutic communication, 93
therapeutic presence, 327–328
therapeutic responses, values in, 106
therapeutic use of self, 92–93
thiazides, 314
threatening behavior, 76, 118, 200
time, cultural concepts, 206–210
timing, of interview, 226
traditional biomedical ethics, 54–55
transcendence, 32, 246, 247
transtheoretical model of change, 268–269
traumatic brain injury, 180
treatment settings, comparison of, 208–209
tricyclic antidepressants, 314
troubled families, 15
trust vs mistrust, developmental stage, 16

uncertainty, 51
unhealthy families, 15, 18–19
United Spinal Association, 274
universal-ethical principle orientation, 37
unsafe environments, 146

values
    activity, awareness through, 38–39
    clarification of, 34, 303, 331
    conflicts, 32–33
    core values, 32
    defining, 31
    detracting from therapeutic presence, 33–34
    ethical consciousness, 34–35
    ethical relativism, 34
    ethical subjectivism, 34
    exercises, 40–47
    integrity, 38
    moral awareness, moral consciousness, distinguished, 37–38
    moral decision making, 35–37
    moral development model, Piaget, 36
    moral development stages, Kohlberg, 36–37
    morals vs nonmoral values, 31
    needs, distinguished, 31
    professional values, 32
    reinforcing healing, 34
    therapeutic responses, 106
veracity, 55
verbal abuse, as bullying, 118
virtue, discernment as, 58–59
virtue ethics, 57–58
visualization, 184, 188
vulnerability, 20, 104, 186

WebMD, as health resource, 274
weight control, 314
women with disability, 293–295
words, power of, 286
work interference, as bullying, 118
work overload, 81
Workforce Investment Act, 292
workplace bullying, 118–119
written materials, evaluating, 273–275

X generation, 22

Y generation, 22

Z generation, 22